D1151773

EYEWITNESS ⬥ HANDBOOKS

HERBS

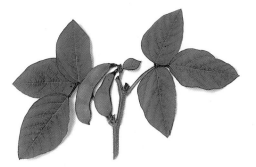

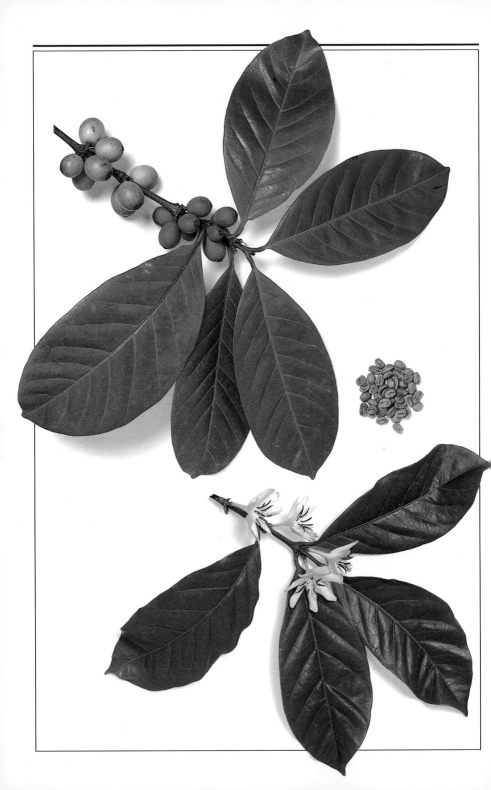

EYEWITNESS ◉ HANDBOOKS

HERBS

LESLEY BREMNESS

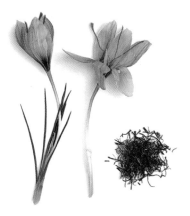

Photography by
NEIL FLETCHER
MATTHEW WARD

Editorial Consultant
DR. PAT GRIGGS

DORLING KINDERSLEY
LONDON • NEW YORK • SYDNEY • MOSCOW

A DORLING KINDERSLEY BOOK

Important Notice
This is not a medical reference book. The information it contains is general, not
specific to individuals. Any plant substance, whether used as food or medicine,
externally or internally, can cause an allergic reaction in some people. Neither
the author nor the publishers can be held responsible for claims arising from
the mistaken identity of any herbs, or the inappropriate use of any remedy.

Project Editor Charlotte Davies
Project Art Editor Colin Walton
Assistant Editors Lucinda Hawksley, Lesley Malkin
Design Assistant Gloria Horsfall
Production Controller Adrian Gathercole
Series Editor Jonathan Metcalf
Series Art Editors Peter Cross, Spencer Holbrook
Illustrations researched and commissioned by Mustafa Sami

First published in Great Britain in 1994
by Dorling Kindersley Limited,
9 Henrietta Street, London WC2E 8PS
Visit us on the World Wide Web at
http://www.dk.com

Reprinted 1997

Copyright © 1994
Dorling Kindersley Limited, London
Text Copyright © 1994 Lesley Bremness

All rights reserved. No part of this publication may be reproduced, stored in
a retrieval system, or transmitted in any form or by any means, electronic,
mechanical, photocopying, recording or otherwise, without the prior written
permission of the copyright owner. The right of Lesley Bremness to be
identified as the author of this work has been asserted by her in accordance
with the Copyright, Designs, and Patents Act 1988.

A CIP catalogue record for this book is available
from the British Library

ISBN 0-7513-1023-9 hardcover
ISBN 0-7513-1022-0 flexibound

Computer page make-up by
Colin Walton Graphic Design, Great Britain

Text film output by
The Right Type, Great Britain

Reproduced by
Colourscan, Singapore

Printed and bound by
Kyodo Printing Co., Singapore

CONTENTS

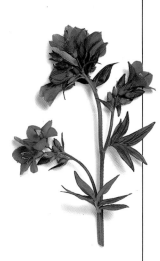

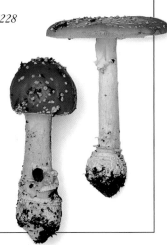

AUTHOR'S INTRODUCTION

Herbs are plants that connect us to the past, present, and future. We associate them with appetizing food, natural scents, gentle healing, peaceful gardens, beneficial crafts, intriguing history, and sacred activities. Each subject in this colourful tapestry enriches the others, but through the threads the background remains green, because the basis of all these delights is the plants themselves.

MORE THAN 20,000 plant varieties with herbal uses grow around the world; of these, 7,500 medicinal plants occur in Indonesia alone. Travel and cookery books have widened our general knowledge of exotic flavourings: garlic, ginger, and lemongrass are now joined by lime leaves, the finger roots of Thailand's kra chaai, the perfumed pandanus leaf which is steamed with rice parcels, and aromatic lotus leaves which can be wrapped around a prepared chicken. Cosmetics and skin-care products continue to appear from unlikely souces. Fresh tomato or pineapple rubbed on the face and left for five minutes will "eat" dead skin cells. Carrot oil and Aloe Vera juice both screen UV-A sun rays, the single most ageing factor for skin. Herbs such as Chamomile and Rhubarb offer safe hair highlights. A rich red hair colouring comes from Henna, and a black dye is derived from Indigo.

ANCIENT CURE
As long as 200,000 years ago, Euryale ferox seeds were eaten by early man in China. Many centuries later its medicinal uses were recognized and it appears in early Chinese herbals.

ESSENTIAL OILS

Essential oils, the aromatic plant essences, continue to inspire new research. Several oils, including peppermint and thyme, have been found to reduce another ageing factor, that is the presence of free radicals in the skin.

Classic French perfumes were once blended from essential oils, musks, and ethyl alcohol, but many manufacturers have now switched over to synthetic substitutes. As extraction methods improve, a greater range of essential oils has become available to the public, making it possible to recreate the traditional, more subtle scents.

COWSLIP
Many wild flowers like Cowslip hold forgotten herbal secrets. It is sedative when taken fresh or in a tea.

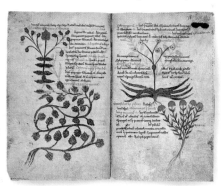

MONASTIC HERBAL
Herbals such as this, an Apuleius text copied by Canterbury monks around AD1100, spread botanical medical knowledge across continents. Despite botanical inaccuracies, recent archaeological finds suggest monastic herbal medicine was highly sophisticated.

FLOATING MARKET

Among the melons in Thailand's floating markets are lime leaves, lemon grass, galangal, and betel leaf bundles. All have medicinal and culinary uses. Also on sale are medicinal centella and lotus root, and jasmine garlands for temple offerings. Some are cultivated; others are collected from the wild.

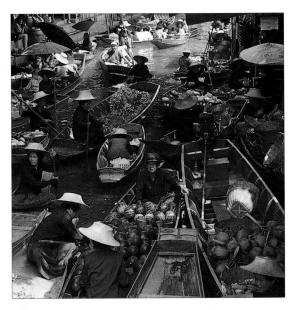

ENHANCED ENVIRONMENT

Plants can also improve the quality of one's living and working environment. Growing Azalea, *Scindapis*, and *Dieffenbachia* species in offices is known to filter out a variety of pollutants from cigarette smoke, cleaning solutions, and spray glue, which might otherwise cause staff illness. Plants also add oxygen to the air, improving alertness and concentration. Large plants reduce office noise, a common source of stress, and some plants, such as Rhapsis Palm, can increase humidity.

POISONOUS PLANTS

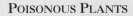

The Glory Lily (*Gloriosa superba* see right) is an Asian suicide herb, but in minute doses it can treat leprosy. Curare arrow poison from *Chondrodendron* 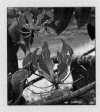 species is also an important muscle relaxant for surgery and now saves lives. However, toxic plants must only be used by experts. To avoid poisoning from an unfamiliar herb, accurate identification is vital – for plants taken from the wild and bought in shops. A herbalist's instructions must be followed precisely. If adverse reactions occur, stop the treatment and consult a qualified herbalist again.

CHINESE HERBALISM

Research into the beneficial qualities of herbs is taken very seriously in China, where a recent publication lists the results of tests on 236 herbs thought to combat cancer. The success of the traditional Chinese treatment of childhood eczema has focused attention on their 2,000 years of trial data. The Chinese system of selecting a suitable balance of herbs for each individual contrasts greatly with methods used in the West, where the emphasis is on creating a standard formula. However, many Chinese herbs are now being "discovered" by the West. Kudzu Vine (*Pueraria lobata*) has long been used in China for alcoholism, and research in the USA has confirmed the presence of ingredients that appear to suppress an individual's appetite for alcohol. But separating the "active" ingredients in a plant may cause adverse side-effects, which do not occur when the whole plant is used. Other components may serve to balance these active ingredients in ways not yet understood.

SCIENCE AND HERBS

Traditional Western scientific thinking maintains that the whole can eventually be understood from the properties of the parts, like a jigsaw puzzle. Thus botany explains the function of plant parts, and chemistry analyses the chemical components and isolates the active ingredients. However, by starting with very narrowly defined hypotheses, Western scientists may have overlooked some of the subtle interactions between plant and human parts. On the other hand herbalists have maintained for a long time that it is the plant as a whole, and not just its active ingredients, that is important. Now quantum physics, which focuses

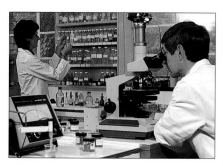

PROCESSING PLANTS
Herbal laboratories use the whole herb to prepare remedies preferred by herbalists. They offer slower-acting, but gentler and safer healing than the potent, patentable drugs made from isolated ingredients that have stronger side-effects.

MORETON BAY CHESTNUT
Unusual alkaloids in the seeds of this plant have stimulated new research into the immune system, AIDS, and cancer.

on the *processes* of nature rather than just its parts, offers some credence to their views, opening up a new understanding of disease and "disharmony" in the body. This shift in the scientific approach to plant research, together with the explosion of popular interest in herbs, offers an exciting and potentially life-enhancing future.

CONSERVATION OF PLANTS FOR THE FUTURE

Only five per cent of all flowering plants have been researched, and yet within the next 50 years a quarter of this number may become extinct. Apart from being a moral issue, the preservation of species also has an economic importance – native communities who have always practised conservation should share in the rewards of any commercialization of their herbal knowledge.

CONSERVATION CHECKLIST
• Identify plants carefully. Never pick rare or endangered species.
• Choose the right plant part and gather plant parts in the correct season.
• Do not take more than you will use.
• Leave some of the reproductive parts (root or seeds) to ensure future growth.
• Avoid disturbing the plant's habitat.

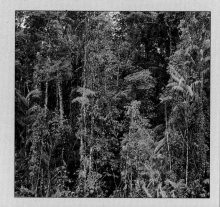

AMAZON RAINFOREST
Full of untapped herbal potential, the rainforests are also the "lungs of the world". Their survival determines our own future.

HOW THIS BOOK WORKS

THIS BOOK is divided into six parts according to major plant type (see p.10): trees, shrubs, herbaceous perennials, annuals and biennials, climbers, and other herbs (including fungi and non-seed-bearing plants). Within each section the entries are arranged alphabetically by their scientific names. The page below shows a typical entry.

scientific family name •

scientific species name •

section name according to plant type •

accepted common species name •

description of plant's appearance •

detailed information about herbal uses •

unusual or notable features, or uses of related species •

related species, forms, varieties, or cultivars shown in many entries •

annotation highlights key identification features or uses •

captions describe related species, forms, varieties, or cultivars •

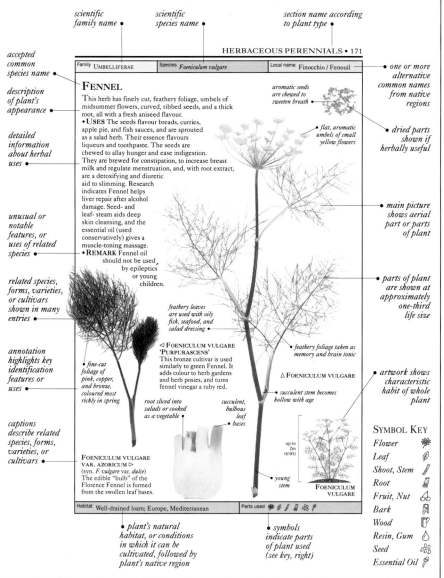

HERBACEOUS PERENNIALS • 171

Family UMBELLIFERAE   Species *Foeniculum vulgare*   Local name Finocchio / Fenouil

FENNEL

This herb has finely cut, feathery foliage, umbels of midsummer flowers, curved, ribbed seeds, and a thick root, all with a fresh aniseed flavour.
• USES The seeds flavour breads, curries, apple pie, and fish sauces, and are sprouted as a salad herb. Their essence flavours liqueurs and toothpaste. The seeds are chewed to allay hunger and ease indigestion. They are brewed for constipation, to increase breast milk and regulate menstruation, and, with root extract, are a detoxifying and diuretic aid to slimming. Research indicates Fennel helps liver repair after alcohol damage. Seed- and leaf- steam aids deep skin cleansing, and the essential oil (used conservatively) gives a muscle-toning massage.
• REMARK Fennel oil should not be used by epileptics or young children.

aromatic seeds are chewed to sweeten breath •

flat, aromatic umbels of small yellow flowers

feathery leaves are used with oily fish, seafood, and salad dressing •

◁ FOENICULUM VULGARE 'PURPURASCENS'
This bronze cultivar is used similarly to green Fennel. It adds colour to herb gardens and herb posies, and turns fennel vinegar a ruby red.

• fine-cut foliage of pink, copper, and bronze, coloured most richly in spring

root sliced into salads or cooked as a vegetable

succulent, bulbous leaf bases

FOENICULUM VULGARE VAR. AZORICUM ▷
(syn. *F. vulgare* var. *dulce*)
The edible "bulb" of the Florence Fennel is formed from the swollen leaf bases.

feathery foliage taken as memory and brain tonic

△ FOENICULUM VULGARE

succulent stem becomes hollow with age

up to 2m (6½ft)

young stem

FOENICULUM VULGARE

Habitat Well-drained loam; Europe, Mediterranean   Parts used 🌼 ⌀ ⫻ 🗘 ⬡ ∮

• one or more alternative common names from native regions

• dried parts shown if herbally useful

• main picture shows aerial part or parts of plant

• parts of plant are shown at approximately one-third life size

• artwork shows characteristic habit of whole plant

• plant's natural habitat, or conditions in which it can be cultivated, followed by plant's native region

• symbols indicate parts of plant used (see key, right)

SYMBOL KEY

Flower	🌼
Leaf	⌀
Shoot, Stem	⫻
Root	🗘
Fruit, Nut	🜊
Bark	🗂
Wood	𝍔
Resin, Gum	⬡
Seed	⬢⬢
Essential Oil	∮

WHAT IS A HERB?

FROM EARLIEST TIMES, humans have divided plants into two groups, the useful and the not useful, the former being the broadest definition of a herb. Those regarded as useful depend on the environment and society in which one lives – an Amazon healer might consider 500 plants to be useful, and therefore "herbs", whereas a city dweller might know only five. Thus "herb" is a cultural rather than a botanical definition.

In this book the widest definition of a herb is not used, as we omit fuel, timber trees, and most food plants (although 100 years ago vegetables were still called "pot herbs"). Exceptions have been made for the growing number of food plants now known to have medicinal or cosmetic benefits; hence several fruits, vegetables, and grains are included.

HERBS IN THE PLANT KINGDOM

Most people assume herbs are annual or herbaceous plants, such as basil, or perhaps ginseng, but in fact herbs span the breadth of the entire plant kingdom, from giant conifers to tiny yeasts. Herb plants are found among mosses, ferns, conifers, and even algae, as well as the more familiar higher flowering plants.

PLANT GROUPS

Botanical divisions within the plant kingdom are based on each plant's method of reproduction. In this book, however, plants have been grouped according to the more easily visible size and shape of growth, rather than according to the formal botanical divisions.

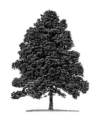

TREES
Woody perennials with a single main stem, usually branching well above the ground to create a crown.

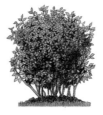

SHRUBS
A loose term for woody perennials with multiple branches from the base; generally smaller than trees.

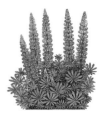

HERBACEOUS PERENNIALS
Perennial plants that die back to roots in autumn and grow new shoots in spring.

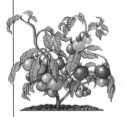

ANNUALS AND BIENNIALS
Annuals germinate, seed, and die in one year. Biennials complete their cycle in two years, flowering in the second year.

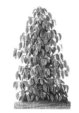

CLIMBERS
Vines and scrambling plants with a tendency to climb (by adaptations of stems, leaves, or roots), to twine, or to grow tendrils or suckers.

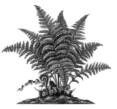
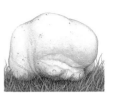

OTHER HERBS
Herbal plants and fungi that do not reproduce by seed: mainly the ferns (above left) and fungi (above right). This group also includes mosses such as Sphagnum, and primitive plants such as Horsetail (which reproduce by means of spores) and seaweeds, such as Bladderwrack.

ALGAE
Some algaes are used in cosmetics.

Whatever family they belong to, all herbs used in this book contain one or more chemically defined active ingredients that have a specific use.

ACTIVE INGREDIENTS

• **ALKALOIDS** are active organic compounds containing at least one nitrogen atom, potent but often toxic (e.g. morphine). Alkaloids provide many important drugs and are the focus of most pharmaceutical research.
• **BITTERS** are diverse compounds which share a bitter taste and stimulate the appetite.
• **ENZYMES** are organic catalysts, essential for biochemical functions, and are found in all plants.

ALKALOIDS
Quinine alkaloids are a cure for malaria.

• **ESSENTIAL OILS** are aromatic plant essences extracted by distillation, organic solvents, or pressing.
• **GUMS** are sticky substances, insoluble in organic solvents, often produced in response to wounding of the plant.
• **GLYCOSIDES** are substances that can be broken down by specific enzymes to yield a sugar and a therapeutically active, often toxic, "aglycone".

△ **GUM**
Liquidambar orientalis is expectorant.

• **MUCILAGE** is a viscous gum which swells into a gel in water. It is used to soothe irritated or inflamed skin.
• **SAPONINS** are emulsifying, often irritating or toxic, glycosides, similar to soap and chemically akin to steroids, which yield sex hormones.
• **TANNINS** are astringent compounds that cause proteins in blood to coagulate.
• **VITAMINS AND MINERALS** are required for various metabolic functions, but, unlike enzymes, are not catalysts.

SCIENTIFIC NAMES

A species is the basic plant group, classified according to the structure of its flowers, fruit, and other organs. Species are grouped into genera and families, and may be subdivided into subspecies, hybrids, varieties, forms, and cultivars.

FAMILY
A family contains a single genus or several related genera. The mints shown here all belong to the Labiatae family.

GENUS
A genus contains one species or several related species. The name appears in italic type, e.g. *Mentha*.

SPECIES
Species members are similar. The name consists of the genus name and the species epithet printed in italic type ◁ e.g. *Mentha aquatica*.

HYBRID
A hybrid is produced when two species cross together. This is indicated by a multiplication sign, e.g. *Mentha x villosa*. ▷

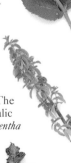

VARIETY, FORM, & SUBSPECIES
Varieties (var.), forms (f.), and subspecies (subsp.) are minor subdivisions of a species. The names are written in italic and roman type, e.g. *Mentha pugelium* var. *erecta*. ▷

CULTIVAR
A cultivar is a type of plant that has been produced artificially, e.g. *Mentha spicata* 'Crispa'. ▷

LEAVES AND STEMS

THE LEAF is the most frequently used part of a herb and its activity, photosynthesis, is fundamental to human existence, forming the basis of our food chain. During photosynthesis, the pigment in leaves, chlorophyll, absorbs red and blue light to convert water and carbon dioxide into sugars and oxygen; green light is reflected, making leaves appear green. Variegated leaves contain less chlorophyll than non-variegated leaves and may contain smaller amounts of active ingredients. Chlorophyll is antiseptic and deodorizing. Its ability to clear toxins formed the basis of an entire healing system. Photosynthesis

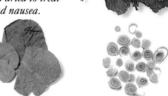

dried leaves keep scent

PERILLA ▷
Perilla frutescens *var.* crispa
antibiotic leaves are used fresh in sushi to reduce seafood poisoning, and dried to treat flu, coughs, and nausea.

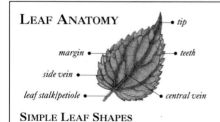

SWEET GRASS
Hierochloe odorata *is a fragrant, sacred native American incense plant.*

PALE CATECHU
In China a decoction of Uncaria rhynchophylla *thorns treats dizziness, hypertension, and children's convulsions.*

COIN LEAF CLOVER
The leaves of Desmodium styracifolium *treat colic, gall-stones, and hepatitis.*

LEMON GRASS
The lemon-flavoured culinary stems of Cymbopogon citratus *also have medicinal and aromatic uses.*

LEAF ANATOMY

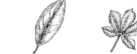

tip
margin
teeth
side vein
leaf stalk/petiole
central vein

LEAF ARRANGEMENTS

WHORL   OPPOSITE   ALTERNATE

SIMPLE LEAF SHAPES

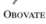

OVATE   OBOVATE   ELLIPTIC

COMPOUND LEAF SHAPES

PALMATE   PINNATE   BIPINNATE

decreases in autumn, and nutrients are exported from the leaves, thus reducing their flavour and therapeutic value. Leaf chemistry gives rise to a variety of culinary flavours, perfumes, and medicines. Leaves also produce oxygen as a by-product of photosynthesis, so indoor plants improve stale air.

Stems transport nutrients and support the plant. Many yield useful sap and supply strong, flexible fibres, such as flax and hemp, used in the manufacture of linen, rope, and paper.

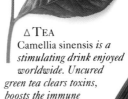

△ TEA
Camellia sinensis *is a stimulating drink enjoyed worldwide. Uncured green tea clears toxins, boosts the immune system, and inhibits some cancers.*

SWEET BAY ▷
Laurus nobilis *has evergreen leaves used all year round as a flavouring and symbol of attainment.*

◁ TRAVELLERS' PALM
Ravenala madagascariensis *aids travellers because the leaves fan out to indicate east and west, and the leaf-stalks hold an emergency water supply.*

STEVIA
Stevia rebaudiana *is a tropical annual with very sweet leaves which yield the substance "stevioside". This white crystalline powder is 250–300 times sweeter than sucrose.*

FIDDLEHEAD FERN
The emerging leaves and stalks of Pteridium aquilinum *are cooked or pickled. Bulk raw enzymes destroy vitamin B1 (thiamine).*

HARVESTING LEAVES

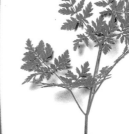

For most species, pick clean, dry, undamaged leaves or sprigs mid-morning, just before flowering, for maximum value. Freeze immediately, or dry in loose bunches in warm, dust-free, circulating air, out of sun, until brittle (4–10 days). Store in dark, airtight jars.

• *hollow at base of leaf-stalks can collect 1–2 litres (2–4 pints) of water*

HEMLOCK △
Conium maculatum *is extremely poisonous, with a mousy, fetid smell. It is used in the witches' brew in Shakespeare's* Macbeth.

FLOWERS

ANSWERING THE CALL to reproduce, many plants evolved a flower, and each flower part can be used herbally. In the centre of a basic flower is the female organ, the pistil, consisting of the ovary below, and style and stigma above, surrounded by a ring of male stamens (each made up of a filament and an anther). Around the centre is the corolla, or petals, whose colour, scent, and nectar evolved to entice bees and other insects to aid pollination. The outer ring – the calyx or sepals – protects the flower when in bud.

Cross-fertilization occurs when pollen released by the stamens of one flower reaches the ripe stigma of another, and travels down into the ovary to fertilize an ovule. This can sometimes create interesting new varieties or, less happily from a herbal point of view, muddy blends.

The flowers of pungent-leaved herbs often have a milder flavour than the leaves, and many flowers, such as mint, rosemary, and chive florets, are delicious eaten raw. Indeed many flowers in this book are enjoyed in cuisines world-wide. However flowers from poisonous plants should be avoided in food and drinks.

Fragrance from flowers is captured in pot-pourri, and in perfumes such as the popular Hindu champac from

△ ELDERFLOWER
The creamy flower clusters of Sambucus nigra *have a muscatel flavour used with gooseberries in fool and in refreshing elderflower "champagne" or "lemonade".*

PASSION FLOWER ▷
The distinctive shapes of Passiflora incarnata *invited symbolism. It is used with the leaf and stem as a non-addictive, non-depressant sedative.*

CALENDULA ▷
The edible golden petals of Calendula officinalis *rejuvenate skin, are anti-septic and anti-fungal. They heal cracked skin, sunburn, and eczema.*

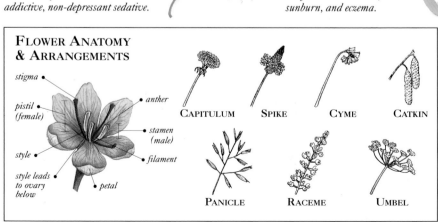

FLOWER ANATOMY & ARRANGEMENTS

stigma •
pistil (female)
• anther
style •
• stamen (male)
• filament
style leads to ovary below
• petal

CAPITULUM   SPIKE   CYME   CATKIN

PANICLE   RACEME   UMBEL

Michelia champaca. Medicinal flowers include the world's largest (*Rafflesia keithii*), a liana parasite, considered to be an aphrodisiac.

HARVESTING FLOWERS

Flowers contain the most active ingredients when they first open fully. Collect unblemished flowers of good shape in dry weather at midday. Pick flowering stems and avoid touching the petals. Discard soiled flowers as washing spoils the texture. Transport loose in open baskets.

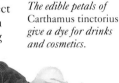

SAFFLOWER
The edible petals of
Carthamus tinctorius
*give a dye for drinks
and cosmetics.*

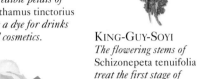

KING-GUY-SOYI
The flowering stems of
Schizonepeta tenuifolia
*treat the first stage of
boils, rashes, and
itching.*

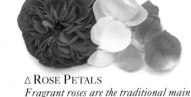

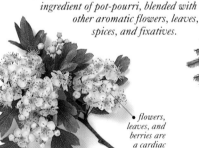

△ **ROSE PETALS**
*Fragrant roses are the traditional main
ingredient of pot-pourri, blended with
other aromatic flowers, leaves,
spices, and fixatives.*

**TEA
CHRYSANTHEMUM**
*Cooling, antibiotic flower
tea from* Chrysanth-
emum morifolium
*reduces blood pressure,
and is a Taoist elixir.*

**ENGLISH
HAWTHORN**
Crataegus monogyna
*flowers improve
damaged heart valves.*

• *flowers,
leaves, and
berries are
a cardiac
tonic*

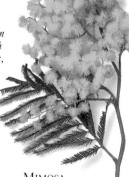

MIMOSA
Acacia dealbata
*is the florist's
Mimosa.*

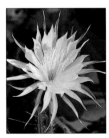

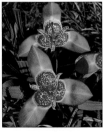

**QUEEN OF
THE NIGHT**
The cactus flower
Selenicereus grandi-
florus *is a stimulant.*

TIGER FLOWER
The beautiful flower of
Tigridia tenuifolia *was
once a valued ancient
Mexican fertility drug.*

DRYING FLOWERS

Spread out whole small flowers or thick petals of large flowers on paper or gauze, in warm, dust-free, circulating air for 1–3 weeks. Turn them once or twice. Dry roses and other large flower-heads upright in mesh. Hang loose bundles of lavender stems and remove the flowers later.

SEEDS, FRUITS, AND NUTS

SEEDS ARE PRODUCED by flowering and some non-flowering plants. Inside every seed is the genetic information for future growth, a store of food, and a dormant embryo that can grow into a seedling. The condensed nutrition in seeds supplies the world's major foods: cereals and pulses, such as rice, wheat and soya beans. Many seeds have an extremely high fatty oil content (different from essential oil), which can be pressed out for cooking, cosmetics, medicines, and for craft and industrial uses.

A fruit is a ripe, developed flower ovary which can be succulent or dry. A

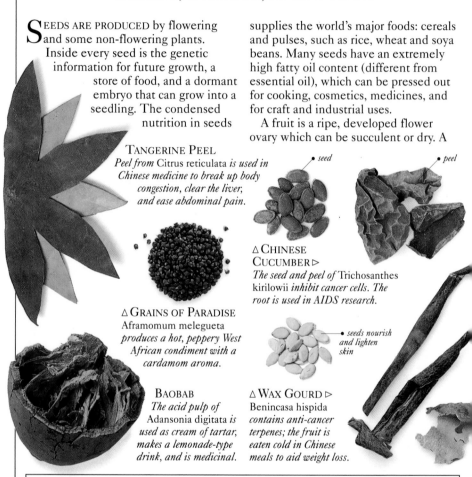

TANGERINE PEEL
Peel from Citrus reticulata *is used in Chinese medicine to break up body congestion, clear the liver, and ease abdominal pain.*

• seed

• peel

△ **GRAINS OF PARADISE**
Aframomum melegueta *produces a hot, peppery West African condiment with a cardamom aroma.*

△ **CHINESE CUCUMBER** ▷
The seed and peel of Trichosanthes kirilowii *inhibit cancer cells. The root is used in AIDS research.*

• seeds nourish and lighten skin

BAOBAB
The acid pulp of Adansonia digitata *is used as cream of tartar, makes a lemonade-type drink, and is medicinal.*

△ **WAX GOURD** ▷
Benincasa hispida *contains anti-cancer terpenes; the fruit is eaten cold in Chinese meals to aid weight loss.*

FRUIT, NUT, AND SEED ANATOMY

Seeds develop in a flower's ovary; the ovary wall then develops into the fruit. In different species the fruit may be fleshy, a narrow pod with a row of seeds, or so thin it appears to be just a husk. A nut is a hard, dry fruit that does not split when ripe, and contains one seed.

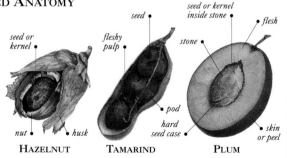

seed or kernel •

fleshy pulp •

seed •

seed or kernel inside stone •

stone •

• flesh

nut •

• husk

HAZELNUT

• pod

hard seed case •

TAMARIND

• skin or peel

PLUM

succulent fruit is fleshy, like a plum or cherry. A nut is a type of dry fruit with a hard or woody pericarp (fruit wall), such as a hazelnut or chestnut.

HERBAL USES

Seeds and seed-pods supply many spices, from anise to vanilla. They also yield the stimulant drinks coffee, cocoa, cola, and guarana; poppy seed capsules are the source of the drugs opium and morphine; beads come from Job's Tears; and Vegetable Ivory provides a carving material. Fruits supply food, flavourings, dyes, cosmetic enzymes, perfumes, wax, and medicines. Fruits are usually used when fresh, but may also be dried, or frozen.

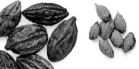

◁△ BILLY GOAT PLUM
Terminalia ferdinandiana
is an Australian fruit rich in
vitamin C. T. chebula
seeds (above left)
stimulate the appetite.

△ MIRACULOUS
BERRY
Dark red berries of the
West African shrub
Synsepalum dulci-
ficum *stimulate the*
tongue so food tastes
sweet for several hours.

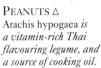

PEANUTS △
Arachis hypogaea *is*
a vitamin-rich Thai
flavouring legume, and
a source of cooking oil.

△ TONKA BEANS
Dipteryx odorata *is an*
aromatic fixative for
pot-pourri; the seed oil
is given for earache.

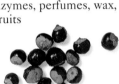

△ GUARANA
Seeds from the Amazon-
ian Paullinia cupana
give a stimulant,
caffeine-rich drink.

◁ PRICKLY PEAR
Opuntia ficus-indica *is*
a Mexican cactus with
succulent fruit which is
nutritious, medicinal,
and a source of alcohol.

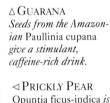

BANANA ▷
The sweet, phosphorous-
and carbohydrate-rich
fruit of this Musa
species is popular
with athletes for its
quick conversion
to energy. Its
pulp in face
masks
softens
skin.

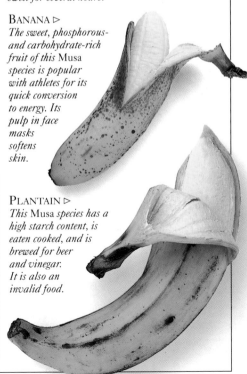

PLANTAIN ▷
This Musa *species has a*
high starch content, is
eaten cooked, and is
brewed for beer
and vinegar.
It is also an
invalid food.

DRYING SEEDS

Pick seeds when ripe from healthy plants on a warm, dry day. Shake into a paper bag, or cut whole stalks. Lay seeds or stalks on paper or hang above an open box in a warm place for two weeks to ensure no moisture re- mains. Rub seeds from their stalks or pods; store in airtight jars.

ROOTS

Roots are the underground parts of a plant. They hold it in the soil, absorb water and nutrients, and some are storage organs, containing concentrated active compounds. For example, the potency of the ginseng root increases each year following the sharp frosts of autumn, when goodness from the aerial parts of the plant returns to the root for storage in winter. Roots are valued for a range of uses: Orris root is enjoyed for its long-lasting fragrance, Marshmallow roots are used in soothing skin creams, and Liquorice for lozenges.

Bulbs, corms, and tubers are all types of underground storage organ – the Early Purple Orchid tuber contains the most nutritious plant substance known. Rhizomes are creeping, horizontal, under-

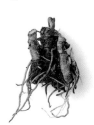

△ GOLDEN SEAL
Hydrastis canadensis *is a strong general tonic for the mucous membranes, liver, and uterus, and for venous circulation.*

◁ HORSERADISH
A pungent condiment, Armoracia rusticana *also stimulates the appetite. A root section left in the ground will regrow.*

△ SKUNK CABBAGE
The roots of Symplocarpus foetidus *treat asthma and headaches and stem blood flow. The root hairs reduce toothache.*

WHITE SQUILL ▷
Urginea maritima *bulbs are expectorant and diuretic. Red Squill is used as a rat poison.*

ROOT ANATOMY

The tiny hairs on roots absorb nutrients and water and may exude protective chemicals. Thick roots act as an anchor and as storage organs in dormant seasons. Root skin or bark may contain a different mixture of active compounds from the interior.

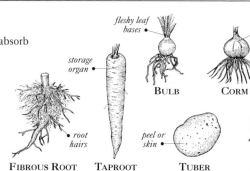

fleshy leaf bases •

• new corm grows above old corm

storage organ •

BULB

CORM

• root hairs

peel or skin •

FIBROUS ROOT   **TAPROOT**   **TUBER**   **RHIZOME**

ground stems from which roots and new shoots grow. Runners and stolons are both horizontal stems, not roots. Runners grow new plants where they touch the soil; stolons grow new plants at nodal joints (points with growing cells).

HARVESTING ROOTS

In seasonal climates, the best quality roots are dug in spring before sap rises, or in autumn. The dry season is best in the tropics. If leaving some root for regrowth, cut cleanly with a knife.

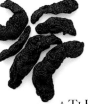

△ TI HUANG
A cooling yin tonic, Rehmannia glutinosa *beautifies hair and nourishes the blood.*

GREENBRIAR ▷
Smilax glabra *is a cooling, purgative tonic. It relieves itching and inflammation, treats boils and syphilitic lesions, and inhibits cancer cells.*

◁ DEVIL'S CLAW
Harpagophytum procumbens *eases arthritic pain and swelling; it is also a liver tonic.*

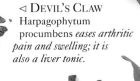

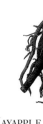

GREATER GALANGAL
Alpina galanga *root has a peppery, ginger flavour. It yields an essential oil,* Essence d'Amali.

MAYAPPLE
The toxic, anti-viral rhizome and resin of Podophyllum peltatum *are used in drugs for venereal warts, verrucas, and some cancers.*

CHINESE FAIRY VINE
Aristolochia debilis *treats poisonous snakebites, stomach pains, sore throats, and coughs. It contains toxic anti-tumour agents, and a painkiller for cancer.*

WHITE FALSE HELLEBORE ▷
The poisonous Veratrum album *treats hypertension, is a heart sedative, an insecticide, and a vet medicine.*

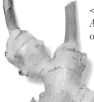

◁ GINGER
A popular spice, Zingiber officinale *reduces nausea from travel and from eating too much garlic.*

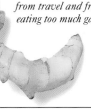

PREPARING ROOTS

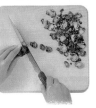

Shake or rub off soil, remove fibrous roots, and scrub clean. Chop, then spread to dry in a cool oven (50–60°C, 120–150°F) for 2–6 hours until brittle. Store in dark, airtight jars and label. Most roots prepared in this way will keep for years without absorbing moisture.

BARK, WOOD, AND RESIN

WOOD AND ITS protective layer of bark are found in the trunk, limbs, and roots of trees and shrubs. In spring, a ring of cells growing under the bark, the cambium layer, begins to divide, creating new sapwood to serve as vertical feeding channels for the plant. This hardens by the autumn. Outer bark, which is composed of dead cells, cracks or peels as the wood expands. Bark is continually replaced by the cambium layer, which means the inner bark stays moist and alive (see box below).

Bark is used in deodorizing charcoals, as cork, for soil improvement, and as a source of tannins and spices. Many bark drugs come from trees native to the

Americas, like the malaria cure quinine (*Cinchona* spp.), and witch-hazel.

Wood is primarily used in construction, and for fuel and paper pulp. But various woods have herbal uses, such as the medicinal Lignum Vitae (*Guaiacum officinale*) and Quassia, which is also an insecticide. Aromatic woods have long been used as incense, and the essential oils they contain are antiseptic and kill airborne disease. Woods such as sandalwood and cedar hold their scent for years, which increases their value as perfumes.

Resins and gums are inflammable, sticky, often aromatic compounds, which are insoluble in water. Trees make them to protect themselves when damaged. Latex is a whitish juice

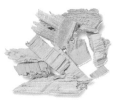

CINNAMON ▽▷
The sweet, spicy quills (below) are the branch bark of Cinnamomum verum, *used in desserts; the robust red-brown trunk bark from C.* aromatica *(right) is known as cassia, and flavours savoury dishes.*
Sliced cassia branches treat poor circulation and fevers.

• sliced branches

• cassia inner bark

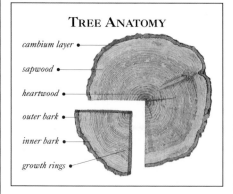

• outer bark

• quills

QUASSIA
The medicinal wood chips of Picrasma excelsa *also yield an insecticide for woolly aphids and greenfly.*

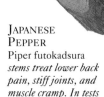

JAPANESE PEPPER
Piper futokadsura *stems treat lower back pain, stiff joints, and muscle cramp. In tests they inhibit cancer cells.*

TREE ANATOMY

cambium layer •

sapwood •

heartwood •

outer bark •

inner bark •

growth rings •

MINDANO GUM
Eucalyptus deglupta *has coloured, camphor-scented bark that peels in ribbons and is a folk medicine for fatigue.*

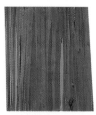

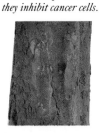

IRONWOOD
A sacred Buddhist tree, Mesua ferrea *has aromatic, astringent bark, given to induce perspiration.*

or sap exuded for the same reason. Resin, gum, and latex are usually collected by cutting the bark (see box bottom right).

HARVESTING BARK AND WOOD

Bark is levered off in the tree's dormant season; wood is chipped and dried. Ring barking kills trees and all bark removal can make trees vulnerable. When gathering bark, brush clean, wash if necessary, then spread out and dry.

COPAL RESIN
The resin of Protium copal *is a sacred, protective, and medicinal Mayan incense.*

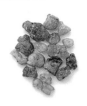

FRANKINCENSE
Boswellia carteri *resin makes a healing incense, which induces a meditative state.*

ALOE WOOD
The prized elusive scent of Aquilaria agallocha *only exists in resin-saturated diseased wood.*

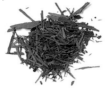

PAU D'ARCO
Tabebuia impetiginosa *is an immune enhancer and fabled cure-all for cancer and candida.*

TRAGACANTH
Astragalus gummifer *gum, scentless until burned, is cosmetic, medicinal, an incense, and a fumigant.*

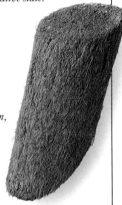

BAOBAB
The spongy wood of Adansonia digitata *stores carbohydrates and water, and is carved as panscrapers (above) and fishing floats. Its acid fruit thickens rubber latex.*

ANGOSTURA
Bitters is made from the resinous inner bark of Galipea officinalis, *a fragrant palm-like tree. It is a stimulant folk medicine, and is added to sherry and gin.*

LIGNUM VITAE
Guaiacum officinale *wood has a laxative resin. The heated wood is aromatic.*

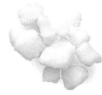

BORNEO CAMPHOR
Dryobalanops camphora *crystals are used in mothballs and are less toxic than camphor.*

RESIN, GUM, AND LATEX EXTRACTION

Resin, gum, and latex are harvested by puncturing or cutting the bark in diagonal grooves, avoiding the cambium layer. It is collected later (as seen right, where latex is being tapped from the Rubber Tree, *Hevea brasiliensis*). Pine, copal, dragon's blood (from *Dracaena* species), dammar (from *Shorea* species), balsams, mastic, and storax are all collected in this way. Resin is also collected as naturally exuded "tears" from frankincense, myrrh, and gum trees.

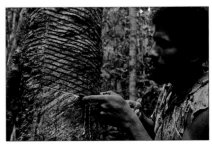

ESSENTIAL OILS

ESSENTIAL OILS, also known as volatile or ethereal oils, are the concentrated aromatic essences of plants. They are found in special cells of flowers, leaves, seeds, peel, and roots, and in the bark, resin, and wood of trees. More than 400 essences have been identified, of which about 50 are available to the public. The most expensive, Tuberose, comes from the flower *Polianthes tuberosa*. These essences provide antiseptic protection to the growing plant. They also give the herb its flavour and part of its health value, but their main attraction is their fragrance. This seductive scent lies behind the appeal of aromatherapy, in which oils are administered mainly via massage. A dramatic increase in public interest in essential oils has led to their greater accessibility, and there is now a growing demand for their use in aromatherapy courses and treatment.

These wonderful substances can be used to uplift, refresh, or relax mind, body, and spirit, to soothe muscles, and to beautify the skin. They may also be used to treat common ailments, in room-sprays, in incenses, and in the bath.

USING ESSENTIAL OILS SAFELY

It is vital that users of essential oils are extremely safety conscious. Essential oils should not be taken internally

ROSE OIL
Rosa damascena is grown mainly in Turkey and Bulgaria for rose essential oil. This is usually extracted by solvents, but in this process valuable components are lost, so the more expensive method of "enfleurage" may be used, creating rose attar.

PATCHOULI OIL
Distilled from leaves and shoots, this exotic fragrance of India became a symbol of the 1960s. The pure oil is less heavy than many Patchouli perfumes.

▽ PAU D'ANGOLA
(*Mespilodaphne pretiosa*)

▽ TUCUMA
(*Astrocaryum tucuma*)

△ PRIPRIOCA
(*Cyperus odoratus*)

AROMATIC POWDERS
When essential oils exist in strong cells, such as in many woods and roots, they keep their scent for years and can be usefully stored in powdered form. Pau D'Angola, Priprioca, and Tucuma are all used in both perfumes and medicines.

EXTRACTING OILS FROM PLANTS

It takes 60,000 roses to make 30g (1oz) of rose oil (see right), hence its extremely high price. Essential oils are extracted by distillation, expression, enfleurage, or by a solvent. The plant part used and the delicacy of the oil determine the method employed. Distillation is the most common, used for flowers less affected by heat, like lavender, and for most leaves, seeds, and wood. Expression is when the oil is pressed out. Enfleurage, in which fat is used to absorb the perfume, is suitable for fragile petals, like jasmine. Alcohol is the usual solvent used, but a non-alcohol solvent system has recently been developed.

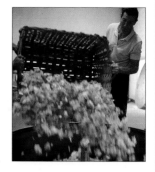

except when prescribed by qualified persons, and training is necessary to learn which oils should be avoided during pregnancy for example, or by sufferers of epilepsy or high blood pressure, or by people with sensitive skin. Essential oils should not be confused with *pressed* oils, usually from seeds, used in cooking.

ESSENTIAL OIL DOSES

Essential oil doses are measured in drops; and for massage, 2 or 3 drops of essential oil are blended with 5ml (1tsp) of pressed or "carrier" oil, such as almond or grape-seed oil. Once mixed, their shelf life is reduced from years to months.

FRANKIN-CENSE
Another source of frankincense resin (see p.21), Boswellia thurifera *is distilled to produce oil used in rejuvenating creams for mature skins.*

COSTUS
The scented root oil of Saussurea lappa *treats skin disease and is added to oriental perfumes and hair dyes.*

◁ MYRRH
An ancient and sacred incense, the antiseptic, anti-inflammatory oil of Commiphora myrrha *was used for embalming. It is now found in toothpaste and perfume.*

LEMON
Lemon peel oil is a bleach and immune system enhancer. Eighty-five lemons yield 30g (1oz) of oil.

CAJAPUT
The antiseptic leaf oil is used in cold treatments and liniments.

JASMINE
Jasmine flowers collected in the early morning yield expensive jasmine oil by enfleurage. It is an anti-depressant and aphrodisiac, used in perfumes, dry skin care, and massage.

BUYING AND STORING OILS

Buy oils that have been tested for purity, and extracted from organically grown plants. They should be sold in dark glass bottles with a dropper, and labelled with the botanic name, country of origin, and safety advice. Keep oils in cool darkness. They may be fatal if ingested, so store securely, away from children.

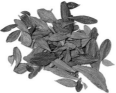

◁ ROUND BUCHU
The leaf of Barosma betulina *is a urinary antiseptic and kidney tonic, and is infused in oil to give perfume.*

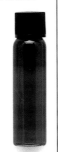

BOLDO ▷
Peumus boldus *is a digestive, liver tonic, diuretic, and a slimming aid. When distilled, its sweet, refreshing leaf oil is popular in soaps and perfumes.*

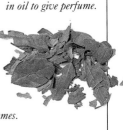

USING HERBS FOR COOKERY

HERBS TASTE GOOD and look good. They are the ingredients that can transform ordinary food and drinks into sumptuous meals. Greater travel opportunities and exotic cookbooks have introduced many new herbs to our diet, and long-forgotten edible flowers, buds, leaves, and roots are creeping back into common usage. Research has shown that culinary herbs can also have digestive, stimulant, or calming effects.

There are three basic ways of cooking with herbs. Some plants, such as borage, are eaten fresh, as a garnish, or in drinks and salads. Mild herbs like parsley are included towards the end of cooking to bring out flavour. Stronger tasting herbs and spices such as garlic and bay are added to dishes as cooking starts.

USEFUL EQUIPMENT

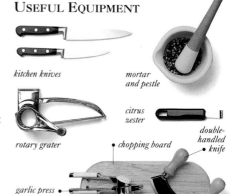

kitchen knives

mortar and pestle

citrus zester

double-handled knife

rotary grater

chopping board

garlic press

wheel

HERB AND SPICE MIXTURES

Every cuisine has its favourite blends. The Chinese have five-spice with star anise, fagara, fennel, cassia, and cloves. Malay blends include chilli, tamarind, coconut, galangal, candle-nuts, and lime leaf. Cajun mixes use paprika, mustard, cumin, chilli, and oregano. Pizza herbs are basil, sweet marjoram, and oregano, and the North American pumpkin pie mix is cinnamon, allspice, nutmeg, and ginger.

BOUQUET GARNI

A herb bundle is used in the cooking of soups and stews. It is tied for easy removal and traditionally comprises three parsley stalks, a small thyme sprig, and a bay leaf, with a range of extras from lemon peel to a celery-stalk wrapping.

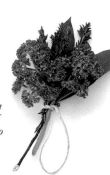

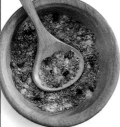

◁ **CHAT MASALA**
An Indian salad mix, made of asafoetida, ajowan, cumin, mint, cayenne, ginger, mango, and pomegranate seeds.

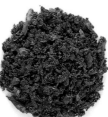

◁ **HARISSA**
A Tunisian paste for couscous stews, with red chillies, coriander seeds, caraway, garlic, cumin, and mint, in olive oil.

QUATRE-EPICES ▷
A French blend for pork dishes with black peppercorns, cloves, ginger, nutmeg, and occasionally cinnamon.

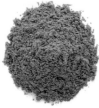

ZAHTAR ▷
An aromatic North African mixture for meatballs, featuring sumac, roasted sesame seeds, and thyme.

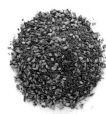

STORING HERBAL FLAVOURS

Many cooking ingredients absorb plant flavours. Unheated vegetable oil, heated vinegar, or warmed honey will assume the flavours of fresh herbs, fragrant flowers, or spices. The plants should be steeped in the liquid for about two weeks. For a stronger flavour, the process may be repeated with fresh herbs. Vanilla sugar is achieved by "dry infusion" with a vanilla pod. Butter rolled in chopped herbs or covered in rose petals overnight will absorb the taste and fragrance.

CAPERS
Pickled buds of Capparis spinosa.

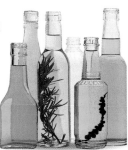

HERBAL VINEGARS
White or red wine vinegars are made by adding fresh herbs and flowers, such as dill, chilli, marjoram, rosemary, elderflower, or lavender, to cider or wine vinegar, in an airtight bottle. They add flavour to dressings and marinades.

DRINKS

From desert nomads to the Arctic Inuit, tribes worldwide find local plants to brew, like Mormon tea (*Ephedra nevadensis*), maté, and guarana. Many of these, such as tea and coffee, are now widely used. Herbs steeped in tonic wines, liqueurs, and syrups create delights such as electuaries, cordials, and robs.

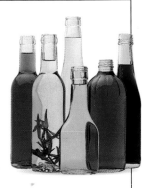

SARSAPARILLA
The roots of Smilax regelii, (*syn.* Smilax officinalis) *flavour soft drinks and root beer; it is also an Amazonian tonic taken for skin disease and to restore virility.*

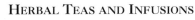

YERBA MATÉ
The leaves of Ilex paraguariensis *are brewed to make a South American, caffeine-rich, stimulant tea.*

ROOIBOSCH
This South African, fermented, red-leaf tea, from Aspalathus linearis, *is low in caffeine, and reduces allergies.*

LABRADOR TEA
The slightly narcotic leaves of the Arctic evergreen shrub Ledum groenlandicum *are brewed as tea (steeped only, as boiling may release a harmful alkaloid) or beer. They are used by Canadian native peoples to expel catarrh and treat colds.*

HERBAL TEAS AND INFUSIONS

Place the fresh or dried leaf, flower, crushed seed, bark, or root in a teapot; add boiling water and brew for 5 minutes. Allow a teaspoon of dried herb or a fresh sprig of about 6–9 leaves per cup. Strain and serve.

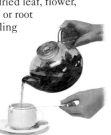

YELLOW GENTIAN
Gentiana lutea *roots and the underground stem make gentian bitters and brandy (to aid digestion and stimulate appetite), and a nerve tonic used by the Ancient Greeks as a poison antidote.*

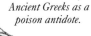

HEALING HERBS

TURNING TO PLANTS for healing is an instinct as old as human history and is mirrored in the behaviour of animals. As humans evolved, so too did a variety of beliefs in what maintained life and the events or forces that could damage it. Many healing remedies that involved plants were selected by observation, inspiration, and experience, and skilled healers became highly valued members of tribes of all races.

CHINESE HERBALISM

Underlying Chinese herbalism is the Taoist philosophy in which all phenomena result from the interplay of yin (feminine, cool, moist) and yang (masculine, hot, dry) as they create a spiral of continuous change. So early Taoists tasted each herb to feel its yin or yang effect, and linked each with a season, taste, emotion, and an

DANG SHEN
Codonopsis pilosula *is a tonic, detoxifying, yin herb, one of 2,000 Chinese herbs tested over 4,500 years.*

element (fire, water, wood, earth, or metal) to symbolize its way of creating change in the body. Taoists sensed three types of body energy: Jing – inherited instinct and growth, nurtured by food and herbs; Qi (Chi) – the life force in all things, adjusted through acupuncture and herbs; and Shen which gives higher consciousness by meditation. All three energies are considered in the Chinese holistic approach to diagnosis. A herb is seldom used alone as a treatment, but is combined with others to reinforce its action and to counter side-effects.

JI ZI
Wolfberries (Lycium chinense) *are a kidney tonic linked to the element earth.*

AYURVEDIC

Ayurveda, "the science of living", is an ancient Hindu healing system working with meditation, yoga, and about 500 herbs. It sees three forces interacting with body systems: prana (breath), agni (fire), and soma (love). It maintains that imbalance causes illness, so uses herbs to re-balance the whole system, as well as to treat specific symptoms. It links energy in the body with the energy of the universe through the chakras – seven points along the spine, each with specific associations. For example, the golden crown chakra is linked to the brain and pineal gland, and is balanced with brain tonic herbs.

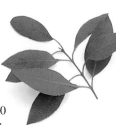

SANDALWOOD
It strengthens the brow chakra and cleanses and cools the blood.

SAFFRON
Saffron tones the heart chakra and benefits both heart and skin.

NATIVE TRIBES OF THE AMERICAS

Each tribe uses local plants for healing, under the guidance of the shaman, or medicine man. He is taught to "listen" to the plants as teachers, and to divine cures, using medicine wheel plant totems and incense. Sauna-like sweat lodges are used for purification.

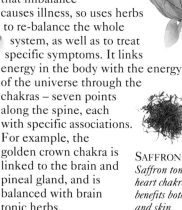

SQUAW VINE
Mitchella repens *was taken by early settlers to ease childbirth.*

WESTERN HERBALISM

Western herbal systems evolved from 3,000BC in Sumer, Crete, Egypt, and Greece. In Greece in 1,300BC, Asklepios developed healing centres which combined music and sport with his visionary diagnostic skills and unrivalled knowledge of herbs. Asklepians

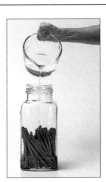

GARLIC
A daily ration for pyramid builders maintained their stamina.

became a noble order of healers, and included Hippocrates, who emphasized self-healing. About AD175 Galen codified Greek ideas of the four elements: earth, water, fire, and air, relating them to four humours and personality types. These formed the basis of European herbalism (and Unani medicine in Pakistan). A Roman "mechanistic" view took over from the Ancient Greek "holistic" ideas, and came to dominate science until recently.

MANDRAKE
Poisonous, man-shaped, narcotic root, as used by Lucrezia Borgia.

HOMEOPATHIC REMEDIES

A recent interpretation of new physics principles suggests that all things, from light waves, to plants and humans, are composed of patterns of energy. This may explain how homeopathy works: minute doses of plants, repeatedly diluted in alcohol, are given as treatment. In the most "potent" doses almost nothing of the plant remains, but as the remedies often work, one theory is that the plant's pattern of energy has left a kind of "echo" in the alcohol. A holistic approach is taken, which considers physical and emotional symptoms and picks plants that cause similar symptoms to stimulate the body's defences. This is called "treating like with like".

Bach Flower Remedies and Californian and Australian Flower Remedies come from wild plants, prescribed to heal inharmonious states of mind.

ARNICA
This immuno-stimulant is used in homeopathy to reduce bruises and jet-lag.

HERBAL PREPARATIONS

Herbal remedies require various preparation methods. Infusions are the most common (see p.25), but compresses, poultices, syrups, and powders can all be made at home, as well as decoctions, ointments, and tinctures. A standard infusion or decoction dose is 5ml (1tsp) of dried herb or a fresh sprig of 6–9 leaves to 225ml (1 cup) of water.

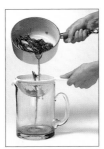

DECOCTION
Bruise the root, bark, or seed; put in cold water in a covered pan. Bring to boil and simmer until a quarter of the volume; strain.

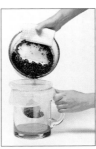

OINTMENT
Melt 250g (10oz) petroleum jelly; add 30g (1oz) dried or 90g (3oz) fresh herbs. Simmer for up to 2 hours; strain.

TINCTURE
Put 100g (4oz) dried or 250g (10oz) fresh herbs in jar; add 500ml (1¼pt) of 60° proof alchohol. Stand for two weeks; strain.

MEDICINAL MEALS

The Chinese have long recognized the therapeutic value of herbs and food combined. A Chinese medicinal meal is designed to rebalance conditions that cause illness, using cooling yin foods, such as barley or cucumber, or warming yang foods, such as ginger or red pepper. Fat-reducing preparations include dates, oats, mung beans, and lotus. Celery, lotus seeds, haws, and parsley are used to slow the ageing process. The ingredients pictured here are for a tonic soup to build Qi and Jing, detoxify the blood, and tone the organs.

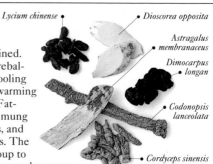

Lycium chinense •

• *Dioscorea opposita*

Astragalus membranaceus

Dimocarpus longan

• *Codonopsis lanceolata*

• *Cordyceps sinensis*

MODERN HERBALISM

Herbs offer hope for cures for modern diseases. Alkaloids that inhibit HIV have been discovered in Australia's Moreton Bay Chestnut tree (see p.43), Amazon Alexa trees, and Hogweed (see p.176). Diseases such as malaria, which are now resistant to some synthetic drugs, have been found to respond to treatment with traditional herb cures. The number of herbs believed to combat cancer grows daily – Suma (*Pfaffia paniculata*), the so-called "Amazon Ginseng", is now a patented cancer treatment – and more people are using tonics like the

PORIA COCOS
This fungus is given in fat-reducing meals in China. It also inhibits cancer cells.

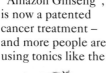

FALSE INDIGO
A North American herb, with indigo flowers and an antiseptic root, Baptista australis *is under research as a potential immune system booster.*

• *leaflets stimulate the appetite and aid digestion*

Chinese Sweet Tea Vine (*Gynostemma pentaphyllum*) to boost energy levels and strengthen the immune system.

The demand for accurate information about new herbal products is growing. In Europe the scientific evaluation of 200 herbs now taking place will enable their medicinal actions to be legally quoted on packaging.

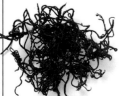

HERBA SARGASSUM
Sargassum fusiforme *is one of 300 Chinese anti-tumour herbs.*

ICELAND MOSS
The lichen Cetraria islandica *gives a brown dye and helps to fight tuberculosis.*

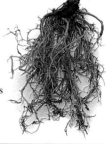

ASTRAGALUS ROOT
Astragalus membranaceus *boosts the immune system and generates anti-cancer cells in the body.*

HERBS FOR OTHER USES

HERBS TOUCH OUR DAILY LIVES in many ways, from the mint in our morning toothpaste to the cotton in our bed sheets. The herb plants in this book are described chiefly in terms of their culinary and medicinal virtues, but there are many more exotic and unusual ways to use plants. Some uses are widespread, others specific to certain countries or areas.

VEGETABLE IVORY
The seeds of Hyphaene benguellensis *replace ivory, for carving and buttons.*

LOCAL SECRETS

Each culture discovers its own cosmetic plants. In Peru dried Rhatany root (*Krameria triandra*) is used as a gum-tightening toothpaste which removes tartar and preserves teeth. The dried leaves of the South American shrub Jaborandi (*Pilocarpus jaborandi*) are used as a powerful but potentially hazardous hair tonic which opens skin pores to combat premature baldness. Sweet-scented carnauba wax from the leaf buds of *Copernicia* species is an ingredient in hair creams and mascaras. Plants are also used in many cultures to decorate

AGAR-AGAR
Gelidium amansii *is used by cooks as a vegetarian thickener.*

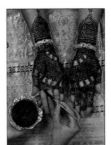

◁ **HENNA**
Lawsonia inermis *is used for bridal hand-painting in India.*

MACADAMIA ▽
Macadamia integrifolia *nuts give supple skin.*

and colour the body. In Peru the sap of the Genipa tree (*Genipa americana*) yields a blue body paint.

Plant aphrodisiacs often appear in the form of energizing herb tonics, such as the bark of Belize's Tree of Togetherness (*Anemopaegma arvense*). In southern USA the berries of Saw Palmetto (*Serenoa repens*) go into love potions with the root of Sweet Anise (*Osmorhiza occidentalis*), and in Ghana the aphrodisiac leaf of Flakwa (*Vernonia conferta*) is added to palm wine.

TATOO PLANT
Eclipta prostrata *leaf-juice makes an indigo skin dye.*

HERBAL PEST CONTROL

Some toxic herbs are used to stupefy fish for easy catching – without any ill-effects when eaten. A few, such as certain *Derris* species, may also be used as organic insecticides. Fish Poison Plant (*Tephrosia vogelii*) has cleared the Bilharzia water snail from Africa's Lake Malawi.

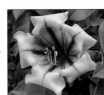

DAMIANA
The aromatic leaf of Turnera aphrodisiaca *is a flavouring, tonic, and aphrodisiac.*

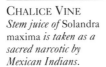

CHALICE VINE
Stem juice of Solandra maxima *is taken as a sacred narcotic by Mexican Indians.*

DEVIL'S TOBACCO
The toxic leaves of Lobelia tupa *are smoked in the Andes as a hallucinogenic intoxicant.*

HERB GARDENS

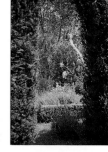

THE CHARM and attraction of herbs are magnified in a herb garden. Herbs will bring grace, fragrance, and flavour to almost every site: herbaceous borders, alpine and wild gardens, conservatories, patios, and interiors. Certain plants grow particularly well alongside others and when they are planted together deliberately this is known as companion planting. Many herbs are suitable companion plants. Some, especially pungent herbs like garlic and mint, deter pests that are attracted by aroma; some, like chamomile, exude a tonic for their neighbours, while others may discourage the growth of weeds.

PRIVATE AND PUBLIC GARDENS

A separate site, where herbs can grow together in profusion, is most desirable for a private garden. It should be located to receive maximum sunlight (this brings out leaf and flower scents) and enclosed to focus attention on the sensory pleasures and enhance the feeling of a special space.

A disciplined, geometric path design is a perfect complement to the "cottage-garden" abundance of herbs, giving a strong pattern in winter and making herb-gathering easier in bad weather. Most herbs are adaptable and easy to grow, flourishing even in confined locations such as patio pots, hanging baskets, and window boxes.

Public herb gardens offer great potential benefit for local communities. The fragrance and soft textures of herbs delight the blind. The subtle shades of silver and pink flowers and foliage, and

◁ HERB POTS
Pots allow you to move aromatic herbs into sunlight or to bring half-hardy and tender plants indoors during cold spells. The soil will drain well, an essential growing condition for many species.

SECRET GARDEN ▷
An enclosed herb garden lures you into its peaceful space, creating a feeling of seclusion and encouraging a closer knowledge of each plant.

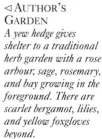

◁ AUTHOR'S GARDEN
A yew hedge gives shelter to a traditional herb garden with a rose arbour, sage, rosemary, and bay growing in the foreground. There are scarlet bergamot, lilies, and yellow foxgloves beyond.

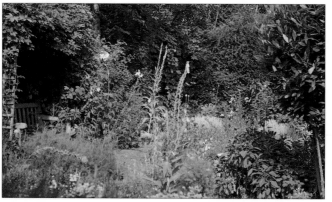

◁ DECORATIVE HERBS ▷
A basket (see left) offers sharp drainage conditions in which this group of thyme, tarragon, sage, and savory flourish. A cartwheel (see right) is an attractive and practical means of displaying herbs. Here, a range of low thymes allow the spokes of the wheel to remain visible.

soothing aromas, can be a tonic to the stressed.

Many herbs are grown in places of worship, as they have sacred associations, and aid contemplation and meditation. Schools, hospitals, and prisons could all benefit from their enriching influence.

PLANT PHARMACIES

Herb gardens in the past were frequently used as community chemists. From as early as AD529, Europe's first monastery at Monte Cassino, Italy, became a centre for herb growing and first-aid. In the 9th century, the usefulness of St. Gall's herb garden in Switzerland so impressed Holy Roman Emperor Charlemagne that he ordered duplicates to be built across his empire. In Asia, in AD657, a Tang dynasty emperor commissioned botanical details and information on how to grow and use 844 medicinal herbs from all over China. This information was printed and distributed to every town, with orders to grow herbs for the local people. A similar system still exists in Vietnamese villages today. The abbey gardens of Bury St. Edmunds, England, supplied plants to pharmacists from the 7th century until 1950. Many botanic gardens, such as two of Europe's first at Padua and Pisa in Italy, began life as herb gardens. Koishikawa, the oldest botanic garden in Tokyo, Japan, was planted as a physic garden, to reduce the need for medicinal imports from China.

The plant labels used by many botanic gardens today list uses, and are a testimony to the role of these ancient herb gardens.

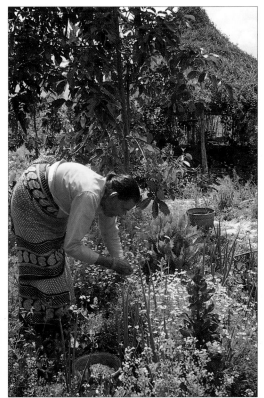

◁ NEPALESE HERB GARDEN
In this garden, Nepalese entomologist Kaminee Vaidya conducts organic pest control experiments. She uses different methods of companion planting based on a combination of Ayurvedic ideas (see p.26), and scientific theories.

TREES

Family PINACEAE	Species *Abies balsamea*	Local name Canada Balsam

BALSAM FIR

The 50 species of *Abies* are tall, evergreen conifers named from the Latin *abire*, to rise up. Balsam Fir has aromatic needles, scented purple cones, and bark covered in bubbles of valuable resin.

• **USES** The liquid resin taken from bark incisions is known variously as Balm of Gilead, Canada Turpentine, and, more recently, Canada Balsam. It has been used in Friar's Balsam and is one of the best gargles for sore throats. The resin is a treatment for catarrh and is applied as a poultice to help arthritis, cuts, and bruises. It has also been used to mount slide specimens and to make fine lacquer. Balsam gum is chewed. The resinous needles, cones, and winter buds are added to pot-pourri.

• **REMARK** *Abies alba* bark resin is distilled to make Strassburg turpentine. The buds and leaves are distilled to make the expectorant and antiseptic Silver Pine needle oil which is used in cough drops, asthma inhalations, and to give pine scent to toiletries.

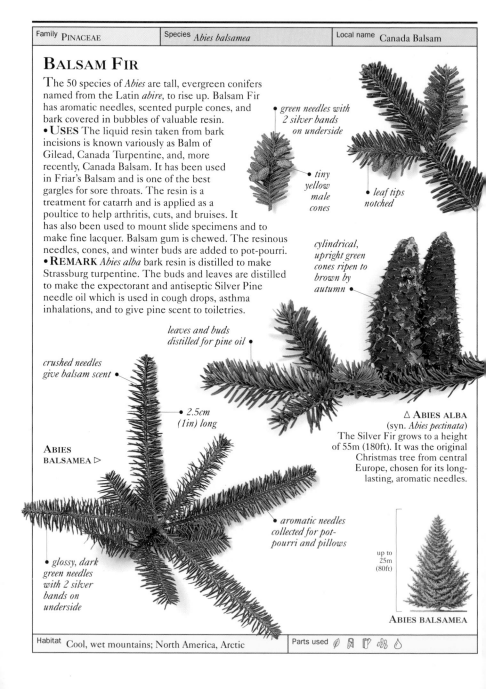

green needles with 2 silver bands on underside •

• tiny yellow male cones

• leaf tips notched

cylindrical, upright green cones ripen to brown by autumn •

leaves and buds distilled for pine oil •

crushed needles give balsam scent •

• 2.5cm (1in) long

ABIES BALSAMEA ▷

△ **ABIES ALBA**
(syn. *Abies pectinata*)
The Silver Fir grows to a height of 55m (180ft). It was the original Christmas tree from central Europe, chosen for its long-lasting, aromatic needles.

• aromatic needles collected for pot-pourri and pillows

up to 25m (80ft)

ABIES BALSAMEA

• glossy, dark green needles with 2 silver bands on underside

Habitat Cool, wet mountains; North America, Arctic	Parts used

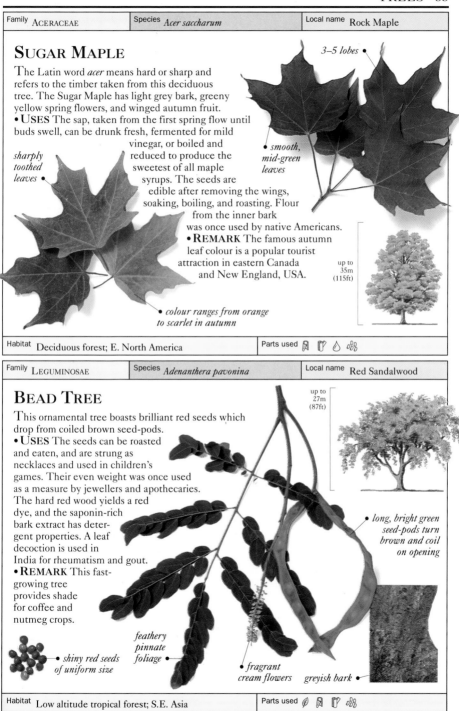

| Family ACERACEAE | Species *Acer saccharum* | Local name Rock Maple |

SUGAR MAPLE

The Latin word *acer* means hard or sharp and refers to the timber taken from this deciduous tree. The Sugar Maple has light grey bark, greeny yellow spring flowers, and winged autumn fruit.
• **USES** The sap, taken from the first spring flow until buds swell, can be drunk fresh, fermented for mild vinegar, or boiled and reduced to produce the sweetest of all maple syrups. The seeds are edible after removing the wings, soaking, boiling, and roasting. Flour from the inner bark was once used by native Americans.
• **REMARK** The famous autumn leaf colour is a popular tourist attraction in eastern Canada and New England, USA.

3–5 lobes •

• smooth, mid-green leaves

sharply toothed leaves •

up to 35m (115ft)

• colour ranges from orange to scarlet in autumn

| Habitat Deciduous forest; E. North America | Parts used |

| Family LEGUMINOSAE | Species *Adenanthera pavonina* | Local name Red Sandalwood |

BEAD TREE

This ornamental tree boasts brilliant red seeds which drop from coiled brown seed-pods.
• **USES** The seeds can be roasted and eaten, and are strung as necklaces and used in children's games. Their even weight was once used as a measure by jewellers and apothecaries. The hard red wood yields a red dye, and the saponin-rich bark extract has detergent properties. A leaf decoction is used in India for rheumatism and gout.
• **REMARK** This fast-growing tree provides shade for coffee and nutmeg crops.

up to 27m (87ft)

• long, bright green seed-pods turn brown and coil on opening

• shiny red seeds of uniform size

feathery pinnate foliage •

• fragrant cream flowers

greyish bark •

| Habitat Low altitude tropical forest; S.E. Asia | Parts used |

| Family BOMBACACEAE | Species *Adansonia digitata* | Local name Cream of Tartar Tree |

BAOBAB

The swollen-trunked Baobab tree is a distinctive feature of the African landscape. It bears carrion-scented, nocturnal white flowers which become long, woody fruit, each containing about 100 seeds.
• USES Baobab fruit has a powdery, acidic white pith, rich in vitamin C, which serves as Africa's equivalent to the lemon in food and drink. The bark is prescribed for fevers, the fruit for dysentery, the seed for gum disease, and the leaves have anti-histamine properties. The inner bark fibres absorb enough water to tap and the fibres are used to scour pans. The leaves are eaten. The tree also provides soap, dye, glue, fodder, and space for storage.
• REMARK The Baobab can live for 2,000 years, but pressure for land and its slow regeneration have put it under threat.

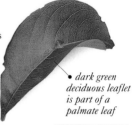

• *dark green deciduous leaflet is part of a palmate leaf*

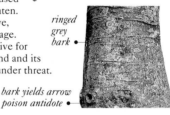

ringed grey bark •

bark yields arrow poison antidote •

up to 20m (65ft)

| Habitat Dry areas of tropics; African & Australian savannah | Parts used ✳ ✎ ⚄ ⚖ ⚘ ⛁ ⚙ |

| Family HIPPOCASTANACEAE | Species *Aesculus hippocastanum* | Local name Conker Tree |

HORSE CHESTNUT

The vigorous Horse Chestnut tree has fragrant cream flowers in early summer. In autumn, spiny green fruit yields up to three seeds or "conkers" and the leaves turn yellow-orange. Winter buds are protected from frost by sticky resin which melts in the spring, allowing shoots to emerge above horseshoe-shaped leaf scars.
• USES Seed compounds help prevent thrombosis by strengthening vein walls, and are an excellent astringent treatment for haemorrhoids. A seed extract is used in bath oils to improve skin tone and suppleness. During food shortages, treated fruit mash has been used as fodder and the protein-rich seeds made into flour and coffee. The tonic bark treats fevers and also gives a yellow dye.
• REMARK The nuts are mildly narcotic and the untreated seeds are toxic.

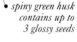

• *spiny green husk contains up to 3 glossy seeds*

• *upright panicles*

• *compound palmate leaf has 4–7 leaflets*

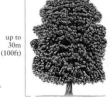

up to 30m (100ft)

• *creamy flowers*

• *unstalked serrated leaflet*

| Habitat Deciduous woodland; Europe | Parts used ✳ ⚖ ⚘ ⛁ ⚙ |

Family EUPHORBIACEAE	Species *Aleurites moluccana*	Local name Kemiri / Buah Keras

CANDLE-NUT TREE

This evergreen has lobed leaves with a rust-coloured fuzzy surface on the underside. Cymes of small white flowers are followed by fruit containing the candle-nuts. The name refers to primitive candles made from the oily nuts which are threaded on to palm leaf ribs.

• USES The Candle-nut seed yields drying oils for varnishes, and artists' paints. In Indonesia the oil treats hair loss, calloused skin, and constipation, while the bark relieves dysentery. The pulped kernel and boiled leaves are prescribed for headaches, ulcers, and swollen joints. The treated nut is cooked in Indonesian curries. The oil is used in wood preservatives, batik work, and soap.

long stalk •

• grey-green bark

mid-green, hand-sized leaf with 3–5 lobes •

up to 20m (65ft)

fresh nuts contain poison which gradually disappears •

Habitat Lime-free & acid soils in tropical forests; S.E. Asia	Parts used

Family BETULACEAE	Species *Alnus glutinosa*	Local name Scottish Mahogany

COMMON ALDER

This fast-growing riverside tree keeps its leaves until late into autumn. Fruit "cones" last through winter and are joined in spring by yellow-green catkins and sticky new shoots. The bark is dark grey and ridged.

• USES The Alder supplies a remarkable range of dyes: the bark colours wool red and with mordants can give black or yellow; the young shoots provide a yellowish grey dye used in tapestries; new shoots give a cinnamon colour; fresh wood makes a pink dye; and catkins make green dye. A leaf poultice relieves pain and swelling and a leaf infusion makes a refreshing bath for sore feet.

up to 25m (80ft)

ALNUS GLUTINOSA

• young, dark green leaves have sticky surface said to capture fleas

• hair tufts on underside of veins

◁ **ALNUS RUBRA**
The Red Alder with double-toothed leaves and small, cone-like fruit yields tannin, dyes, and medicine.

• young catkins

△ **ALNUS GLUTINOSA**

• small ripe fruit "cones"

Habitat Riverbanks & damp areas; Europe, N. Africa	Parts used

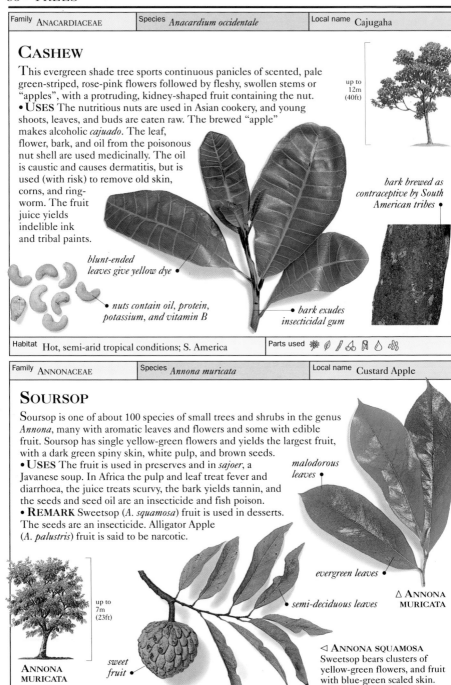

Family ANACARDIACEAE	Species *Anacardium occidentale*	Local name Cajugaha

CASHEW

This evergreen shade tree sports continuous panicles of scented, pale green-striped, rose-pink flowers followed by fleshy, swollen stems or "apples", with a protruding, kidney-shaped fruit containing the nut.
• **USES** The nutritious nuts are used in Asian cookery, and young shoots, leaves, and buds are eaten raw. The brewed "apple" makes alcoholic *cajuado*. The leaf, flower, bark, and oil from the poisonous nut shell are used medicinally. The oil is caustic and causes dermatitis, but is used (with risk) to remove old skin, corns, and ringworm. The fruit juice yields indelible ink and tribal paints.

up to 12m (40ft)

bark brewed as contraceptive by South American tribes •

blunt-ended leaves give yellow dye •

• nuts contain oil, protein, potassium, and vitamin B

• bark exudes insecticidal gum

Habitat Hot, semi-arid tropical conditions; S. America	Parts used

Family ANNONACEAE	Species *Annona muricata*	Local name Custard Apple

SOURSOP

Soursop is one of about 100 species of small trees and shrubs in the genus *Annona*, many with aromatic leaves and flowers and some with edible fruit. Soursop has single yellow-green flowers and yields the largest fruit, with a dark green spiny skin, white pulp, and brown seeds.
• **USES** The fruit is used in preserves and in *sajoer*, a Javanese soup. In Africa the pulp and leaf treat fever and diarrhoea, the juice treats scurvy, the bark yields tannin, and the seeds and seed oil are an insecticide and fish poison.
• **REMARK** Sweetsop (*A. squamosa*) fruit is used in desserts. The seeds are an insecticide. Alligator Apple (*A. palustris*) fruit is said to be narcotic.

malodorous leaves

evergreen leaves •

△ **ANNONA MURICATA**

semi-deciduous leaves •

up to 7m (23ft)

ANNONA MURICATA

sweet fruit •

◁ **ANNONA SQUAMOSA**
Sweetsop bears clusters of yellow-green flowers, and fruit with blue-green scaled skin.

Habitat Hot, moist, tropical conditions; tropical USA	Parts used

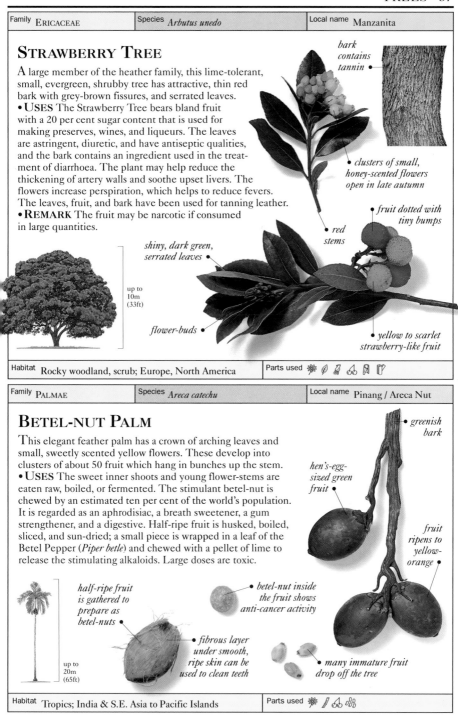

| Family ERICACEAE | Species *Arbutus unedo* | Local name Manzanita |

STRAWBERRY TREE

A large member of the heather family, this lime-tolerant, small, evergreen, shrubby tree has attractive, thin red bark with grey-brown fissures, and serrated leaves.
• USES The Strawberry Tree bears bland fruit with a 20 per cent sugar content that is used for making preserves, wines, and liqueurs. The leaves are astringent, diuretic, and have antiseptic qualities, and the bark contains an ingredient used in the treatment of diarrhoea. The plant may help reduce the thickening of artery walls and soothe upset livers. The flowers increase perspiration, which helps to reduce fevers. The leaves, fruit, and bark have been used for tanning leather.
• REMARK The fruit may be narcotic if consumed in large quantities.

bark contains tannin •

• clusters of small, honey-scented flowers open in late autumn

• fruit dotted with tiny bumps

• red stems

shiny, dark green, serrated leaves •

up to 10m (33ft)

flower-buds •

• yellow to scarlet strawberry-like fruit

| Habitat Rocky woodland, scrub; Europe, North America | Parts used ❊ ⊘ 🖊 ⚖ 🗚 🍃 |

| Family PALMAE | Species *Areca catechu* | Local name Pinang / Areca Nut |

BETEL-NUT PALM

This elegant feather palm has a crown of arching leaves and small, sweetly scented yellow flowers. These develop into clusters of about 50 fruit which hang in bunches up the stem.
• USES The sweet inner shoots and young flower-stems are eaten raw, boiled, or fermented. The stimulant betel-nut is chewed by an estimated ten per cent of the world's population. It is regarded as an aphrodisiac, a breath sweetener, a gum strengthener, and a digestive. Half-ripe fruit is husked, boiled, sliced, and sun-dried; a small piece is wrapped in a leaf of the Betel Pepper (*Piper betle*) and chewed with a pellet of lime to release the stimulating alkaloids. Large doses are toxic.

• greenish bark

hen's-egg-sized green fruit •

fruit ripens to yellow-orange •

half-ripe fruit is gathered to prepare as betel-nuts •

• betel-nut inside the fruit shows anti-cancer activity

• fibrous layer under smooth, ripe skin can be used to clean teeth

• many immature fruit drop off the tree

up to 20m (65ft)

| Habitat Tropics; India & S.E. Asia to Pacific Islands | Parts used ❊ 🖊 🍃 🎋 |

Family PALMAE	Species *Arenga pinnata*	Local name Gomuti Palm

SUGAR PALM

The Sugar Palm tree is crowned with a spray of feathery leaves. The ringed trunk is clothed with the fibrous black sheaths of old leaves.

• **USES** Palm sugar is produced by tapping the tree's sap. The sap is collected and evaporated to a thick syrup which cools to a toffee-like sugar. The stem pith is used as sago. Juice from the developing flower is fermented into palm wine, or "toddy", which is used medicinally to treat menstrual disorders and vertigo, or distilled to make the spirit *arrack*. The root is used in local medicine to treat kidney stones. The young leaf sheaths produce useful fibres and the trunks are made into water pipes.

up to 20m (65ft)

glossy leaflets up to 1.5m (5ft) long

• fronds up to 8.5m (28ft) long, with irregularly shaped tips

Habitat Rainforests; Malaysia, Indonesia	Parts used ✳ ∅ 🔏 🏹 ◊

Family MORACEAE	Species *Artocarpus heterophyllus*	Local name Nangka

JACKFRUIT

This evergreen shade tree is cultivated mainly for its massive, oval green fruit which can grow directly from the trunk.

• **USES** The white flesh is eaten raw, cooked, or preserved, or made into a flavouring paste. Young leaves are eaten as a vegetable, and the small fruit added to soup. In Java, young flower clusters are eaten with syrup and agar-agar, and the seeds are added to curries. In Thailand, the roots are used to treat diarrhoea, the flowers to combat diabetes, and the fruit as an astringent or laxative.

• **REMARK** The tree means good fortune to Thais and the trunk yields a yellow dye for monks' robes.

• rounded, glossy green leaves, spirally arranged

grey-brown bark with green lichen •

fruit can weigh up to 30kg (66lb)

up to 15m (50ft)

Habitat Tropical forests & riverbanks; S.E. Asia	Parts used ✳ ∅ 🔏 🍃 🏹 ⚘

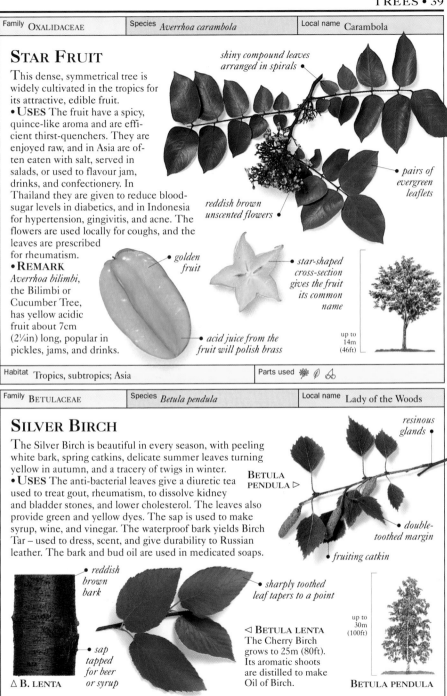

| Family OXALIDACEAE | Species *Averrhoa carambola* | Local name Carambola |

STAR FRUIT

This dense, symmetrical tree is widely cultivated in the tropics for its attractive, edible fruit.
• **USES** The fruit have a spicy, quince-like aroma and are efficient thirst-quenchers. They are enjoyed raw, and in Asia are often eaten with salt, served in salads, or used to flavour jam, drinks, and confectionery. In Thailand they are given to reduce blood-sugar levels in diabetics, and in Indonesia for hypertension, gingivitis, and acne. The flowers are used locally for coughs, and the leaves are prescribed for rheumatism.
• **REMARK** *Averrhoa bilimbi*, the Bilimbi or Cucumber Tree, has yellow acidic fruit about 7cm (2¼in) long, popular in pickles, jams, and drinks.

shiny compound leaves arranged in spirals

pairs of evergreen leaflets

reddish brown unscented flowers

golden fruit

star-shaped cross-section gives the fruit its common name

acid juice from the fruit will polish brass

up to 14m (46ft)

| Habitat Tropics, subtropics; Asia | Parts used |

| Family BETULACEAE | Species *Betula pendula* | Local name Lady of the Woods |

SILVER BIRCH

The Silver Birch is beautiful in every season, with peeling white bark, spring catkins, delicate summer leaves turning yellow in autumn, and a tracery of twigs in winter.
• **USES** The anti-bacterial leaves give a diuretic tea used to treat gout, rheumatism, to dissolve kidney and bladder stones, and lower cholesterol. The leaves also provide green and yellow dyes. The sap is used to make syrup, wine, and vinegar. The waterproof bark yields Birch Tar – used to dress, scent, and give durability to Russian leather. The bark and bud oil are used in medicated soaps.

BETULA PENDULA ▷

resinous glands

double-toothed margin

fruiting catkin

reddish brown bark

sharply toothed leaf tapers to a point

◁ **BETULA LENTA**
The Cherry Birch grows to 25m (80ft). Its aromatic shoots are distilled to make Oil of Birch.

sap tapped for beer or syrup

△ **B. LENTA**

up to 30m (100ft)

BETULA PENDULA

| Habitat Young woods; N. Asia, Europe | Parts used |

Family BIXACAE	Species *Bixa orellana*	Local name Annatto or Urucú

LIPSTICK TREE

This small tree, popular with bees, bears panicles of white or pink flowers, similar to wild roses, and a hairy, reddish fruit capsule containing 30–50 seeds.
• **USES** The red seed coats (arils) are scraped off for use as an orange-red dye. The dye colours cheese, butter, and chocolate, and is used locally to flavour rice. Amazonians use the dye on their bodies, weapons, and fabric, and eat it as an antidote to prussic acid poisoning caused by poorly treated Cassava (see p.115). The root is used locally as a digestive and to make rope fibre, and the seeds are prescribed as an expectorant.
• **REMARK** Taken internally the seed dye tints skin bronze and is now available in commercial tanning capsules.

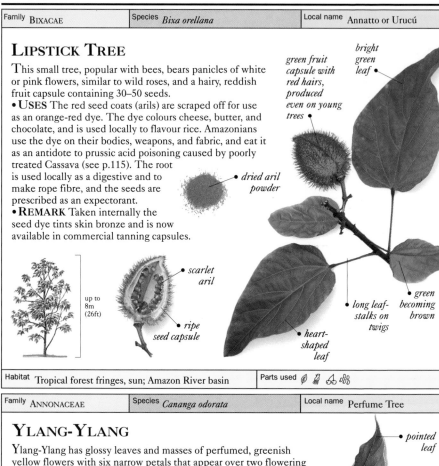

bright green leaf

green fruit capsule with red hairs, produced even on young trees

dried aril powder

up to 8m (26ft)

scarlet aril

ripe seed capsule

long leaf-stalks on twigs

green becoming brown

heart-shaped leaf

Habitat Tropical forest fringes, sun; Amazon River basin	Parts used

Family ANNONACEAE	Species *Cananga odorata*	Local name Perfume Tree

YLANG-YLANG

Ylang-Ylang has glossy leaves and masses of perfumed, greenish yellow flowers with six narrow petals that appear over two flowering periods. These are followed by oblong fruit with several seeds.
• **USES** The spicy, jasmine-scented flowers are picked for personal adornment, worn as an aphrodisiac, and used to scent linen. The essential oil is distilled by steam and features in many perfumes, soaps, skin lotions, and to balance sebum in Macasser hair oil. Aromatherapists consider the oil to have calming and relaxing properties.
• **REMARK** Ylang-Ylang means "flower of flowers".

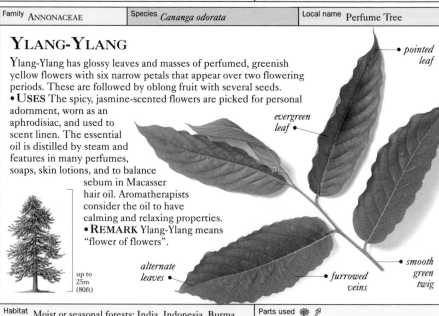

pointed leaf

evergreen leaf

up to 25m (80ft)

alternate leaves

furrowed veins

smooth green twig

Habitat Moist or seasonal forests; India, Indonesia, Burma	Parts used

Family BURSERACEAE	Species *Canarium commune*	Local name Elemi

JAVA ALMOND

This deciduous tree has panicles of pale yellow fragrant flowers and fleshy fruit with an edible seed.
• USES The pale yellow resin collected from bark incisions is known as "brea" or "manila elemi". The sharp lemon-scented resin is used in incense and its distilled oil is added to perfumes, cosmetics, and soaps. The edible seeds are used locally to treat beri-beri and in confectionery. The seed oil is used for cooking. In Indonesia the bark is prescribed for malaria and the leaves for vertigo.
• REMARK *Canarium edule* resin is used as perfume, incense, and to treat skin complaints.

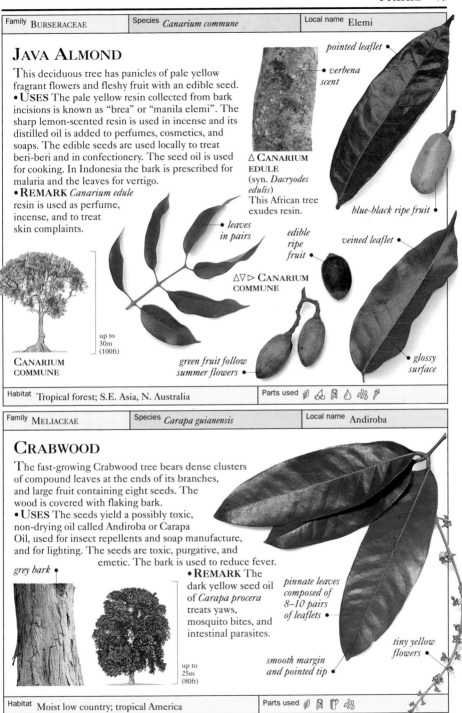

pointed leaflet •

• *verbena scent*

△ CANARIUM EDULE (syn. *Dacryodes edulis*) This African tree exudes resin.

blue-black ripe fruit •

leaves in pairs •

edible ripe fruit •

veined leaflet •

△▽▷ CANARIUM COMMUNE

up to 30m (100ft)

CANARIUM COMMUNE

green fruit follow summer flowers •

• *glossy surface*

Habitat Tropical forest; S.E. Asia, N. Australia	Parts used

Family MELIACEAE	Species *Carapa guianensis*	Local name Andiroba

CRABWOOD

The fast-growing Crabwood tree bears dense clusters of compound leaves at the ends of its branches, and large fruit containing eight seeds. The wood is covered with flaking bark.
• USES The seeds yield a possibly toxic, non-drying oil called Andiroba or Carapa Oil, used for insect repellents and soap manufacture, and for lighting. The seeds are toxic, purgative, and emetic. The bark is used to reduce fever.

grey bark •

• REMARK The dark yellow seed oil of *Carapa procera* treats yaws, mosquito bites, and intestinal parasites.

pinnate leaves composed of 8–10 pairs of leaflets •

tiny yellow flowers •

up to 25m (80ft)

smooth margin and pointed tip •

Habitat Moist low country; tropical America	Parts used

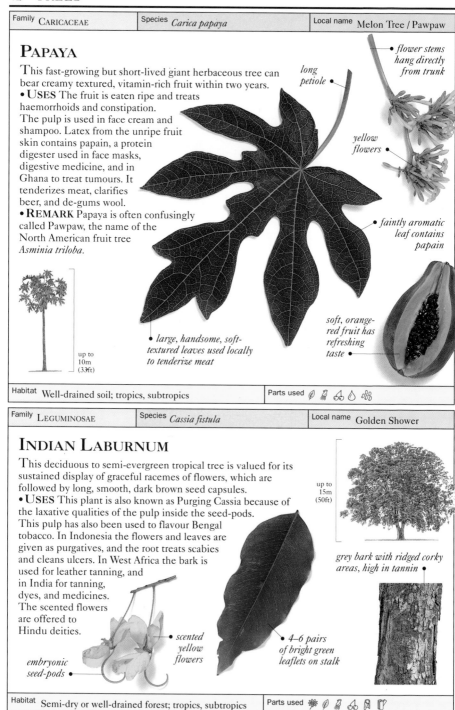

| Family CARICACEAE | Species *Carica papaya* | Local name Melon Tree / Pawpaw |

PAPAYA

This fast-growing but short-lived giant herbaceous tree can bear creamy textured, vitamin-rich fruit within two years.
• USES The fruit is eaten ripe and treats haemorrhoids and constipation. The pulp is used in face cream and shampoo. Latex from the unripe fruit skin contains papain, a protein digester used in face masks, digestive medicine, and in Ghana to treat tumours. It tenderizes meat, clarifies beer, and de-gums wool.
• REMARK Papaya is often confusingly called Pawpaw, the name of the North American fruit tree *Asminia triloba*.

long petiole

flower stems hang directly from trunk

yellow flowers

faintly aromatic leaf contains papain

up to 10m (33ft)

large, handsome, soft-textured leaves used locally to tenderize meat

soft, orange-red fruit has refreshing taste

| Habitat Well-drained soil; tropics, subtropics | Parts used |

| Family LEGUMINOSAE | Species *Cassia fistula* | Local name Golden Shower |

INDIAN LABURNUM

This deciduous to semi-evergreen tropical tree is valued for its sustained display of graceful racemes of flowers, which are followed by long, smooth, dark brown seed capsules.
• USES This plant is also known as Purging Cassia because of the laxative qualities of the pulp inside the seed-pods. This pulp has also been used to flavour Bengal tobacco. In Indonesia the flowers and leaves are given as purgatives, and the root treats scabies and cleans ulcers. In West Africa the bark is used for leather tanning, and in India for tanning, dyes, and medicines. The scented flowers are offered to Hindu deities.

up to 15m (50ft)

grey bark with ridged corky areas, high in tannin

scented yellow flowers

4–6 pairs of bright green leaflets on stalk

embryonic seed-pods

| Habitat Semi-dry or well-drained forest; tropics, subtropics | Parts used |

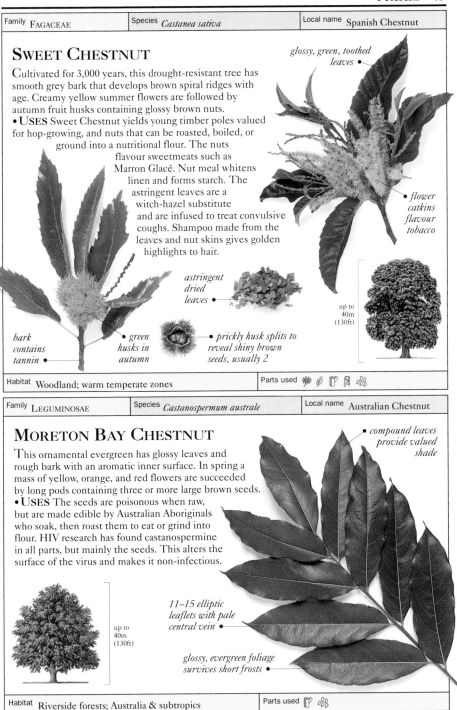

Family FAGACEAE	Species *Castanea sativa*	Local name Spanish Chestnut

SWEET CHESTNUT

Cultivated for 3,000 years, this drought-resistant tree has smooth grey bark that develops brown spiral ridges with age. Creamy yellow summer flowers are followed by autumn fruit husks containing glossy brown nuts.
• USES Sweet Chestnut yields young timber poles valued for hop-growing, and nuts that can be roasted, boiled, or ground into a nutritional flour. The nuts flavour sweetmeats such as Marron Glacé. Nut meal whitens linen and forms starch. The astringent leaves are a witch-hazel substitute and are infused to treat convulsive coughs. Shampoo made from the leaves and nut skins gives golden highlights to hair.

glossy, green, toothed leaves •

• flower catkins flavour tobacco

astringent dried leaves •

up to 40m (130ft)

bark contains tannin •

• green husks in autumn

• prickly husk splits to reveal shiny brown seeds, usually 2

Habitat Woodland; warm temperate zones	Parts used

Family LEGUMINOSAE	Species *Castanospermum australe*	Local name Australian Chestnut

MORETON BAY CHESTNUT

This ornamental evergreen has glossy leaves and rough bark with an aromatic inner surface. In spring a mass of yellow, orange, and red flowers are succeeded by long pods containing three or more large brown seeds.
• USES The seeds are poisonous when raw, but are made edible by Australian Aboriginals who soak, then roast them to eat or grind into flour. HIV research has found castanospermine in all parts, but mainly the seeds. This alters the surface of the virus and makes it non-infectious.

• compound leaves provide valued shade

up to 40m (130ft)

11–15 elliptic leaflets with pale central vein •

glossy, evergreen foliage survives short frosts •

Habitat Riverside forests; Australia & subtropics	Parts used

Family PINACEAE	Species *Cedrus libani*	Local name Tree of the Lord

CEDAR OF LEBANON

This noble conifer, with tiers of horizontal branches shading its dark, fissured bark, is famed for its aromatic wood.

• **USES** The fragrant resin has been used since ancient times: in incense and cosmetics, for embalming, and to treat leprosy and parasites. Today the wood of the Atlas Cedar subspecies is steam-distilled for its essential oil. This oil repels pests and is valued by aromatherapists to soothe chronic anxiety and to treat cystitis, problem skin, and bronchial conditions. Cedar Oil may inhibit the division of tumour cells.

• **REMARK** The extravagant use of Cedar in the building of the Hanging Gardens of Babylon and Solomon's Temple nearly brought about the tree's extinction.

dark green to blue needles in dense whorls

△ **CEDRUS LIBANI**

◁ **CEDRUS LIBANI SUBSP. ATLANTICA**
The flat-topped Atlas Cedar grows to 50m (164ft) and bears barrel-shaped cones.

grey to blue-green slender needles on side-shoots •

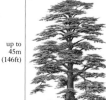

up to 45m (146ft)

CEDRUS LIBANI

Habitat Mountain forests; Lebanon, S.W. Turkey	Parts used 🍃 💧 🌱

Family BOMBACACEAE	Species *Ceiba pentandra*	Local name Silk Cotton Tree

KAPOK

The Kapok has a spiny trunk with buttress wings. It sports cup-shaped, pale yellow or pink flowers that become large, shiny capsules containing many seeds. The seeds are embedded in cream silky fibres, known as kapok.

• **USES** Kapok is buoyant and water-resistant and is used in life-jackets and pillows, for sound and temperature insulation, and as cotton wool. The edible seed oil is also used for soap and paint making. In West Africa the leaves treat colic, the bark is emetic, and the roots treat leprosy.

• kapok, the silky down from the seed-pod

young reddish leaves are • edible

circle of 5–9 leaflets •

up to 70m (230ft)

• dark green deciduous leaflet

Habitat Moist tropics; Africa, S. America, S.E. Asia	Parts used 🌰 🍂 🌿 🌾 🍃 🌸

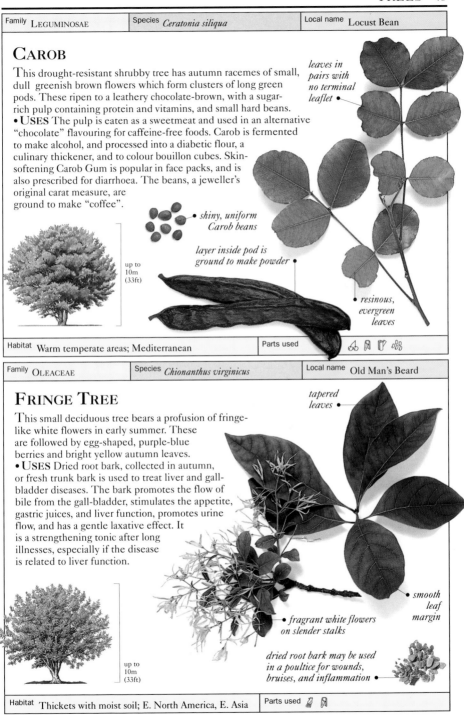

Family LEGUMINOSAE	Species *Ceratonia siliqua*	Local name Locust Bean

CAROB

This drought-resistant shrubby tree has autumn racemes of small, dull greenish brown flowers which form clusters of long green pods. These ripen to a leathery chocolate-brown, with a sugar-rich pulp containing protein and vitamins, and small hard beans.
• **USES** The pulp is eaten as a sweetmeat and used in an alternative "chocolate" flavouring for caffeine-free foods. Carob is fermented to make alcohol, and processed into a diabetic flour, a culinary thickener, and to colour bouillon cubes. Skin-softening Carob Gum is popular in face packs, and is also prescribed for diarrhoea. The beans, a jeweller's original carat measure, are ground to make "coffee".

leaves in pairs with no terminal leaflet

shiny, uniform Carob beans

layer inside pod is ground to make powder

resinous, evergreen leaves

up to 10m (33ft)

Habitat Warm temperate areas; Mediterranean	Parts used

Family OLEACEAE	Species *Chionanthus virginicus*	Local name Old Man's Beard

FRINGE TREE

This small deciduous tree bears a profusion of fringe-like white flowers in early summer. These are followed by egg-shaped, purple-blue berries and bright yellow autumn leaves.
• **USES** Dried root bark, collected in autumn, or fresh trunk bark is used to treat liver and gall-bladder diseases. The bark promotes the flow of bile from the gall-bladder, stimulates the appetite, gastric juices, and liver function, promotes urine flow, and has a gentle laxative effect. It is a strengthening tonic after long illnesses, especially if the disease is related to liver function.

tapered leaves

smooth leaf margin

fragrant white flowers on slender stalks

dried root bark may be used in a poultice for wounds, bruises, and inflammation

up to 10m (33ft)

Habitat Thickets with moist soil; E. North America, E. Asia	Parts used

Family RUTACEAE	Species *Citrus* species	Local name Various

CITRUS

The Citrus genus includes about 16 species of evergreen trees and shrubs, with perfumed flowers and segmented, aromatic fruit.
• **USES** The fruit, juice, and peel of Citrus fruits flavour food and drink and provide vitamin C. Essential oils from the peel scent food, cosmetics, and perfume; the seed oils are used in soaps. Bitter Orange flowers yield Neroli oil for perfumes and aromatherapy, the leaves and young shoots give the lighter petit-grain oil; both treat anxiety and depression. Bitter Orange seed oil reduces cholesterol, and Bergamot fruit essential oil is used in perfumes and aromatherapy. Lemon juice is antiseptic, astringent, and lightens hair; the essential oil is a stimulant and helps purify water.
• **REMARK** Untreated essential oils of some citrus fruits, especially Bergamot, increase skin photo-sensitivity and require cautious use.

up to 7m (23ft)

CITRUS LIMON

orange peel is used as a diuretic and digestive

fragrant flowers

◁ △ ▽ **CITRUS LIMON**

richly fragrant, white flowers

small toothed leaves

fruit ripens to bright orange

◁ **CITRUS AURANTIUM** (syn. *Citrus bigaradia*)
Bitter Orange is a 10m (33ft) tree with leathery leaves. The flowers, shoots, fruit, and seeds yield essential oils, and the by-product orange flower water.

Lemon fruit ripens to yellow

pale green fruit

slices of the pear-shaped, wrinkly fruit

double leaves

◁ ▽ **CITRUS HYSTRIX**
The Kaffir Lime is a small tree with double leaves and a clean, lemon taste; they are used with fruit peel in Thai and Indonesian cooking and medicine.

fresh and dried leaves have culinary uses

aromatic, warty rind

grated peel

Habitat Well-drained, moist soil; S.E. Asia, Pacific Islands	Parts used

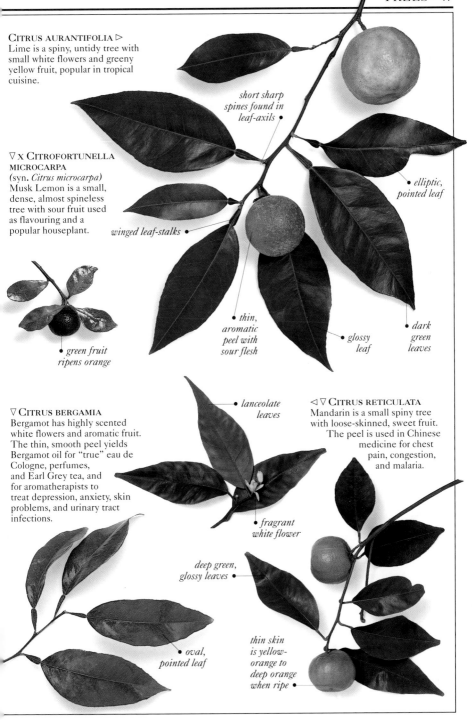

CITRUS AURANTIFOLIA ▷
Lime is a spiny, untidy tree with small white flowers and greeny yellow fruit, popular in tropical cuisine.

short sharp spines found in leaf-axils •

▽ x **CITROFORTUNELLA MICROCARPA**
(syn. *Citrus microcarpa*)
Musk Lemon is a small, dense, almost spineless tree with sour fruit used as flavouring and a popular houseplant.

winged leaf-stalks •

• *elliptic, pointed leaf*

• *green fruit ripens orange*

• *thin, aromatic peel with sour flesh*

• *glossy leaf*

• *dark green leaves*

• *lanceolate leaves*

▽ **CITRUS BERGAMIA**
Bergamot has highly scented white flowers and aromatic fruit. The thin, smooth peel yields Bergamot oil for "true" eau de Cologne, perfumes, and Earl Grey tea, and for aromatherapists to treat depression, anxiety, skin problems, and urinary tract infections.

◁ ▽ **CITRUS RETICULATA**
Mandarin is a small spiny tree with loose-skinned, sweet fruit. The peel is used in Chinese medicine for chest pain, congestion, and malaria.

• *fragrant white flower*

deep green, glossy leaves •

• *oval, pointed leaf*

thin skin is yellow-orange to deep orange when ripe •

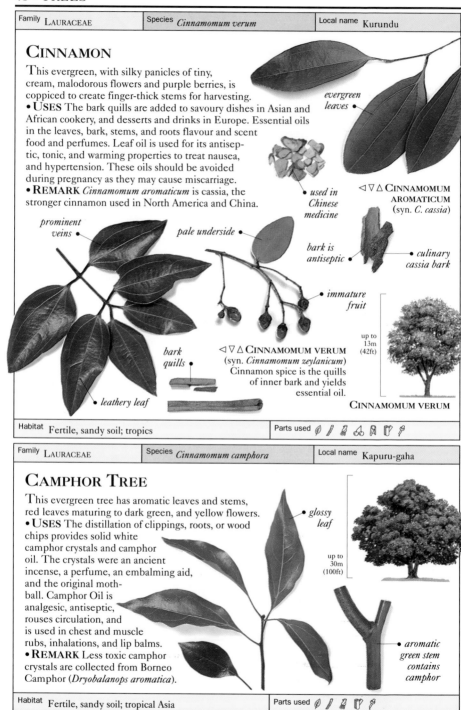

Family LAURACEAE	Species *Cinnamomum verum*	Local name Kurundu

CINNAMON

This evergreen, with silky panicles of tiny, cream, malodorous flowers and purple berries, is coppiced to create finger-thick stems for harvesting.
• USES The bark quills are added to savoury dishes in Asian and African cookery, and desserts and drinks in Europe. Essential oils in the leaves, bark, stems, and roots flavour and scent food and perfumes. Leaf oil is used for its antiseptic, tonic, and warming properties to treat nausea, and hypertension. These oils should be avoided during pregnancy as they may cause miscarriage.
• REMARK *Cinnamomum aromaticum* is cassia, the stronger cinnamon used in North America and China.

evergreen leaves •

◁ ▽ △ **CINNAMOMUM AROMATICUM** (syn. *C. cassia*)

• used in Chinese medicine

prominent veins •

pale underside •

bark is antiseptic •

• culinary cassia bark

• immature fruit

bark quills •

◁ ▽ △ **CINNAMOMUM VERUM** (syn. *Cinnamomum zeylanicum*) Cinnamon spice is the quills of inner bark and yields essential oil.

up to 13m (42ft)

CINNAMOMUM VERUM

• leathery leaf

Habitat Fertile, sandy soil; tropics	Parts used 🌿 🍴 🌰 ⚗ 🎀 🥄

Family LAURACEAE	Species *Cinnamomum camphora*	Local name Kapuru-gaha

CAMPHOR TREE

This evergreen tree has aromatic leaves and stems, red leaves maturing to dark green, and yellow flowers.
• USES The distillation of clippings, roots, or wood chips provides solid white camphor crystals and camphor oil. The crystals were an ancient incense, a perfume, an embalming aid, and the original mothball. Camphor Oil is analgesic, antiseptic, rouses circulation, and is used in chest and muscle rubs, inhalations, and lip balms.
• REMARK Less toxic camphor crystals are collected from Borneo Camphor (*Dryobalanops aromatica*).

• glossy leaf

up to 30m (100ft)

• aromatic green stem contains camphor

Habitat Fertile, sandy soil; tropical Asia	Parts used 🌿 🍴 🌰 🎀 🥄

Family PALMAE	Species *Cocos nucifera*	Local name Tennai or Thenga

COCONUT PALM

This graceful,
leaning palm is
topped by a spray of pinnate leaves,
6m (20ft) long, an inflorescence of cream
flowers, and large, single-seeded fruit. The husk
under the ripe skin houses the hard-shelled coconut.

• USES The most valuable of all the palms, the trunk
is used as building material, the leaves for thatch and
weaving, and the palm heart (stem tip) is cooked. The
sap is tapped for palm sugar, fermented for toddy, or
distilled to make the spirit *arrack*. The coconut shell
contains the white meat layer of edible coconut, and
refreshing coconut "milk". The milk is gradually
absorbed by the ripening meat which, when dried
yields Coconut Oil for soap, synthetic rubber,
glycerine, cosmetics, and special diets for
disorders where normal fat is not absorbed.

• REMARK The name "coco" is
Spanish for a grinning face,
referring to the
eyes on the
coconut base.

*fruit ranges from green to orange and
pale yellow, and hangs in clusters
at top of trunk •*

*• shells
provide utensils,
fuel, and charcoal to
absorb poisons*

*outer layer
matures to
fibrous husk,
sold as coir
and compost •*

*very small, unripe
fruit cooked in curries •*

*• nutritious
milky coconut
juice taken for
fever and
urinary
disorders*

*"King Coconut"
yields aromatic hair,
skin, and sun oils •*

*"Nawasi" is the
edible-husked coco-
nut, eaten young •*

up to
30m
(100ft)

*when dried, meat is
called copra, and
yields Coconut Oil •*

*• grey trunk with
crescent scars*

*• ripe white meat is shredded
into desiccated coconut or
macerated to make milk*

Habitat Salty, sandy soil; tropics, subtropics	Parts used 🌿 ⬯ ⚘ 🏺 📜 ⚙

Family STERCULIACEAE	Species *Cola nitida*	Local name Kola

COLA NUT

Cola is a dense evergreen with ornamental, pale yellow, purple-lined flowers, star-shaped compound fruit, and large, woody seed-pods containing six to ten red or white seeds.
• **USES** Cola seeds were one of the original ingredients of cola drinks. They are also used as a food flavouring, to improve digestion, and to give a red dye. Fresh cola nuts contain theo-bromine and caffeine, which act as a mild stim-ulant to the heart and nerves. Locals chew the seeds to enable them to do heavy work for long periods. They are taken for headaches and depression and as a diuretic.

COLA
NITIDA ▷

shiny oblong leaf •

• *leathery leaf*

△ **COLA ACUMINATA**
This dense evergreen is also grown commercially for Cola nuts.

• *bitter red or white seeds preferred fresh*

up to 20m (65ft)

COLA NITIDA

Habitat Coastal and estuary forests; Africa, Brazil, W. Indies	Parts used 🍃 🌰

Family HYPERICACEAE	Species *Cratoxylum formosum*	Local name Derum

PINK MEMPAT

The tropical Pink Mempat has an airy crown, and rough grey bark with rich brown patches. Every four to six months the leaves fall; pink flowers like cherry blossom emerge, followed by reddish leaves, which become green.
• **USES** In Indonesia a bark decoction treats abdominal complaints; the yellow to black resin from young branches treats scabies, scurvy, wounds, and burns. Crushed leaves are also used as a burn treatment.

CRATOXYLUM FORMOSUM ▽ ▷

bark yields resin •

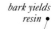

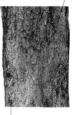

• *fragrant pink blossom*

• *peeling bark*

• *leaf clusters*

• *young leaves emerge reddish*

up to 15m (45ft)

◁ **CRATOXYLUM COCHINCHINESE**
The Kemutong is a tropical forest tree with small, pink to crimson flowers. The root, leaf, bark, and resin are medicinal.

• *yellow-brown bark*

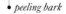

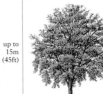

CRATOXYLUM FORMOSUM

Habitat Tropical conditions; S.E. Asia	Parts used 🌿 ⚬ 🍃 🍃 💧

Family CUPRESSACEAE	Species *Cupressus sempervirens*	Local name Cemetery Cypress

ITALIAN CYPRESS

This tall evergreen has grey-brown bark, and tiny, dark green leaves. It bears yellowish male cones and green female cones, which ripen to brown.
• USES Cypress Oil, distilled from the leaves, branches, and cones, has a refreshing, camphor-resinous scent, popular in perfumes, after-shaves, and soaps. Aromatherapists use its astringency and vein-constricting properties to treat broken capillaries and excess fluid conditions, such as cellulite and heavy menstruation; as a circulation tonic for varicose veins and haemorrhoids; and as an anti-spasmodic to reduce cough spasms.

'SWANE'S GOLDEN' ▽
This is a small, slow-growing, compact cultivar with gold-tipped foliage.

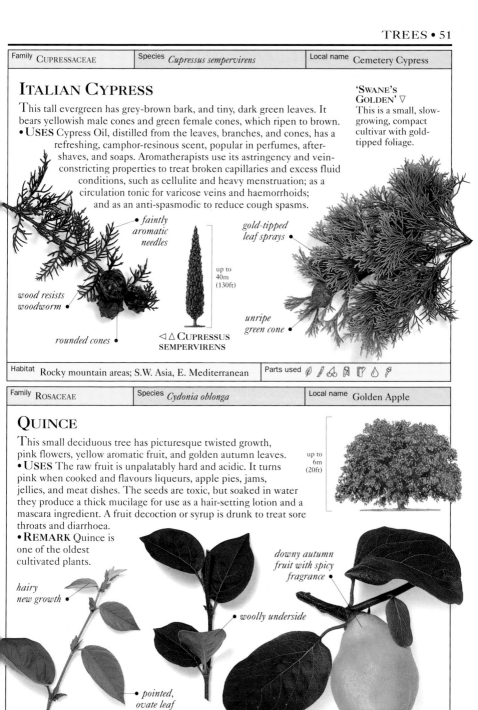

faintly aromatic needles

gold-tipped leaf sprays

wood resists woodworm

up to 40m (130ft)

unripe green cone

rounded cones

◁ △ CUPRESSUS SEMPERVIRENS

Habitat Rocky mountain areas; S.W. Asia, E. Mediterranean	Parts used

Family ROSACEAE	Species *Cydonia oblonga*	Local name Golden Apple

QUINCE

This small deciduous tree has picturesque twisted growth, pink flowers, yellow aromatic fruit, and golden autumn leaves.
• USES The raw fruit is unpalatably hard and acidic. It turns pink when cooked and flavours liqueurs, apple pies, jams, jellies, and meat dishes. The seeds are toxic, but soaked in water they produce a thick mucilage for use as a hair-setting lotion and a mascara ingredient. A fruit decoction or syrup is drunk to treat sore throats and diarrhoea.
• REMARK Quince is one of the oldest cultivated plants.

up to 6m (20ft)

hairy new growth

downy autumn fruit with spicy fragrance

woolly underside

pointed, ovate leaf

Habitat Damp soil; temperate Mediterranean, C. Asia, Crete	Parts used

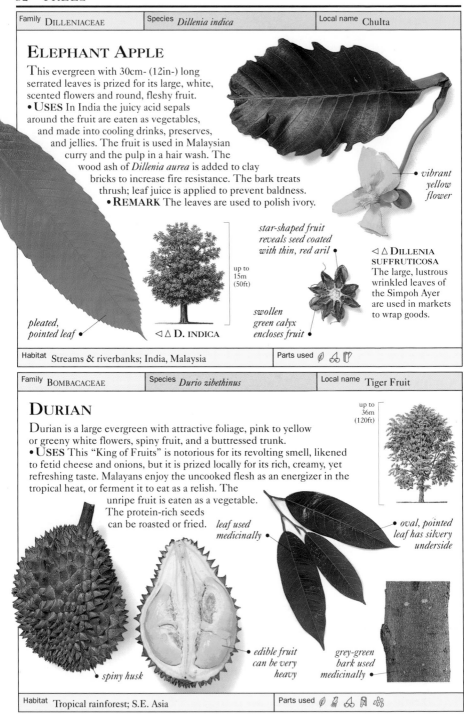

| Family DILLENIACEAE | Species *Dillenia indica* | Local name Chulta |

ELEPHANT APPLE

This evergreen with 30cm- (12in-) long
serrated leaves is prized for its large, white,
scented flowers and round, fleshy fruit.
• USES In India the juicy acid sepals
around the fruit are eaten as vegetables,
and made into cooling drinks, preserves,
and jellies. The fruit is used in Malaysian
curry and the pulp in a hair wash. The
wood ash of *Dillenia aurea* is added to clay
bricks to increase fire resistance. The bark treats
thrush; leaf juice is applied to prevent baldness.
• REMARK The leaves are used to polish ivory.

*vibrant
yellow
flower*

*star-shaped fruit
reveals seed coated
with thin, red aril* •

up to
15m
(50ft)

◁ △ DILLENIA
SUFFRUTICOSA
The large, lustrous
wrinkled leaves of
the Simpoh Ayer
are used in markets
to wrap goods.

*pleated,
pointed leaf* •

◁ △ D. INDICA

*swollen
green calyx
encloses fruit* •

| Habitat Streams & riverbanks; India, Malaysia | Parts used |

| Family BOMBACACEAE | Species *Durio zibethinus* | Local name Tiger Fruit |

DURIAN

up to
36m
(120ft)

Durian is a large evergreen with attractive foliage, pink to yellow
or greeny white flowers, spiny fruit, and a buttressed trunk.
• USES This "King of Fruits" is notorious for its revolting smell, likened
to fetid cheese and onions, but it is prized locally for its rich, creamy, yet
refreshing taste. Malayans enjoy the uncooked flesh as an energizer in the
tropical heat, or ferment it to eat as a relish. The
unripe fruit is eaten as a vegetable.
The protein-rich seeds
can be roasted or fried. *leaf used
medicinally* •

*oval, pointed
leaf has silvery
underside*

*edible fruit
can be very
heavy*

*grey-green
bark used
medicinally* •

• *spiny husk*

| Habitat Tropical rainforest; S.E. Asia | Parts used |

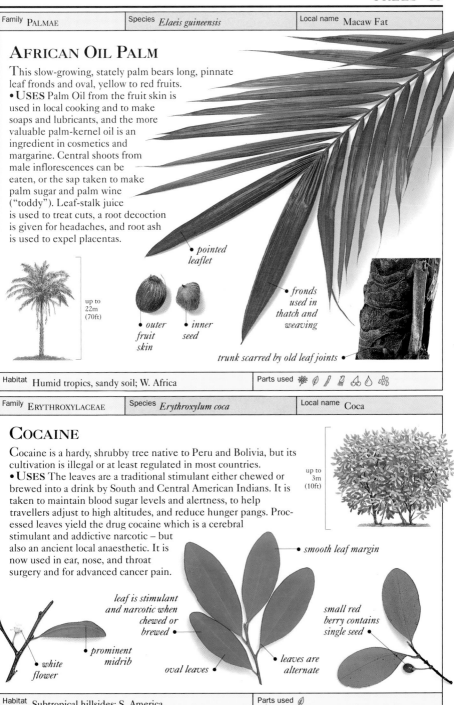

Family PALMAE	Species *Elaeis guineensis*	Local name Macaw Fat

AFRICAN OIL PALM

This slow-growing, stately palm bears long, pinnate leaf fronds and oval, yellow to red fruits.
• **USES** Palm Oil from the fruit skin is used in local cooking and to make soaps and lubricants, and the more valuable palm-kernel oil is an ingredient in cosmetics and margarine. Central shoots from male inflorescences can be eaten, or the sap taken to make palm sugar and palm wine ("toddy"). Leaf-stalk juice is used to treat cuts, a root decoction is given for headaches, and root ash is used to expel placentas.

• *pointed leaflet*

up to 22m (70ft)

• *outer fruit skin*

• *inner seed*

• *fronds used in thatch and weaving*

trunk scarred by old leaf joints •

Habitat Humid tropics, sandy soil; W. Africa	Parts used 🌼 🖊 ⬟ 🍃 △◌ 🦴

Family ERYTHROXYLACEAE	Species *Erythroxylum coca*	Local name Coca

COCAINE

Cocaine is a hardy, shrubby tree native to Peru and Bolivia, but its cultivation is illegal or at least regulated in most countries.
• **USES** The leaves are a traditional stimulant either chewed or brewed into a drink by South and Central American Indians. It is taken to maintain blood sugar levels and alertness, to help travellers adjust to high altitudes, and reduce hunger pangs. Processed leaves yield the drug cocaine which is a cerebral stimulant and addictive narcotic – but also an ancient local anaesthetic. It is now used in ear, nose, and throat surgery and for advanced cancer pain.

up to 3m (10ft)

• *smooth leaf margin*

leaf is stimulant and narcotic when chewed or brewed •

• *white flower*

• *prominent midrib*

oval leaves •

• *leaves are alternate*

small red berry contains single seed •

Habitat Subtropical hillsides; S. America	Parts used 🍃

Family MYRTACEAE	Species *Eucalyptus* species	Local name Gum Tree

EUCALYPTUS

The *Eucalyptus* genus comprises over 500 species of aromatic trees and shrubs with deciduous bark. The most common species, Tasmanian Blue Gum (*Eucalyptus globulus*), has a blue-grey trunk, blue-green juvenile leaves, green adult leaves, and white flower stamens.
• **USES** Eucalyptus leaves, scented of balsamic camphor, are used by Aboriginals to bind wounds; the flower nectar gives honey; and the oil, distilled from the leaves and twigs, is used in medicines, aromatherapy, and perfumes. Eucalyptus Oil is antiseptic, expectorant, and anti-viral, treats pulmonary tuberculosis, lowers blood sugar levels, and is useful for burns, catarrh, and flu.
• **REMARK** Eucalyptus trees inhibit the growth of nearby plants, as their roots secrete a poisonous chemical.

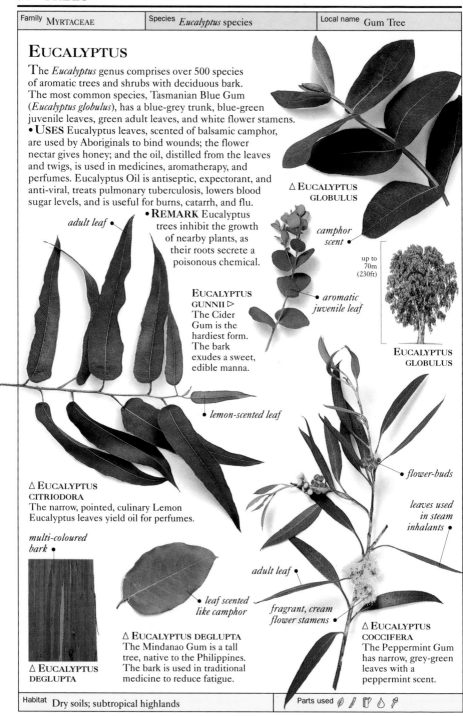

adult leaf •

△ **EUCALYPTUS GLOBULUS**

camphor scent •

• *aromatic juvenile leaf*

up to 70m (230ft)

EUCALYPTUS GUNNII ▷
The Cider Gum is the hardiest form. The bark exudes a sweet, edible manna.

EUCALYPTUS GLOBULUS

• *lemon-scented leaf*

• *flower-buds*

leaves used in steam inhalants •

△ **EUCALYPTUS CITRIODORA**
The narrow, pointed, culinary Lemon Eucalyptus leaves yield oil for perfumes.

multi-coloured bark •

adult leaf •

• *leaf scented like camphor*

fragrant, cream flower stamens •

△ **EUCALYPTUS COCCIFERA**
The Peppermint Gum has narrow, grey-green leaves with a peppermint scent.

△ **EUCALYPTUS DEGLUPTA**

△ **EUCALYPTUS DEGLUPTA**
The Mindanao Gum is a tall tree, native to the Philippines. The bark is used in traditional medicine to reduce fatigue.

Habitat Dry soils; subtropical highlands	Parts used 🌿 🍃 🏵 △ ⚘

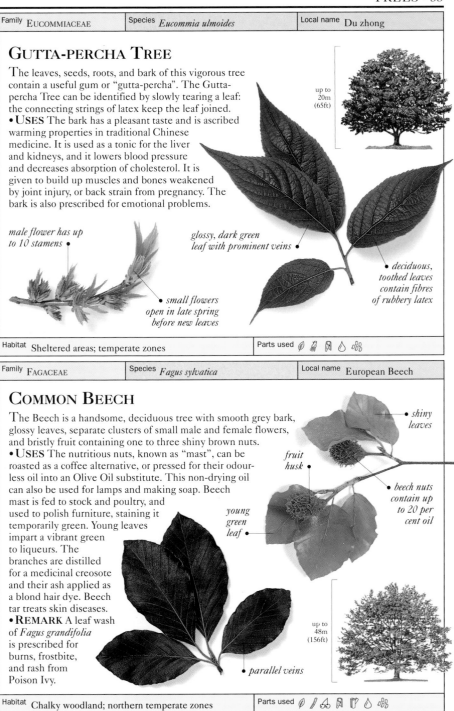

Family EUCOMMIACEAE	Species *Eucommia ulmoides*	Local name Du zhong

GUTTA-PERCHA TREE

The leaves, seeds, roots, and bark of this vigorous tree contain a useful gum or "gutta-percha". The Gutta-percha Tree can be identified by slowly tearing a leaf: the connecting strings of latex keep the leaf joined.
• **USES** The bark has a pleasant taste and is ascribed warming properties in traditional Chinese medicine. It is used as a tonic for the liver and kidneys, and it lowers blood pressure and decreases absorption of cholesterol. It is given to build up muscles and bones weakened by joint injury, or back strain from pregnancy. The bark is also prescribed for emotional problems.

up to
20m
(65ft)

male flower has up to 10 stamens •

glossy, dark green leaf with prominent veins •

• *deciduous, toothed leaves contain fibres of rubbery latex*

• *small flowers open in late spring before new leaves*

Habitat Sheltered areas; temperate zones	Parts used

Family FAGACEAE	Species *Fagus sylvatica*	Local name European Beech

COMMON BEECH

The Beech is a handsome, deciduous tree with smooth grey bark, glossy leaves, separate clusters of small male and female flowers, and bristly fruit containing one to three shiny brown nuts.
• **USES** The nutritious nuts, known as "mast", can be roasted as a coffee alternative, or pressed for their odour-less oil into an Olive Oil substitute. This non-drying oil can also be used for lamps and making soap. Beech mast is fed to stock and poultry, and used to polish furniture, staining it temporarily green. Young leaves impart a vibrant green to liqueurs. The branches are distilled for a medicinal creosote and their ash applied as a blond hair dye. Beech tar treats skin diseases.
• **REMARK** A leaf wash of *Fagus grandifolia* is prescribed for burns, frostbite, and rash from Poison Ivy.

• *shiny leaves*

fruit husk •

young green leaf •

• *beech nuts contain up to 20 per cent oil*

up to
48m
(156ft)

• *parallel veins*

Habitat Chalky woodland; northern temperate zones	Parts used

Family LOGANIACEAE	Species *Fagraea fragrans*	Local name Tembusu

TEMBUSA

This tropical shade and ornamental street tree produces large bunches of scented, funnel-shaped flowers both in the middle and at the end of the year. The tree is "gregarious" which means all Tembusas flower together and follow with clusters of small berries.
• USES The leaves and branches are used in Indonesian medicine. The highly fragrant flowers open in the evening and are gathered by women for garlands and personal adornment.
• REMARK Tembusa is planted as a shade tree and to check soil erosion, as it tolerates low soil fertility.

small, red, pulpy berries contain many tiny seeds •

• fragrant creamy white flowers turn yellow

narrow oval leaves with leathery texture •

small evergreen leaves provide constant shade •

up to 25m (80ft)

Habitat Open tropical forest, sandy coasts; S.E. Asia, India	Parts used ❋ ⌀ ∥ ☂

Family MORACEAE	Species *Ficus religiosa*	Local name Pipal Tree / Sacred Fig

SACRED BO TREE

The Sacred Bo Tree, with its pairs of small, flecked purple figs and large, rustling leaves, is sacred to Hindus and Buddhists, representing knowledge and enlightenment.
• USES In India the astringent bark is used for toothache and cracked, inflamed feet. Leaves and shoots are prescribed for skin diseases. The fruit (only a famine food) is a mild laxative and is given powdered in water for asthma. The latex is used as a sealing wax and to mend pottery, and bark fibres have been used in Burma to make paper.

tiny seeds •

• nourishing ripe flesh

purple skin •

△ FICUS CARICA
The rich edible fruit of the Common Fig is a mild laxative. The leaves yield a yellow dye.

heart-shaped leaf •

• long, elegant point

△ FICUS RELIGIOSA

• large leaves sometimes painted with images of Krishna

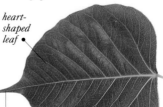

up to 8m (26ft)

FICUS RELIGIOSA

Habitat Humid tropics to subtropics; S.E. Asia	Parts used ⌀ ∥ ⚘ ⚬ ⌂ ◇ ⁂

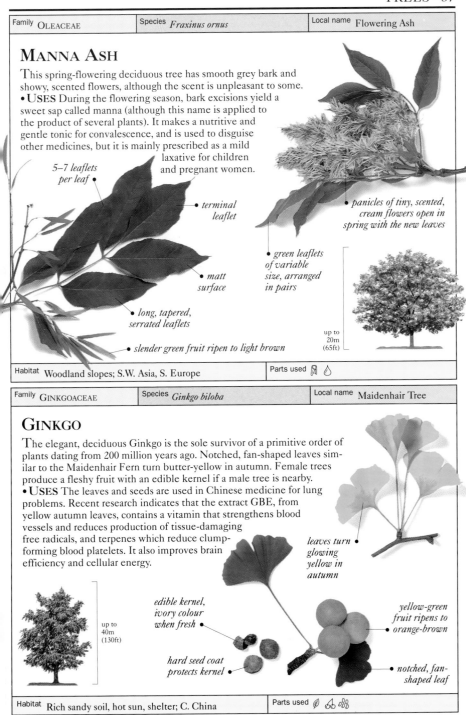

Family OLEACEAE	Species *Fraxinus ornus*	Local name Flowering Ash

MANNA ASH

This spring-flowering deciduous tree has smooth grey bark and showy, scented flowers, although the scent is unpleasant to some.
• USES During the flowering season, bark excisions yield a sweet sap called manna (although this name is applied to the product of several plants). It makes a nutritive and gentle tonic for convalescence, and is used to disguise other medicines, but it is mainly prescribed as a mild laxative for children and pregnant women.

5–7 leaflets per leaf •

• terminal leaflet

• matt surface

• long, tapered, serrated leaflets

• slender green fruit ripen to light brown

• panicles of tiny, scented, cream flowers open in spring with the new leaves

• green leaflets of variable size, arranged in pairs

up to 20m (65ft)

Habitat Woodland slopes; S.W. Asia, S. Europe	Parts used

Family GINKGOACEAE	Species *Ginkgo biloba*	Local name Maidenhair Tree

GINKGO

The elegant, deciduous Ginkgo is the sole survivor of a primitive order of plants dating from 200 million years ago. Notched, fan-shaped leaves similar to the Maidenhair Fern turn butter-yellow in autumn. Female trees produce a fleshy fruit with an edible kernel if a male tree is nearby.
• USES The leaves and seeds are used in Chinese medicine for lung problems. Recent research indicates that the extract GBE, from yellow autumn leaves, contains a vitamin that strengthens blood vessels and reduces production of tissue-damaging free radicals, and terpenes which reduce clump-forming blood platelets. It also improves brain efficiency and cellular energy.

leaves turn glowing yellow in autumn

up to 40m (130ft)

edible kernel, ivory colour when fresh •

hard seed coat protects kernel •

yellow-green fruit ripens to • orange-brown

• notched, fan-shaped leaf

Habitat Rich sandy soil, hot sun, shelter; C. China	Parts used

Family GNETACEAE	Species *Gnetum gnemon*	Local name Spinach Joint Fir

GNEMON TREE

The Gnemon Tree is a tropical evergreen with short, drooping branches and a grey trunk with rings created by the scars of old leaf joints. Small "flowers" yield yellow "fruit" which ripen to orange-red and contain a large kernel.

• USES Edible young leaves, shoots, and inflorescences are steamed and served hot with coconut milk, or in vegetable soup. The seeds are ground into a flour and made into frying crackers, called "emping". In Indonesia, the leaves and seeds are given for anaemia and fluid retention, and the root as an antidote for poison and a treatment for malaria.

• REMARK The *Gnetum* genus is thought to be a botanical link between conifers and flowering plants.

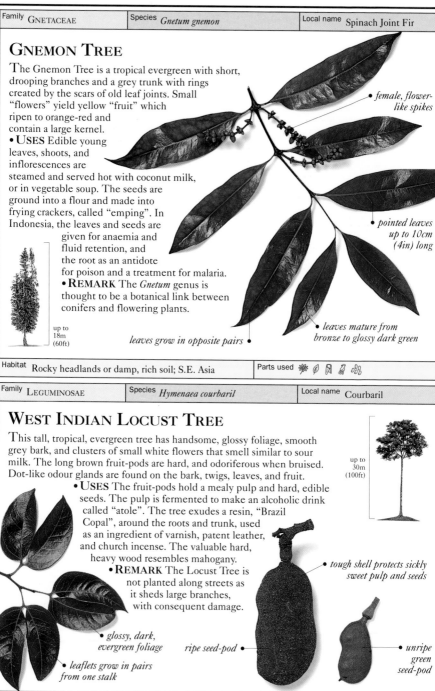

• *female, flower-like spikes*

• *pointed leaves up to 10cm (4in) long*

• *leaves mature from bronze to glossy dark green*

up to 18m (60ft)

leaves grow in opposite pairs •

Habitat Rocky headlands or damp, rich soil; S.E. Asia	Parts used

Family LEGUMINOSAE	Species *Hymenaea courbaril*	Local name Courbaril

WEST INDIAN LOCUST TREE

This tall, tropical, evergreen tree has handsome, glossy foliage, smooth grey bark, and clusters of small white flowers that smell similar to sour milk. The long brown fruit-pods are hard, and odoriferous when bruised. Dot-like odour glands are found on the bark, twigs, leaves, and fruit.

up to 30m (100ft)

• USES The fruit-pods hold a mealy pulp and hard, edible seeds. The pulp is fermented to make an alcoholic drink called "atole". The tree exudes a resin, "Brazil Copal", around the roots and trunk, used as an ingredient of varnish, patent leather, and church incense. The valuable hard, heavy wood resembles mahogany.

• REMARK The Locust Tree is not planted along streets as it sheds large branches, with consequent damage.

• *tough shell protects sickly sweet pulp and seeds*

• *glossy, dark, evergreen foliage*

ripe seed-pod •

• *unripe green seed-pod*

• *leaflets grow in pairs from one stalk*

Habitat Tropical rainforest; the Americas, W. Indies	Parts used

Family ILLICIACEAE	Species *Illicium verum*	Local name Chinese Anise

STAR ANISE

All parts of this small, evergreen tree are aromatic: the smooth, grey-white bark; narrow to elliptic, shiny green leaves; solitary, yellow flowers; and glossy brown seeds.
• USES The distinctive seeds and pods are used as a spice in Asian cookery, notably as an ingredient of Chinese five-spice powder. The fruit and foliage yield essential oil, used as a substitute aniseed flavouring, or, medicinally, to promote appetite and digestion and to relieve chest complaints, rheumatism, and flatulence. The oil appears in soaps, hair oils, and Oriental perfumes.
• REMARK *Illicium anisatum*, Japanese Star Anise, has cardamom-scented, poisonous fruit, used externally in Oriental medicine. Its flowers lack scent and the leaves are a poison. This Star Anise is revered in Japan and planted near Buddhist temples, where the bark is burned as incense.

◁ ILLICIUM VERUM

• *each point of the star-shaped seed-pod contains a seed*

ILLICIUM ANISATUM ▽

smooth, aromatic, evergreen leaves are poisonous •

up to 18m (60ft)

ILLICIUM VERUM

Habitat Lime-free soils, light tropics; China, Vietnam	Parts used

Family JUGLANDACEAE	Species *Juglans regia*	Local name Persian Walnut

ENGLISH WALNUT

The deciduous English Walnut has smooth silver bark that fissures with age, dark green leaves, and male catkins in spring or early summer. The autumn fruit appears singly, in pairs, or in threes.
• USES English Walnut consumption reduces cholesterol. The nuts are enjoyed fresh in salads and sweets, or are pickled before their shells harden. They give edible Walnut Oil which is a non-drying oil also used in soap production. In China the nuts treat wheezing, back and leg pain, and constipation. The bark, leaves, and husks yield a brown dye. Crushed leaves treat skin eruptions and repel insects.
• REMARK In India the Walnut and Chestnut trees are symbols of longevity.

5–9 pointed leaflets on leaf-stalk •

edible kernel •

hard-shelled walnut develops inside fruit •

up to 30m (100ft)

smooth, dark green leaflets, aromatic when bruised •

• *green leaf-stalk*

• *green fruit on sturdy, short stalk*

Habitat Open woodland; S.E. Europe, Himalayas, China	Parts used

Family CUPRESSACEAE	Species *Juniperus communis*	Local name Common Juniper

JUNIPER

Juniper is an evergreen tree or shrub with needle-like leaves in threes and berry-like cones that ripen to blue-black in their second or third year.
• **USES** The ripe cones or "berries" flavour gin, Chartreuse, pâtés, and game. The "berries" yield a brown dye and the antiseptic, diuretic, and detoxifying Juniper Oil, a treatment for cystitis, acne, eczema, cellulite, and rheumatism. Native Americans boiled the "berries" to treat colds and burned the needles as incense.
• **REMARK** Pencil Cedar (*Juniperus virginiana*) yields Red Cedarwood oil used for its medicinal and insecticide properties.

• *ripe cones*

• *white-banded leaves*

• *ripe cones*

△ JUNIPERUS COMMUNIS

up to 10m (33ft)

◁ JUNIPERUS VIRGINIANA
A North American tree reaching 30m (100ft), with paired leaves.

• *fresh leaves treat blisters*

JUNIPERUS COMMUNIS

Habitat Mountains & scrubland; northern temperate zones	Parts used

Family BIGNONIACEAE	Species *Kigelia africana*	Local name Kigeli-keia

SAUSAGE TREE

This deciduous tree has long panicles of large, nocturnal, bell-shaped, scented flowers of deep velvety red, which become pendulous, bean-pod-shaped, woody brown fruit up to 50cm (20in) long hanging on 1m (39in) stalks.
• **USES** Grown as an ornamental shade tree, the Sausage Tree is also used in West African medicine. The bark is prescribed for rheumatism, wounds, and sores, and the leaves for dysentery. The bark and leaves treat bladder and kidney trouble and stomach pains. The root is taken to expel worms. The fibrous, pulpy fruit is poisonous, but has been used medicinally.
• **REMARK** The Sausage Tree is held sacred by some Africans and associated with magic practices. The fruit is regarded as a charm to bring wealth.

compound leaf up to 50cm (20in) long •

• *wavy margin*

• *leaflets in opposite pairs*

up to 20m (65ft)

Habitat Fertile, well-drained soil; tropical Africa	Parts used

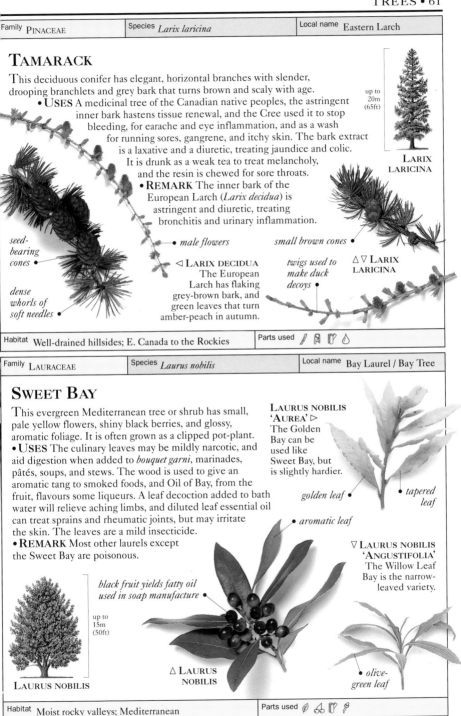

Family PINACEAE	Species *Larix laricina*	Local name Eastern Larch

TAMARACK

This deciduous conifer has elegant, horizontal branches with slender, drooping branchlets and grey bark that turns brown and scaly with age.
• **USES** A medicinal tree of the Canadian native peoples, the astringent inner bark hastens tissue renewal, and the Cree used it to stop bleeding, for earache and eye inflammation, and as a wash for running sores, gangrene, and itchy skin. The bark extract is a laxative and a diuretic, treating jaundice and colic. It is drunk as a weak tea to treat melancholy, and the resin is chewed for sore throats.
• **REMARK** The inner bark of the European Larch (*Larix decidua*) is astringent and diuretic, treating bronchitis and urinary inflammation.

up to 20m (65ft)

LARIX LARICINA

seed-bearing cones •

• male flowers

small brown cones •

◁ **LARIX DECIDUA**
The European Larch has flaking grey-brown bark, and green leaves that turn amber-peach in autumn.

twigs used to make duck decoys •

△▽ **LARIX LARICINA**

dense whorls of soft needles •

Habitat Well-drained hillsides; E. Canada to the Rockies	Parts used 🌿 🍂 ❦ ◊

Family LAURACEAE	Species *Laurus nobilis*	Local name Bay Laurel / Bay Tree

SWEET BAY

This evergreen Mediterranean tree or shrub has small, pale yellow flowers, shiny black berries, and glossy, aromatic foliage. It is often grown as a clipped pot-plant.
• **USES** The culinary leaves may be mildly narcotic, and aid digestion when added to *bouquet garni*, marinades, pâtés, soups, and stews. The wood is used to give an aromatic tang to smoked foods, and Oil of Bay, from the fruit, flavours some liqueurs. A leaf decoction added to bath water will relieve aching limbs, and diluted leaf essential oil can treat sprains and rheumatic joints, but may irritate the skin. The leaves are a mild insecticide.
• **REMARK** Most other laurels except the Sweet Bay are poisonous.

LAURUS NOBILIS 'AUREA' ▷
The Golden Bay can be used like Sweet Bay, but is slightly hardier.

golden leaf •

• tapered leaf

• aromatic leaf

▽ **LAURUS NOBILIS 'ANGUSTIFOLIA'**
The Willow Leaf Bay is the narrow-leaved variety.

black fruit yields fatty oil used in soap manufacture •

up to 15m (50ft)

LAURUS NOBILIS

△ **LAURUS NOBILIS**

• olive-green leaf

Habitat Moist rocky valleys; Mediterranean	Parts used ∅ 🍂 ❦ 🌸

| Family OLEACEAE | Species *Ligustrum lucidum* | Local name White Wax Tree |

CHINESE GLOSSY PRIVET

This evergreen tree or shrub bears bronze leaves that
mature to green, with cream flowers and black berries.
• USES Glossy Privet is a Chinese yin
nourishment. The fruit helps kidney
functions, strengthens muscles and
bones, and is prescribed for
rheumatic pain, back and knee
weakness, palpitations, and
insomnia, and to aid clear vision
and hearing. The fruit is also
prescribed for
premature greying,
dryness, and loss of
hair. The leaves and young
shoots give a strong yellow
fabric dye, and ripe berries
produce a grey-green dye. The
flowers of Common Privet
(*Ligustrum vulgare*) yield a toilet
water, and an oil infusion to
reduce wind- and sunburn.
The bark gives a yellow dye.
• REMARK The local name "White Wax Tree" is from
an industrial wax, produced when insects feed on the stems.

• *long-lasting
panicles of
fragrant cream
flowers*

• *pale
green
underside*

• *flowers
appear in
late summer*

• *opposite
pairs of
leathery
leaves*

• *glossy dark
green leaf*

• *smooth grey-
green stem*

up to
10m
(33ft)

| Habitat Wooded hills & valleys; China, Korea, Japan | Parts used |

| Family HAMAMELIDACEAE | Species *Liquidambar orientalis* | Local name Levant Storax |

ORIENTAL SWEET GUM

This deciduous tree or shrub has tiny, yellow-green, spring flowers,
small brown fruit capsules, and orange-brown balsamic bark.
• USES The leaves release a fragrance when crushed, but the
bark has the most perfume as it contains "storax" resin.
The bark is burned as an incense and for fumigation.
The balsamic resin is an expectorant, and is used in
inhalants for bronchial infections and to treat skin
diseases and parasites. Mixed with rose-
water and witch-hazel, it makes a cosmetic
astringent. Storax is a fixative for scents
and pot-pourri and is included in Oriental
perfumes and scented soaps.
• REMARK All *Liquidambar*
species yield a storax resin.

• *deeply cut leaves
with 3–5 lobes*

up to
30m
(100ft)

• *Levant Storax, a
semi-solid gum*

*gum has
balsamic scent* •

• *matt green leaves
turn orange in autumn*

| Habitat Lime-free moist woodland; Asia | Parts used |

Family MAGNOLIACEAE	Species *Magnolia officinalis*	Local name Chuan how-pow

MAGNOLIA

The deciduous Magnolia has purplish grey bark, long, wavy-edged, light green leaves, and large, fragrant, solitary, cream-white flowers.
• **USES** Magnolia species are used for their aromatic, stimulant, and tonic properties. The bark contains an essential oil and a muscle paralyzer, and is used to treat stomach spasms, peptic ulcers, diarrhoea, vomiting, coughs, and asthma. It is an antiseptic treatment for typhoid, malaria, and salmonella.
• **REMARK** The shape of Magnolia flowers indicates that this native Chinese tree has stayed almost unchanged for 100 million years.

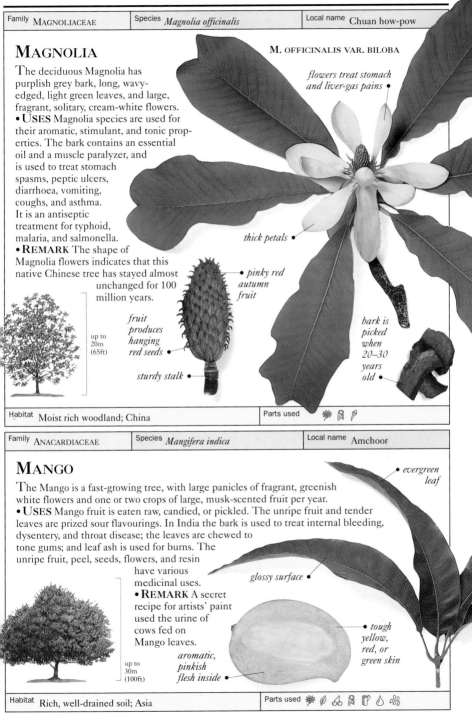

M. OFFICINALIS VAR. BILOBA

flowers treat stomach and liver-gas pains •

thick petals •

• *pinky red autumn fruit*

fruit produces hanging red seeds •

sturdy stalk •

bark is picked when 20–30 years old •

up to 20m (65ft)

Habitat Moist rich woodland; China	Parts used ❋ 🗎 ✍

Family ANACARDIACEAE	Species *Mangifera indica*	Local name Amchoor

MANGO

The Mango is a fast-growing tree, with large panicles of fragrant, greenish white flowers and one or two crops of large, musk-scented fruit per year.
• **USES** Mango fruit is eaten raw, candied, or pickled. The unripe fruit and tender leaves are prized sour flavourings. In India the bark is used to treat internal bleeding, dysentery, and throat disease; the leaves are chewed to tone gums; and leaf ash is used for burns. The unripe fruit, peel, seeds, flowers, and resin have various medicinal uses.
• **REMARK** A secret recipe for artists' paint used the urine of cows fed on Mango leaves.

• *evergreen leaf*

glossy surface •

• *tough yellow, red, or green skin*

aromatic, pinkish flesh inside •

up to 30m (100ft)

Habitat Rich, well-drained soil; Asia	Parts used ❋ ⌀ ⚮ 🗎 ❏ ◊ ⁘

| Family MYRTACEAE | Species *Melaleuca bracteata* | Local name Feathery Ti Tree |

BLACK TEA TREE

The Black Tea Tree is an elegant small tree or shrub with gnarled, twisting branches, feathery, light and dark green foliage, and small flowers with conspicuous stamens and woody seed-pods. The *Melaleuca* genus includes over 150 species of evergreen trees and shrubs, many of which yield important essential oils.

• USES Although the essential oil from this species is not known to have the powerful medicinal applications of its more famous cousins, the light oil, extracted mainly from the aromatic leaves, is a mild stimulant with insect-repellent properties and a clean, refreshing, sweet fragrance used in perfumery. This oil's potential awaits further investigation by scientists.

• **REMARK** Many species are called Tea Tree because their growing tips resemble the tea plant, although they are not related.

up to 2m (6½ft)

• *aromatic leaves*

| Habitat Coastal soils; Australia to Malaysia | Parts used 🍃 🌿 |

| Family MYRTACEAE | Species *Melaleuca cajuputi* | Local name Paper Bark Tree |

CAJUPUT

This evergreen has a dense, grey-green crown on a stout, often twisted, trunk covered with pink, papery, fibrous bark.

• USES Antiseptic Cajuput Oil is extracted from the leaves and twigs. Most commercial Cajuput Oil comes from the leaves and twigs of *Melaleuca leucadendron*, almost identical to *M. cajuputi* and said to be the same species by some authorities. It is an insecticide, a stimulant, a gastrointestinal antiseptic, a painkiller, and combats airborne infections. Tea Tree Oil from *M. alternifolia* is the most important product of the genus and has huge healing potential. It is a powerful antiseptic and immunostimulant, active against bacteria, viruses, and fungi such as athlete's foot and thrush. It helps treat colds, flu, veruccas, warts, and acne. Niaouli Oil is distilled from the leaves and shoots of *M. viridiflora*. It strengthens the immune system, is an antiseptic for chest infections, and a tissue stimulant for wounds and acne. A layer applied before cobalt radiation for cancer reduces burns.

MELALEUCA
LEUCADENDRON ▷

MELALEUCA
CAJUPUTI ▽

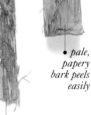

• *pale, papery bark peels easily*

• *pink-fawn fibrous bark in layers*

△ **MELALEUCA LEUCADENDRON**
Woody fruit capsules appear after flowers.

grey-green young shoots •

• *leaves prepared as tea*

crushed leaf applied as painkiller and inhaled for headaches •

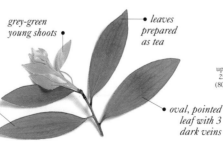

• *oval, pointed leaf with 3 dark veins*

up to 25m (80ft)

◁ △ **M. CAJUPUTI**

| Habitat Coastal swampland; Australia to Malaysia | Parts used 🍃 🌱 🪵 🌿 🌾 |

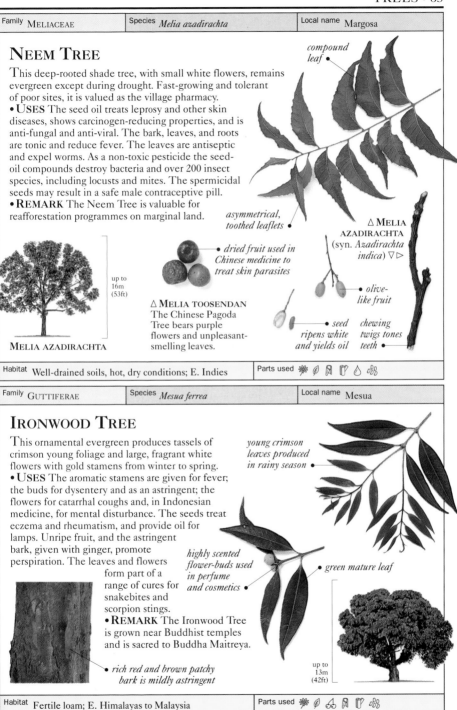

| Family MELIACEAE | Species *Melia azadirachta* | Local name Margosa |

NEEM TREE

compound leaf

This deep-rooted shade tree, with small white flowers, remains evergreen except during drought. Fast-growing and tolerant of poor sites, it is valued as the village pharmacy.
• **USES** The seed oil treats leprosy and other skin diseases, shows carcinogen-reducing properties, and is anti-fungal and anti-viral. The bark, leaves, and roots are tonic and reduce fever. The leaves are antiseptic and expel worms. As a non-toxic pesticide the seed-oil compounds destroy bacteria and over 200 insect species, including locusts and mites. The spermicidal seeds may result in a safe male contraceptive pill.
• **REMARK** The Neem Tree is valuable for reafforestation programmes on marginal land.

asymmetrical, toothed leaflets •

△ **MELIA AZADIRACHTA** (syn. *Azadirachta indica*) ▽ ▷

up to 16m (53ft)

• *dried fruit used in Chinese medicine to treat skin parasites*

• *olive-like fruit*

△ **MELIA TOOSENDAN** The Chinese Pagoda Tree bears purple flowers and unpleasant-smelling leaves.

MELIA AZADIRACHTA

seed ripens white and yields oil •

chewing twigs tones teeth •

| Habitat Well-drained soils, hot, dry conditions; E. Indies | Parts used ❀ 🌿 📋 🍃 💧 🌾 |

| Family GUTTIFERAE | Species *Mesua ferrea* | Local name Mesua |

IRONWOOD TREE

This ornamental evergreen produces tassels of crimson young foliage and large, fragrant white flowers with gold stamens from winter to spring.
• **USES** The aromatic stamens are given for fever; the buds for dysentery and as an astringent; the flowers for catarrhal coughs and, in Indonesian medicine, for mental disturbance. The seeds treat eczema and rheumatism, and provide oil for lamps. Unripe fruit, and the astringent bark, given with ginger, promote perspiration. The leaves and flowers form part of a range of cures for snakebites and scorpion stings.
• **REMARK** The Ironwood Tree is grown near Buddhist temples and is sacred to Buddha Maitreya.

young crimson leaves produced in rainy season •

highly scented flower-buds used in perfume and cosmetics •

• *green mature leaf*

up to 13m (42ft)

• *rich red and brown patchy bark is mildly astringent*

| Habitat Fertile loam; E. Himalayas to Malaysia | Parts used ❀ 🌿 🌾 📋 🍃 🌾 |

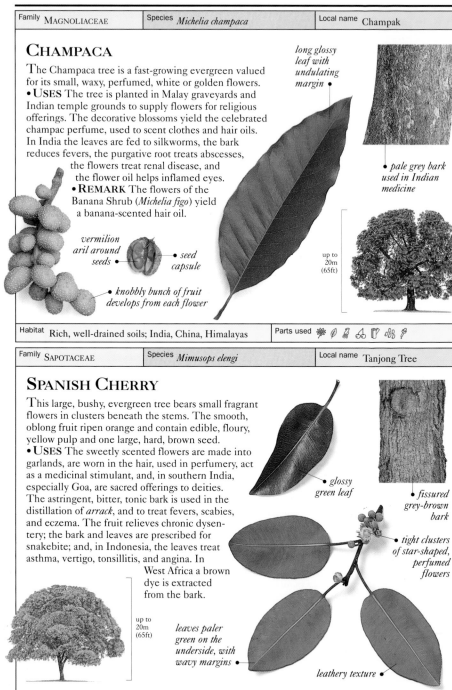

Family MAGNOLIACEAE	Species *Michelia champaca*	Local name Champak

CHAMPACA

The Champaca tree is a fast-growing evergreen valued for its small, waxy, perfumed, white or golden flowers.
• USES The tree is planted in Malay graveyards and Indian temple grounds to supply flowers for religious offerings. The decorative blossoms yield the celebrated champac perfume, used to scent clothes and hair oils. In India the leaves are fed to silkworms, the bark reduces fevers, the purgative root treats abscesses, the flowers treat renal disease, and the flower oil helps inflamed eyes.
• REMARK The flowers of the Banana Shrub (*Michelia figo*) yield a banana-scented hair oil.

long glossy leaf with undulating margin •

• pale grey bark used in Indian medicine

vermilion aril around seeds •

• seed capsule

• knobbly bunch of fruit develops from each flower

up to 20m (65ft)

Habitat Rich, well-drained soils; India, China, Himalayas	Parts used ✿ ∅ 🌿 🍂 🎋 ⚘ 🌾

Family SAPOTACEAE	Species *Mimusops elengi*	Local name Tanjong Tree

SPANISH CHERRY

This large, bushy, evergreen tree bears small fragrant flowers in clusters beneath the stems. The smooth, oblong fruit ripen orange and contain edible, floury, yellow pulp and one large, hard, brown seed.
• USES The sweetly scented flowers are made into garlands, are worn in the hair, used in perfumery, act as a medicinal stimulant, and, in southern India, especially Goa, are sacred offerings to deities. The astringent, bitter, tonic bark is used in the distillation of *arrack*, and to treat fevers, scabies, and eczema. The fruit relieves chronic dysentery; the bark and leaves are prescribed for snakebite; and, in Indonesia, the leaves treat asthma, vertigo, tonsillitis, and angina. In West Africa a brown dye is extracted from the bark.

• glossy green leaf

• fissured grey-brown bark

• tight clusters of star-shaped, perfumed flowers

up to 20m (65ft)

leaves paler green on the underside, with wavy margins •

leathery texture •

Habitat Tropical areas; India to Malaysia & Pacific Islands	Parts used ✿ ∅ 🌿 🍂 🎋 🌾

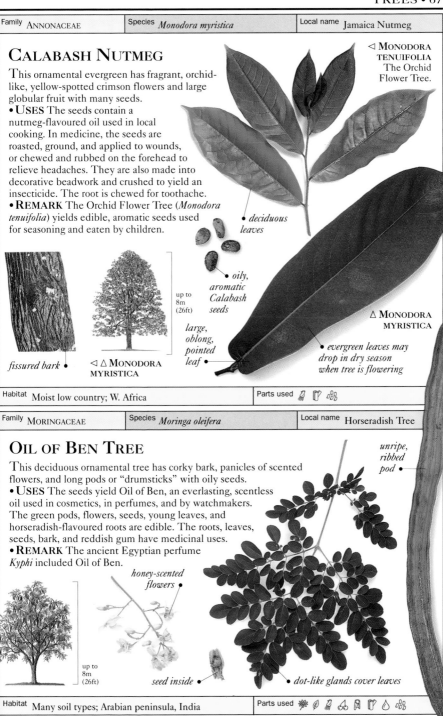

| Family ANNONACEAE | Species *Monodora myristica* | Local name Jamaica Nutmeg |

CALABASH NUTMEG

This ornamental evergreen has fragrant, orchid-like, yellow-spotted crimson flowers and large globular fruit with many seeds.
• **USES** The seeds contain a nutmeg-flavoured oil used in local cooking. In medicine, the seeds are roasted, ground, and applied to wounds, or chewed and rubbed on the forehead to relieve headaches. They are also made into decorative beadwork and crushed to yield an insecticide. The root is chewed for toothache.
• **REMARK** The Orchid Flower Tree (*Monodora tenuifolia*) yields edible, aromatic seeds used for seasoning and eaten by children.

◁ **MONODORA TENUIFOLIA**
The Orchid Flower Tree.

• *deciduous leaves*

• *oily, aromatic Calabash seeds*

up to 8m (26ft)

large, oblong, pointed leaf •

△ **MONODORA MYRISTICA**

• *evergreen leaves may drop in dry season when tree is flowering*

fissured bark •

◁ △ **MONODORA MYRISTICA**

| Habitat Moist low country; W. Africa | Parts used |

| Family MORINGACEAE | Species *Moringa oleifera* | Local name Horseradish Tree |

OIL OF BEN TREE

This deciduous ornamental tree has corky bark, panicles of scented flowers, and long pods or "drumsticks" with oily seeds.
• **USES** The seeds yield Oil of Ben, an everlasting, scentless oil used in cosmetics, in perfumes, and by watchmakers. The green pods, flowers, seeds, young leaves, and horseradish-flavoured roots are edible. The roots, leaves, seeds, bark, and reddish gum have medicinal uses.
• **REMARK** The ancient Egyptian perfume *Kyphi* included Oil of Ben.

unripe, ribbed pod •

honey-scented flowers •

up to 8m (26ft)

seed inside •

• *dot-like glands cover leaves*

| Habitat Many soil types; Arabian peninsula, India | Parts used |

| Family MORACEAE | Species *Morus alba* | Local name Sang Shen-tzu |

WHITE MULBERRY

Cultivated for more than 5,000 years, White Mulberry is a deciduous tree with serrated leaves, edible but bland fruit, and rugged brown bark.
• **USES** It is grown for its leaves, which are famous as silkworm food, as the rubbery, milky sap is thought to give tenacity to silk filaments. The young shoots are edible. The leaves and root bark are diuretic, expectorant, and lower blood pressure. Extracts decrease blood sugar and inhibit tumours in tests.
• **REMARK** Hallucinogens are present in the uncooked shoots and unripe fruit of White and Black Mulberry.

toothed margin •

• *white fruit ripens pink to red*

• *heart-shaped leaf*

◁ MORUS NIGRA
The Black Mulberry is a deciduous tree, grown for its delicious fruit.

△ MORUS ALBA

up to 15m (50ft)

• *hairy underside to leaves*

• *fruit yields purple juice used to soothe sore throats*

• *male flowers*

MORUS ALBA

| Habitat Sheltered, sunny positions; China | Parts used |

| Family MYRISTICACEAE | Species *Myristica fragrans* | Local name Sadhika |

NUTMEG AND MACE

This bushy evergreen has scented leaves and tiny yellow flowers. The fruit holds the seed – nutmeg – and its aril, a red, lacy shell coating – mace.
• **USES** Nutmeg and mace are culinary spices used in sweet and savoury dishes in a variety of cuisines. Nutmeg increases the intoxicating and soporific effect of alcoholic drinks, and is claimed to be an aphrodisiac. It is prescribed for flatulence and nausea. The essential oil is added to perfumes, soaps, hair oils, tobacco, and fumigants. The nuts yield an oil, "nutmeg butter", used in skin creams.
• **REMARK** Large doses of nutmeg are toxic, due to the presence of the hallucinogen myristicin.

• *aromatic leaves*

• *outer part of fruit fermented into an alcoholic drink*

yellow fruit splits to reveal nutmeg and mace •

• *mace is dried shell covering*

nutmeg is inside shell •

grey-green bark •

up to 10m (33ft)

• *scarlet aril*

| Habitat Coastal humid tropics; the Moluccas | Parts used |

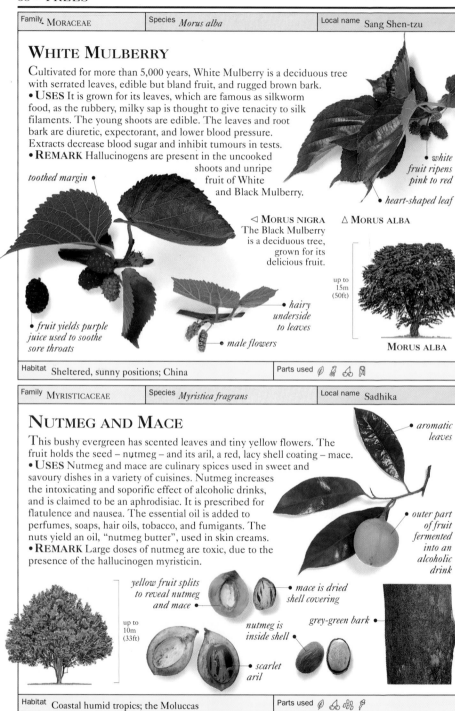

Family LEGUMINOSAE	Species *Myroxylon balsamum*	Local name Balsam Tree

BALSAM OF TOLU

All parts of this handsome, straight-trunked tree are aromatic: the resinous bark, gland-dotted leaves, small white flowers, winged fruit, and the beans.
• USES Bark incisions yield Balsam of Tolu, a balsamic resin with a cinnamon-vanilla scent and sweet citrus taste, used as a flavouring, antiseptic, and expectorant in cold and cough medicines, including Friar's Balsam. It is also a perfume fixative used in soap and hair tonics. The finest scent is extracted from the flower calyces, and a less active "White Balsam" from the fruit.
• REMARK A gum resin from Balsam of Peru (*Myroxylon balsamum* var. *pereirae*) treats skin diseases.

up to 12m (40ft)

MYROXYLON BALSAMUM
(syn. *M. peruiferum*)

• *alternate leaflets*

• *pale, curved bean contains "coumarin"*

• *young shoots*

resinous grey bark •

• *glossy, dark green, oblong leaves, covered in oil glands*

• *winged fruit, papery when mature*

Habitat Tropical regions; Americas	Parts used ✳ ⌀ 🗚 🍶 ◊ ⚘

Family OLEACEAE	Species *Olea europaea* var. *europaea*	Local name Oliva

OLIVE

The Olive is a long-lived, gnarled, drought-resistant evergreen tree, cultivated for over 4,000 years for its oil-yielding fruit.
• USES Green olives are picked unripe, black olives when ripe, and both are then cured for eating. Ripe olives are repeatedly pressed for Olive Oil. Cold-pressed virgin oil is the best quality, with a high anti-oxidant content. It is valued in salad oils and Mediterranean cookery, and for preserving food; it is used medicinally as a laxative, liniment, and carrier oil, and in cosmetics for skin creams. Inferior oil is used in soap, lubricants, and as lamp oil. The leaves are antiseptic. Wood resin is used in bronchial inhalants and perfumes.
• REMARK The flowers of *Olea fragrans* scent Chinese *Chulan* tea. The Olive branch is a symbol of peace.

fragrant cream flowers •

green olives have more acidic flavour •

black olives are brine-cured to remove bitterness •

up to 7m (23ft)

• *opposite pairs of narrow leaves*

Habitat Frost-free hillsides; Mediterranean	Parts used ⌀ ⚘ 🍶 ◊

Family PANDANACEAE	Species *Pandanus odoratissimus*	Local name Umbrella Tree / Kewra

FRAGRANT SCREWPINE

The name "Screwpine" reflects the spiral arrangement of the leaves of plants in this genus, which often have stilt roots and are grown for their unusual appearance. Mature trees bear scented white bracts around the male flower, and pineapple-like fruit.

up to 6m (20ft)

• **USES** The fragrant leaves are used fresh or dried in Asian cookery. The bracts around the male flower contain a strong rose-scented essential oil, used in Indian dishes, fragrant waters, and popular Hindu perfumes. The leaves are used in local medicine as a cure for leprosy, syphilis, and scabies. The essential oil is a stimulant and antiseptic, and is prescribed in Nepal for headaches and rheumatism.

• **REMARK** In India the leaves are sacred and offered to the god Shiva. The flowers are tossed into wells to scent the water.

PANDANUS ODORATISSIMUS (syn. *P. tectorius*)

evergreen leaf

sweetly scented leaf

bright green, young leaves

savoury, evergreen leaf used to flavour curry

segments of fruit

leaves are aromatic

leaves grow in spiral tufts at end of branches

◁ △ **PANDANUS ODORATISSIMUS**

• *pleated leaf*

◁ **PANDANUS LATIFOLIUS** (syn. *P. rhumpii*) Known as Rampe or Curry Leaf, this shrubby tree is grown in Sri Lanka for its aromatic young leaves.

PANDANUS VEITCHII ▽ ▷ A variegated shrub with bark given for dysentery and enteritis.

root-tip becomes sucker

brown stilt root

green-striped, cream leaf with long points

• *dark green mature leaf used in craft work*

Habitat Marshy & coastal areas; S.E. Asia	Parts used ✿ ∅ ෴ ஃ

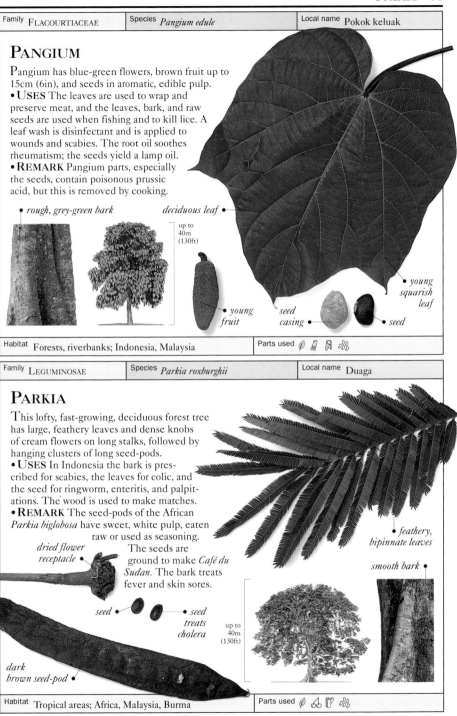

Family FLACOURTIACEAE	Species *Pangium edule*	Local name Pokok keluak

PANGIUM

Pangium has blue-green flowers, brown fruit up to 15cm (6in), and seeds in aromatic, edible pulp.
• **USES** The leaves are used to wrap and preserve meat, and the leaves, bark, and raw seeds are used when fishing and to kill lice. A leaf wash is disinfectant and is applied to wounds and scabies. The root oil soothes rheumatism; the seeds yield a lamp oil.
• **REMARK** Pangium parts, especially the seeds, contain poisonous prussic acid, but this is removed by cooking.

• rough, grey-green bark

deciduous leaf •

up to 40m (130ft)

• young squarish leaf

• young fruit

seed casing •

• seed

Habitat Forests, riverbanks; Indonesia, Malaysia	Parts used

Family LEGUMINOSAE	Species *Parkia roxburghii*	Local name Duaga

PARKIA

This lofty, fast-growing, deciduous forest tree has large, feathery leaves and dense knobs of cream flowers on long stalks, followed by hanging clusters of long seed-pods.
• **USES** In Indonesia the bark is prescribed for scabies, the leaves for colic, and the seed for ringworm, enteritis, and palpitations. The wood is used to make matches.
• **REMARK** The seed-pods of the African *Parkia biglobosa* have sweet, white pulp, eaten raw or used as seasoning. The seeds are ground to make *Café du Sudan*. The bark treats fever and skin sores.

dried flower receptacle •

• feathery, bipinnate leaves

smooth bark •

seed •

• seed treats cholera

up to 40m (130ft)

dark brown seed-pod •

Habitat Tropical areas; Africa, Malaysia, Burma	Parts used

Family LAURACEAE	Species *Persea americana*	Local name Alligator Pear

AVOCADO TREE

This evergreen tree or shrub has panicles of tiny green-ish flowers and pear-shaped green fruit. The Mexican varieties of this plant have aniseed-scented leaves.
• **USES** The delicious edible avocado pulp has the highest protein content of any fruit. Extracted oil from the fruit is used in skin creams and massage oils for its penetrative powers, which improve dull and lifeless skin. The infused diuretic leaves are drunk to cleanse the liver and reduce high blood pressure. The bark and leaves are used to treat stomach and chest ailments and control menstruation. The seeds help treat dysentery.

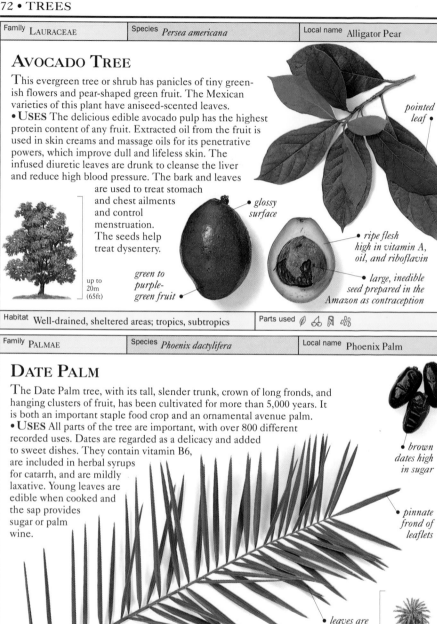

pointed leaf

glossy surface

ripe flesh high in vitamin A, oil, and riboflavin

up to 20m (65ft)

green to purple-green fruit

large, inedible seed prepared in the Amazon as contraception

Habitat Well-drained, sheltered areas; tropics, subtropics	Parts used

Family PALMAE	Species *Phoenix dactylifera*	Local name Phoenix Palm

DATE PALM

The Date Palm tree, with its tall, slender trunk, crown of long fronds, and hanging clusters of fruit, has been cultivated for more than 5,000 years. It is both an important staple food crop and an ornamental avenue palm.
• **USES** All parts of the tree are important, with over 800 different recorded uses. Dates are regarded as a delicacy and added to sweet dishes. They contain vitamin B6, are included in herbal syrups for catarrh, and are mildly laxative. Young leaves are edible when cooked and the sap provides sugar or palm wine.

brown dates high in sugar

pinnate frond of leaflets

leaves are used for thatching

up to 30m (100ft)

leaf fibres are used for ropes and mats

Habitat Warm temperate zones, dry heat; tropics, subtropics	Parts used

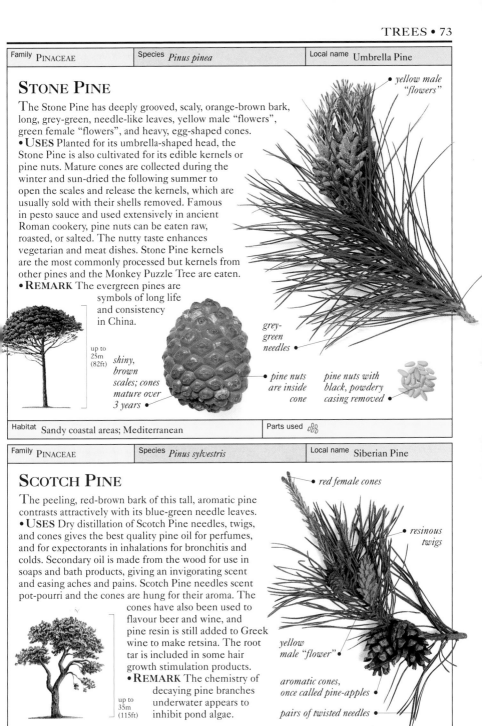

| Family PINACEAE | Species *Pinus pinea* | Local name Umbrella Pine |

• yellow male "flowers"

STONE PINE

The Stone Pine has deeply grooved, scaly, orange-brown bark, long, grey-green, needle-like leaves, yellow male "flowers", green female "flowers", and heavy, egg-shaped cones.
• USES Planted for its umbrella-shaped head, the Stone Pine is also cultivated for its edible kernels or pine nuts. Mature cones are collected during the winter and sun-dried the following summer to open the scales and release the kernels, which are usually sold with their shells removed. Famous in pesto sauce and used extensively in ancient Roman cookery, pine nuts can be eaten raw, roasted, or salted. The nutty taste enhances vegetarian and meat dishes. Stone Pine kernels are the most commonly processed but kernels from other pines and the Monkey Puzzle Tree are eaten.
• REMARK The evergreen pines are symbols of long life and consistency in China.

up to 25m (82ft)

grey-green needles •

shiny, brown scales; cones mature over 3 years •

• pine nuts are inside cone

pine nuts with black, powdery casing removed •

| Habitat Sandy coastal areas; Mediterranean | Parts used |

| Family PINACEAE | Species *Pinus sylvestris* | Local name Siberian Pine |

SCOTCH PINE

The peeling, red-brown bark of this tall, aromatic pine contrasts attractively with its blue-green needle leaves.
• USES Dry distillation of Scotch Pine needles, twigs, and cones gives the best quality pine oil for perfumes, and for expectorants in inhalations for bronchitis and colds. Secondary oil is made from the wood for use in soaps and bath products, giving an invigorating scent and easing aches and pains. Scotch Pine needles scent pot-pourri and the cones are hung for their aroma. The cones have also been used to flavour beer and wine, and pine resin is still added to Greek wine to make retsina. The root tar is included in some hair growth stimulation products.
• REMARK The chemistry of decaying pine branches underwater appears to inhibit pond algae.

up to 35m (115ft)

• red female cones

• resinous twigs

yellow male "flower" •

aromatic cones, once called pine-apples •

pairs of twisted needles •

| Habitat Mountain areas; northern temperate regions | Parts used |

Family MYRTACEAE	Species *Pimenta dioica*	Local name Pimento

ALLSPICE

This tropical evergreen has aromatic bark, leaves, and berries and bunches of greenish white flowers with a pervading scent.
• **USES** The berries, picked when mature but green, are dried to give a peppery flavouring of clove, cinnamon, and nutmeg used in sweet and savoury dishes. Allspice is also a warming medicine given for chills and to ease flatulence. The berries and leaves yield carnation-scented Pimento Oil, used to scent cosmetics.
• **REMARK** The leaves of *Pimenta racemosa* give Bay Oil which is mixed with rum to make Bay Rum, a famous hair and scalp preparation. The variety *P. racemosa* var. *citrifolia* has lemon-scented leaves.

◁▽ **PIMENTA DIOICA** (syn. *Pimenta officinalis*)

• *glossy, leathery leaves*

glossy leaves •

• *oil glands underneath*

shell of dry berries contains most flavour •

◁ **PIMENTA RACEMOSA** (syn. *Pimenta acris*) A small, erect, West Indian tree with aromatic, evergreen leaves distilled to make Bay Oil.

up to 9m (30ft)

PIMENTA DIOICA

Habitat Hot, dry sites; tropical America, W. Indies	Parts used

Family ANACARDIACEAE	Species *Pistacia lentiscus*	Local name Lentisco

MASTIC TREE

This aromatic, evergreen, shrubby tree has scented, pale green spring flowers in clusters, and red to black berries.
• **USES** The bark is tapped for mastic, which is its resin, chewed in the eastern Mediterranean as a breath freshener and employed as a flavouring for bread, pastries, and the liqueur Mastiche. The mastic is also used as an expectorant and in temporary tooth fillings, incense, theatrical glue, varnishes, and antique restoration.
• **REMARK** Pistachio (*Pistacia vera*) is grown for its delicately flavoured nuts, eaten roasted and used in sweets and in savoury dishes. The resin from Cyprus Turpentine (*P. terebinthus*) is used as a perfume base.

up to 4m (13ft)

PISTACIA LENTISCUS

• *deep, central vein on glossy, leathery leaflet*

seed coat •

pinnate leaf •

• *leaflets in opposite pairs become larger towards tip*

◁ **PISTACIA VERA** A small Mediterranean tree which yields the edible pistachio nuts.

bark yields mastic •

△ **PISTACIA LENTISCUS**

Habitat Well-drained soil, sun; Mediterranean, N.W. Africa	Parts used

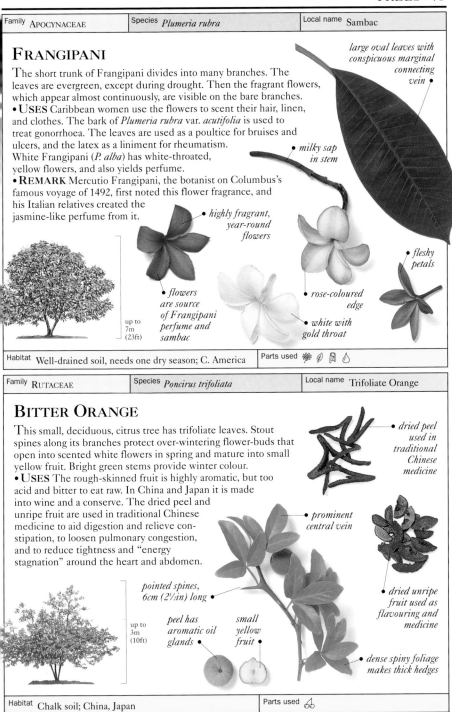

Family APOCYNACEAE	Species *Plumeria rubra*	Local name Sambac

FRANGIPANI

The short trunk of Frangipani divides into many branches. The leaves are evergreen, except during drought. Then the fragrant flowers, which appear almost continuously, are visible on the bare branches.

• **USES** Caribbean women use the flowers to scent their hair, linen, and clothes. The bark of *Plumeria rubra* var. *acutifolia* is used to treat gonorrhoea. The leaves are used as a poultice for bruises and ulcers, and the latex as a liniment for rheumatism. White Frangipani (*P. alba*) has white-throated, yellow flowers, and also yields perfume.

• **REMARK** Mercutio Frangipani, the botanist on Columbus's famous voyage of 1492, first noted this flower fragrance, and his Italian relatives created the jasmine-like perfume from it.

large oval leaves with conspicuous marginal connecting vein •

• milky sap in stem

• highly fragrant, year-round flowers

• fleshy petals

• flowers are source of Frangipani perfume and sambac

• rose-coloured edge

• white with gold throat

up to 7m (23ft)

Habitat Well-drained soil, needs one dry season; C. America	Parts used ❋ ∅ 🗄 ⬦

Family RUTACEAE	Species *Poncirus trifoliata*	Local name Trifoliate Orange

BITTER ORANGE

This small, deciduous, citrus tree has trifoliate leaves. Stout spines along its branches protect over-wintering flower-buds that open into scented white flowers in spring and mature into small yellow fruit. Bright green stems provide winter colour.

• **USES** The rough-skinned fruit is highly aromatic, but too acid and bitter to eat raw. In China and Japan it is made into wine and a conserve. The dried peel and unripe fruit are used in traditional Chinese medicine to aid digestion and relieve constipation, to loosen pulmonary congestion, and to reduce tightness and "energy stagnation" around the heart and abdomen.

• dried peel used in traditional Chinese medicine

• prominent central vein

• dried unripe fruit used as flavouring and medicine

pointed spines, 6cm (2¼in) long •

up to 3m (10ft)

peel has aromatic oil glands •

small yellow fruit •

• dense spiny foliage makes thick hedges

Habitat Chalk soil; China, Japan	Parts used 🍊

Family ROSACEAE	Species *Prunus* species	Local name Various

PRUNUS

Prunus trees have attractive spring flowers and bark, and bear finely toothed, deciduous leaves and various single-stoned fruit.
• **USES** The sweet fruits of Peach, Plum, and Apricot are eaten fresh, dried, or as jam. With the bitter fruits of Sloe, Bullace, Black Cherry, and Chokecherry, they flavour alcoholic drinks and preserves. Almonds (whole and ground) flavour many dishes. Almond essence is a flavouring distilled from the seeds of Bitter Almond (*Prunus dulcis* var. *amara*); Almond Oil is a fixed oil, pressed from Sweet Almond seeds and, like Peach and Apricot seed oils, is used in cosmetics, massage oils, and medicines. Peach and Apricot fruits are used as nourishing face masks. Chokecherry bark tea is used to clear the throats of singers and public speakers.
• **REMARK** The seed, bark, and leaves of Black Cherry, Bullace, Chokecherry, and Bitter Almond contain prunasin which converts into toxic hydrocyanic acid during digestion or on contact with water. Most need treatment before they are safe to use.

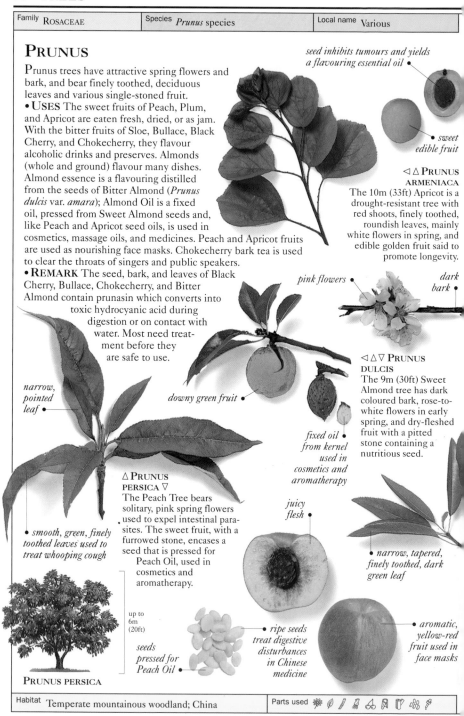

seed inhibits tumours and yields a flavouring essential oil •

• sweet edible fruit

◁ △ **PRUNUS ARMENIACA**
The 10m (33ft) Apricot is a drought-resistant tree with red shoots, finely toothed, roundish leaves, mainly white flowers in spring, and edible golden fruit said to promote longevity.

pink flowers •

dark bark

◁ △ ▽ **PRUNUS DULCIS**
The 9m (30ft) Sweet Almond tree has dark coloured bark, rose-to-white flowers in early spring, and dry-fleshed fruit with a pitted stone containing a nutritious seed.

narrow, pointed leaf •

downy green fruit •

fixed oil • from kernel used in cosmetics and aromatherapy

juicy flesh •

△ **PRUNUS PERSICA** ▽
The Peach Tree bears solitary, pink spring flowers used to expel intestinal parasites. The sweet fruit, with a furrowed stone, encases a seed that is pressed for Peach Oil, used in cosmetics and aromatherapy.

• smooth, green, finely toothed leaves used to treat whooping cough

• narrow, tapered, finely toothed, dark green leaf

up to 6m (20ft)

seeds pressed for Peach Oil •

• ripe seeds treat digestive disturbances in Chinese medicine

• aromatic, yellow-red fruit used in face masks

PRUNUS PERSICA

Habitat Temperate mountainous woodland; China	Parts used

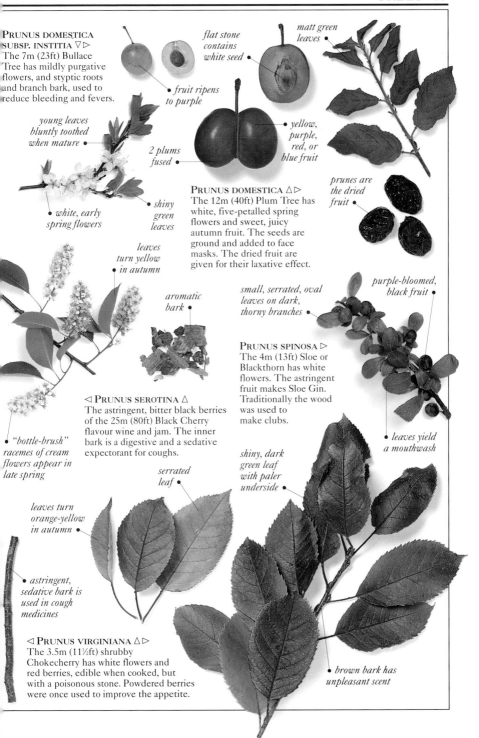

PRUNUS DOMESTICA SUBSP. INSTITIA ▽ ▷
The 7m (23ft) Bullace Tree has mildly purgative flowers, and styptic roots and branch bark, used to reduce bleeding and fevers.

flat stone contains white seed

matt green leaves

fruit ripens to purple

young leaves bluntly toothed when mature •

2 plums fused •

yellow, purple, red, or blue fruit

• white, early spring flowers

shiny green leaves

PRUNUS DOMESTICA △ ▷
The 12m (40ft) Plum Tree has white, five-petalled spring flowers and sweet, juicy autumn fruit. The seeds are ground and added to face masks. The dried fruit are given for their laxative effect.

prunes are the dried fruit •

leaves turn yellow in autumn

aromatic bark •

small, serrated, oval leaves on dark, thorny branches •

purple-bloomed, black fruit •

PRUNUS SPINOSA ▷
The 4m (13ft) Sloe or Blackthorn has white flowers. The astringent fruit makes Sloe Gin. Traditionally the wood was used to make clubs.

◁ **PRUNUS SEROTINA** △
The astringent, bitter black berries of the 25m (80ft) Black Cherry flavour wine and jam. The inner bark is a digestive and a sedative expectorant for coughs.

• "bottle-brush" racemes of cream flowers appear in late spring

serrated leaf •

leaves yield a mouthwash

shiny, dark green leaf with paler underside •

leaves turn orange-yellow in autumn •

• astringent, sedative bark is used in cough medicines

◁ **PRUNUS VIRGINIANA** △ ▷
The 3.5m (11½ft) shrubby Chokecherry has white flowers and red berries, edible when cooked, but with a poisonous stone. Powdered berries were once used to improve the appetite.

brown bark has unpleasant scent •

Family SALICACEAE	Species *Populus balsamifera*	Local name Tacamahac

BALSAM POPLAR

Balsam Poplar has smooth grey bark, resinous, fragrant, sticky buds that unfold into fine-toothed leaves, and spring catkins that release tiny seeds in cotton wool-like hairs.

deciduous, heart-shaped leaf

• **USES** Resin is collected from the unopened leaf-buds of the Balsam Poplar, and its hybrid Balm of Gilead (*Populus × candicans*), for use in pot-pourri, soaps, and as a perfume fixative. The resin is used for its antiseptic, expectorant, stimulant, fever-reducing, and painkilling properties – mostly in cough mixtures and ointments for cuts, skin diseases, and rheumatism. The bark is used in the treatment of rheumatic pain and urinary complaints.

coarse teeth

• **REMARK** Native Americans used the resin to treat skin sores, and in the 1970s Soviet doctors had great success with it in clinical tests to heal bed sores, resistant infections, and post-operative abscesses.

shoot develops from resinous bud

long leaf-stalk

△ **POPULUS BALSAMIFERA**

P. × CANDICANS ▽
(syn. *P. × jackii* 'Giladensis')
Balm of Gilead is a similar tree to the Balsam Poplar and its buds have the same uses.

long-stalked leaves appear to tremble

△ **POPULUS TREMULA**
The European Quaking Aspen is used to make the Bach Flower Remedy for irrational fears and anxiety.

sticky, resinous coating has long-lasting, balsamic fragrance

leaf-buds

up to 30m (100ft)

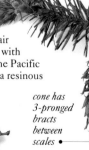

POPULUS BALSAMIFERA

Habitat Moist woodlands; temperate North America	Parts used

Family PINACEAE	Species *Pseudotsuga menziesii*	Local name Oregon Pine

DOUGLAS FIR

One of the tallest trees in the world, this conifer has thick, fissured, reddish brown bark, aromatic leaves, and brownish cones with distinctive projecting bracts.

beginning of female cones

• **USES** The balsamic-scented leaves are used to freshen air and have been boiled into a drink, sometimes with the young twigs, by the native Americans of the Pacific northwest. Tannin is taken from the bark and a resinous product, Oregon Balsam, with medicinal and industrial uses, is extracted from the trunk.

• **REMARK** Douglas Fir is an important cultivated timber.

cone has 3-pronged bracts between scales

up to 100m (330ft)

hanging, yellow, male "flower" clusters in spring

Habitat Moist mountain forests; W. North America	Parts used

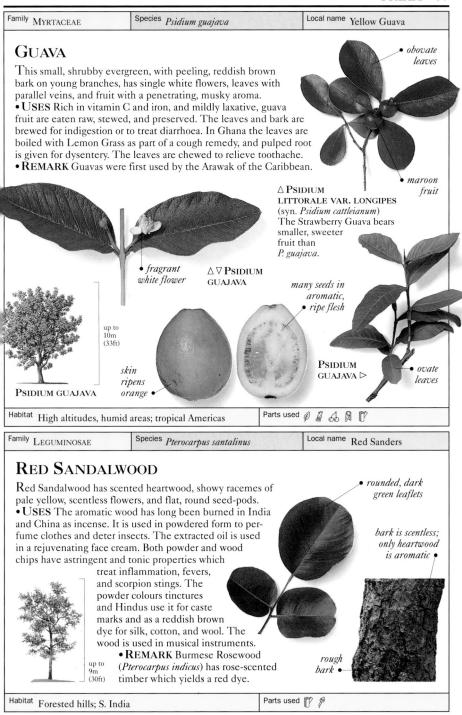

Family MYRTACEAE	Species *Psidium guajava*	Local name Yellow Guava

GUAVA

This small, shrubby evergreen, with peeling, reddish brown bark on young branches, has single white flowers, leaves with parallel veins, and fruit with a penetrating, musky aroma.
• USES Rich in vitamin C and iron, and mildly laxative, guava fruit are eaten raw, stewed, and preserved. The leaves and bark are brewed for indigestion or to treat diarrhoea. In Ghana the leaves are boiled with Lemon Grass as part of a cough remedy, and pulped root is given for dysentery. The leaves are chewed to relieve toothache.
• REMARK Guavas were first used by the Arawak of the Caribbean.

obovate leaves

maroon fruit

△ PSIDIUM LITTORALE VAR. LONGIPES (syn. *Psidium cattleianum*) The Strawberry Guava bears smaller, sweeter fruit than *P. guajava.*

fragrant white flower

△ ▽ PSIDIUM GUAJAVA

many seeds in aromatic, ripe flesh

up to 10m (33ft)

skin ripens orange

PSIDIUM GUAJAVA

PSIDIUM GUAJAVA ▷

ovate leaves

Habitat High altitudes, humid areas; tropical Americas	Parts used

Family LEGUMINOSAE	Species *Pterocarpus santalinus*	Local name Red Sanders

RED SANDALWOOD

Red Sandalwood has scented heartwood, showy racemes of pale yellow, scentless flowers, and flat, round seed-pods.
• USES The aromatic wood has long been burned in India and China as incense. It is used in powdered form to perfume clothes and deter insects. The extracted oil is used in a rejuvenating face cream. Both powder and wood chips have astringent and tonic properties which treat inflammation, fevers, and scorpion stings. The powder colours tinctures and Hindus use it for caste marks and as a reddish brown dye for silk, cotton, and wool. The wood is used in musical instruments.
• REMARK Burmese Rosewood (*Pterocarpus indicus*) has rose-scented timber which yields a red dye.

rounded, dark green leaflets

bark is scentless; only heartwood is aromatic

up to 9m (30ft)

rough bark

Habitat Forested hills; S. India	Parts used

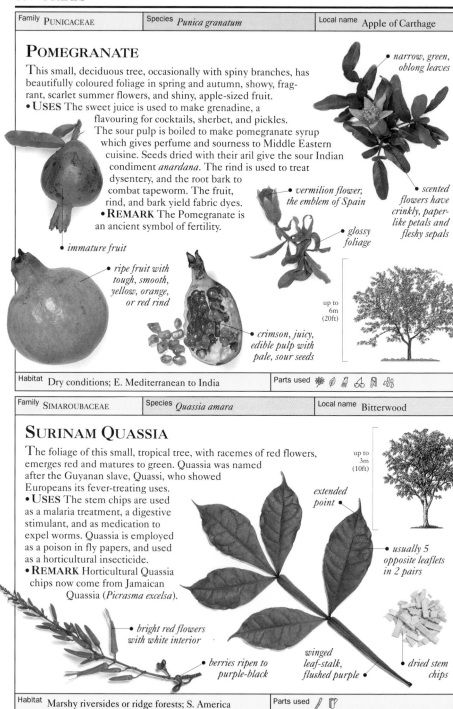

Family PUNICACEAE	Species *Punica granatum*	Local name Apple of Carthage

POMEGRANATE

This small, deciduous tree, occasionally with spiny branches, has beautifully coloured foliage in spring and autumn, showy, fragrant, scarlet summer flowers, and shiny, apple-sized fruit.

• **USES** The sweet juice is used to make grenadine, a flavouring for cocktails, sherbet, and pickles. The sour pulp is boiled to make pomegranate syrup which gives perfume and sourness to Middle Eastern cuisine. Seeds dried with their aril give the sour Indian condiment *anardana*. The rind is used to treat dysentery, and the root bark to combat tapeworm. The fruit, rind, and bark yield fabric dyes.

• **REMARK** The Pomegranate is an ancient symbol of fertility.

• *narrow, green, oblong leaves*

• *vermilion flower, the emblem of Spain*

• *scented flowers have crinkly, paper-like petals and fleshy sepals*

• *glossy foliage*

• *immature fruit*

• *ripe fruit with tough, smooth, yellow, orange, or red rind*

• *crimson, juicy, edible pulp with pale, sour seeds*

up to 6m (20ft)

Habitat Dry conditions; E. Mediterranean to India	Parts used ❁ 🍃 🌰 ⚘ 🍂 ✿

Family SIMAROUBACEAE	Species *Quassia amara*	Local name Bitterwood

SURINAM QUASSIA

The foliage of this small, tropical tree, with racemes of red flowers, emerges red and matures to green. Quassia was named after the Guyanan slave, Quassi, who showed Europeans its fever-treating uses.

• **USES** The stem chips are used as a malaria treatment, a digestive stimulant, and as medication to expel worms. Quassia is employed as a poison in fly papers, and used as a horticultural insecticide.

• **REMARK** Horticultural Quassia chips now come from Jamaican Quassia (*Picrasma excelsa*).

up to 3m (10ft)

• *extended point*

• *usually 5 opposite leaflets in 2 pairs*

• *bright red flowers with white interior*

• *berries ripen to purple-black*

winged leaf-stalk, flushed purple •

• *dried stem chips*

Habitat Marshy riversides or ridge forests; S. America	Parts used 🍃 🗒

Family FAGACEAE	Species *Quercus robur*	Local name Pedunculate Oak

COMMON OAK

This noble, deciduous tree, once a powerful pagan symbol, has large, spreading branches, lobed leaves, and male catkins.

up to 40m (130ft)

• **USES** Oak bark and galls are astringent, antiseptic, and they reduce bleeding. A decoction is drunk to treat acute diarrhoea, gargled for sore throats, applied as a compress for burns and cuts, added to ointments for cuts and piles, and taken powdered as snuff for nose-bleeds. Acorns are roasted as a coffee substitute, and fed to pigs. The shrubby *Quercus infectoria* yields Oak galls for medicine, and a remarkable permanent ink.

• **REMARK** Oak bark provides a leather tan, and as tanners seemed immune to tuberculosis, the bark was used for treatment of the disease.

• *new leaves unfold as flowers open*

mature, dark green leaf •

"Oak Apple" gall formed by larvae of gall wasp •

• *long-stalked, shiny acorns ripen green to brown*

• *acorns were a famine food*

flowering male catkins appear in spring •

fissured bark yields dye •

• *red-brown inner surface*

Habitat Woodland; Europe	Parts used

Family LEGUMINOSAE	Species *Robinia pseudoacacia*	Local name Black Locust Tree

FALSE ACACIA

This thorny, deciduous tree displays attractive foliage, clusters of fragrant flowers, and flat brown seed-pods.

up to 25m (80ft)

• **USES** The flower clusters are made into fritters, flavour jam, and supply nectar for bees and essence for perfumes. Native Americans ate the boiled seeds and used the roots in a red dye recipe. The poisonous bark and roots were once used as purgatives. The timber ages to yield fence posts that are harder than Oak.

• *soft, pollution-tolerant, oval leaflets*

△ ▽ **ROBINIA PSEUDOACACIA**

• **REMARK** The fast-growing False Acacia is used to reclaim arid land as its roots bind the soil, it spreads readily, and the bark is poisonous to foraging animals.

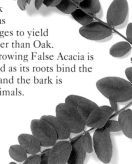

• *bright green, elliptic to ovate leaflets*

◁ **ROBINIA PSEUDOACACIA 'FRISIA'**
This small cultivar bears scarlet thorns and golden lime leaflets on short stalks.

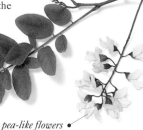

pea-like flowers •

Habitat Well-drained temperate woodland; S.E. USA	Parts used

Family SALICACEAE	Species *Salix alba*	Local name European Willow

WHITE WILLOW

silvery, hairy underside •

Deeply fissured, dark grey bark, elegant branches, and spring catkins mark this deciduous waterside tree.
• **USES** The stem-bark is a painkiller, a fever-reducer, and an original source of salicylic acid for aspirins. Various bark extracts are used as a sore throat gargle, for heartburn, stomach problems, and food poisoning, to relieve arthritic pain, and to remove corns. Infused leaves make a tea for nervous insomnia and are added to baths to ease rheumatism. Pussy Willow (*Salix caprea*) has similar medicinal uses. *S. babylonica* root bark treats leukaemia and restores bone marrow function after chemotherapy.

male catkins with yellow anthers •

The *Salix* species provide the best quality artists' charcoal, branches are used for weaving, and the White Willow var. *caerulea* is the source of wood for cricket bats.
• **REMARK** The genus name *Salix* comes from the Celtic *sal-lis*, "near-water".

up to 25m (80ft)

• important spring food for bumblebees

Habitat Temperate wetland; Europe, W. Asia	Parts used 🌿 ∥ 🍃 🌳

Family CAPRIFOLIACEAE	Species *Sambucus nigra*	Local name Bore Tree

ELDER

This is a common, deciduous, shrub-like tree with musk-scented wood and leaves, creamy white early summer flowers, and wine-coloured berries.
• **USES** The muscatel-scented flowers flavour sweet and savoury dishes, and are made into alcoholic drinks and elder-flower water for eye, skin, and aftershave lotions. The berries give a port-like wine, and add flavour, colour, and vitamin C to cordials, jams, and pies; the buds are pickled. The flowers treat colds, hay fever, sore throats, arthritis, and act as a mild laxative. The leaves are applied to bruises and sprains; the bark is given for epilepsy; and the roots treat lymphatic and kidney ailments. In Chinese medicine, the leaves, stems, and roots are used to treat fractures and muscle spasms. The Elder yields green, violet, and black dyes. A leaf brew is an insecticide.

• upright berry clusters tip down when ripe in autumn

• **REMARK** Named the "country medicine-chest" for its many health uses, the Elder is also rich in European folklore.

• flat heads of star-shaped flowers

• serrated, foxy scented leaflets

up to 10m (33ft)

Habitat Temperate regions; northern hemisphere	Parts used ✳ 🌿 ∥ 🍃 🌿 🌳

Family SANTALACEAE	Species *Santalum album*	Local name Indian Sandalwood

SANDALWOOD

Processed for its fragrant reddish heartwood, the Sandalwood is a slow-growing, semi-parasitic evergreen, with slender, drooping branches, panicles of small pale yellow to purple flowers, and pea-sized fruit containing one seed.
• USES All parts yield Sandalwood Oil, particularly the heartwood and the roots which yield about 61 per cent essential oil. The distilled oil is used in many perfumes, in aftershaves to soothe shaving rash, and in cosmetics – where it is of special benefit to mature skins. Recorded in Ayurvedic medicine and Egyptian embalming, the oil is now used as an inhalant for its expectorant and sedative effect on coughs, and as a powerful antiseptic for lung infections and the urinary tract. The essential oil is distilled from the wood and used in aromatherapy for tension, anxiety, and as an aphrodisiac.
• REMARK Sandalwood gives a popular incense, as its calming effect aids meditation. It is commonly used for funeral pyres in India, where devotees believe the scent protects places from evil spirits.

• *grey-brown bark yields 2 per cent Sandalwood Oil*

• *oval, tapering, evergreen leaves*

• *leaves in opposite pairs*

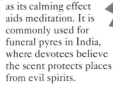

up to 18m (60ft)

leaves and shoots yield 4 per cent Sandalwood Oil •

Habitat Well-drained soil, forests; S.E. Asia	Parts used 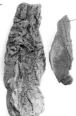

Family LAURACEAE	Species *Sassafras albidum*	Local name Fennel Wood

SASSAFRAS

This aromatic tree has red and gold autumn leaves, yellow spring flowers, and small blue fruit on red stalks.
• USES Ground leaves, called "Filé powder", are used to thicken Cajun soups and make "Filé Gumbo". Root bark oil contains safrole, which is dangerous in large amounts but gives flavour to root beer, toothpaste, and tobacco, and fruit oil is used in perfumes. The safrole in Sassafras root beer, now banned in the USA, is only one fourteenth as carcinogenic as the ethanol in ordinary beer.
• REMARK The leaf, twig, bark, and root were tonic blood purifiers. Sassafras was perhaps the first native American herb to be exported to Europe.

yellow flower clusters •

• *aromatic leaves may be lobed or ovate*

• *inner root bark contains Sassafras essential oil*

• *ground bark gives orange dye*

up to 20m (65ft)

• *deciduous ovate leaf*

Habitat Thickly wooded areas; E. North America	Parts used 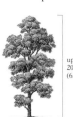

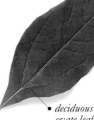

Family LEGUMINOSAE	Species *Sophora japonica*	Local name Chinese Scholar Tree

PAGODA TREE

When mature, this attractive legume has panicles of fragrant, cream, pea-like summer flowers and fruit-pods which are pinched between the seeds.
• USES In China the buds, flowers, and fruit-pods are used to clear fevers, stop bleeding, and control nervousness and dizziness; the flowers are also used to treat high blood pressure. The pods yield a yellow fabric dye.
• REMARK Beans from the Mescal Bean Tree (*Sophora secundiflora*) contain cytisine, which can cause intoxication and death. Once used by native American tribes to induce visions the beans were superseded by the safer Peyote.

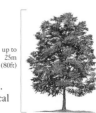

up to
25m
(80ft)

SOPHORA
JAPONICA

deciduous foliage may remain green until it falls •

• notched at tip

• pointed ovate leaflet

• obovate leaflets

△ SOPHORA SECUNDIFLORA
Mescal Bean Tree is a small evergreen with fragrant, violet-blue flowers and a long, woody fruit-pod with up to eight bright red beans.

glossy green stem •

leaflets in opposite pairs •

△ SOPHORA JAPONICA

Habitat Tolerates drought & poor soils; China, Korea	Parts used 🌼 ✎ 🍂

Family ROSACEAE	Species *Sorbus aucuparia*	Local name Mountain Ash

ROWAN

The deciduous Rowan bears flat clusters of cream flowers in spring and bright red berries in autumn, when the leaves may turn red.
• USES Rowan berries, rich in vitamin C, can be made into a tart jelly, ground into flour, fermented into wine, or distilled into spirit. The seeds should be removed as they can contain hydrocyanic acid. The berries are also made into a face mask or a sore throat gargle. The bark and leaves are used in a gargle for thrush.
• REMARK Rowan is a traditional country charm against witchcraft.

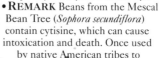

dense clusters of berries •

• cream flowers

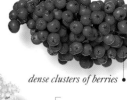

up to
15m
(50ft)

deciduous serrated leaflets have asymmetrical base •

• opposite pairs

Habitat Woodland & upland; northern hemisphere	Parts used ✎ 🍂 📖 🌿

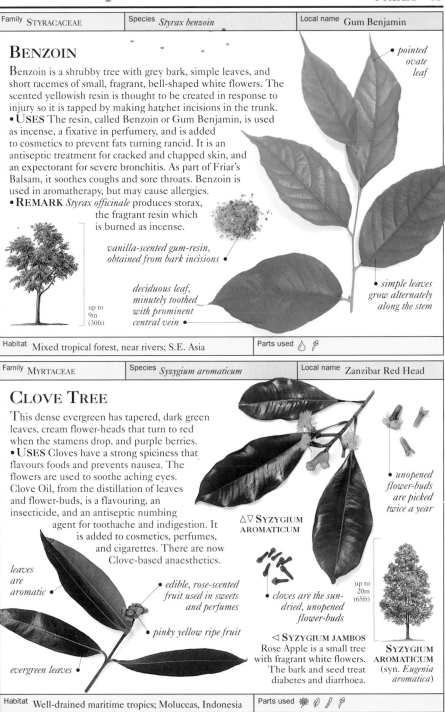

Family STYRACACEAE	Species *Styrax benzoin*	Local name Gum Benjamin

BENZOIN

Benzoin is a shrubby tree with grey bark, simple leaves, and short racemes of small, fragrant, bell-shaped white flowers. The scented yellowish resin is thought to be created in response to injury so it is tapped by making hatchet incisions in the trunk.
• **USES** The resin, called Benzoin or Gum Benjamin, is used as incense, a fixative in perfumery, and is added to cosmetics to prevent fats turning rancid. It is an antiseptic treatment for cracked and chapped skin, and an expectorant for severe bronchitis. As part of Friar's Balsam, it soothes coughs and sore throats. Benzoin is used in aromatherapy, but may cause allergies.
• **REMARK** *Styrax officinale* produces storax, the fragrant resin which is burned as incense.

pointed ovate leaf

vanilla-scented gum-resin, obtained from bark incisions

deciduous leaf, minutely toothed with prominent central vein

simple leaves grow alternately along the stem

up to 9m (30ft)

Habitat Mixed tropical forest, near rivers; S.E. Asia	Parts used 💧 🌿

Family MYRTACEAE	Species *Syzygium aromaticum*	Local name Zanzibar Red Head

CLOVE TREE

This dense evergreen has tapered, dark green leaves, cream flower-heads that turn to red when the stamens drop, and purple berries.
• **USES** Cloves have a strong spiciness that flavours foods and prevents nausea. The flowers are used to soothe aching eyes. Clove Oil, from the distillation of leaves and flower-buds, is a flavouring, an insecticide, and an antiseptic numbing agent for toothache and indigestion. It is added to cosmetics, perfumes, and cigarettes. There are now Clove-based anaesthetics.

△▽ **SYZYGIUM AROMATICUM**

unopened flower-buds are picked twice a year

leaves are aromatic

edible, rose-scented fruit used in sweets and perfumes

pinky yellow ripe fruit

cloves are the sun-dried, unopened flower-buds

evergreen leaves

up to 20m (65ft)

◁ **SYZYGIUM JAMBOS**
Rose Apple is a small tree with fragrant white flowers. The bark and seed treat diabetes and diarrhoea.

SYZYGIUM AROMATICUM (syn. *Eugenia aromatica*)

Habitat Well-drained maritime tropics; Moluccas, Indonesia	Parts used 🌸 🍃 ⚗ 🌿

Family LEGUMINOSAE	Species *Tamarindus indica*	Local name Indian Date

TAMARIND

The Tamarind is a long-lived evergreen, with elegant foliage on arching branches and hanging racemes of fragrant, rose-veined cream flowers.

• **USES** The ripe fruit-pods contain a pleasantly sour pulp used to flavour Indian curries and chutneys, Malay satays, Caribbean sweetmeats, and a refreshing drink for Ramadan. In Thailand the flowers and leaves are flavourings, and in India the seed pectin is used in jam-making. The aerial parts have laxative, astringent, and fever-reducing properties; the bark treats asthma; a seed- or leaf-paste reduces boils; the seeds help diarrhoea; and the flowers reduce blood pressure. The vitamin- and mineral-rich pulp is used in Chinese medicine.

• **REMARK** Tamarind is used in many commercial products, including Worcestershire sauce and Angostura bitters.

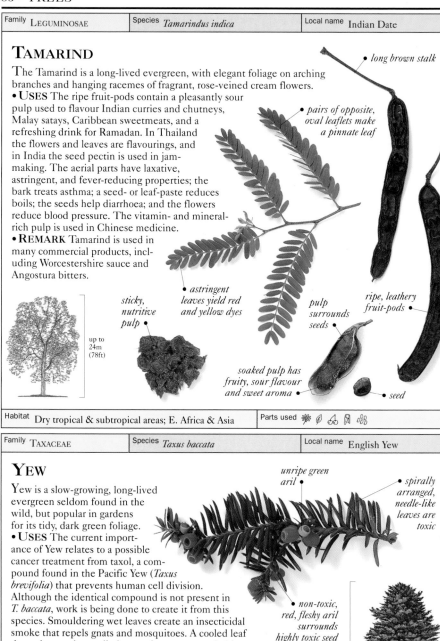

long brown stalk

pairs of opposite, oval leaflets make a pinnate leaf

up to 24m (78ft)

sticky, nutritive pulp

astringent leaves yield red and yellow dyes

pulp surrounds seeds

ripe, leathery fruit-pods

soaked pulp has fruity, sour flavour and sweet aroma

seed

Habitat Dry tropical & subtropical areas; E. Africa & Asia	Parts used ✿ ⬭ ⚶ ⌂ ⣿

Family TAXACEAE	Species *Taxus baccata*	Local name English Yew

YEW

Yew is a slow-growing, long-lived evergreen seldom found in the wild, but popular in gardens for its tidy, dark green foliage.

• **USES** The current import-ance of Yew relates to a possible cancer treatment from taxol, a compound found in the Pacific Yew (*Taxus brevifolia*) that prevents human cell division. Although the identical compound is not present in *T. baccata*, work is being done to create it from this species. Smouldering wet leaves create an insecticidal smoke that repels gnats and mosquitoes. A cooled leaf decoction can be applied to soothe nervous, twitching stock animals, as it has a mild paralyzing effect.

• **REMARK** Yew is valued for bows and axe handles. Both were found with the 5,000 year-old "Ice Man" in the European Alps.

unripe green aril

spirally arranged, needle-like leaves are toxic

non-toxic, red, fleshy aril surrounds highly toxic seed

up to 25m (80ft)

Habitat Limey woodland; temperate northern hemisphere	Parts used ⬭ 🌲

Family STERCULIACEAE	Species *Theobroma cacao*	Local name Chocolate Nut Tree

COCOA TREE

The Cocoa Tree has evergreen leaves, scented
flowers, and fruit growing directly from the trunk.
The fruit contains pink pulp and pale pink beans.
• USES Cocoa beans are fermented and roasted
to develop the chocolate flavour and colour,
and then made into block chocolate or
powder to flavour food and drinks. Cocoa
contains caffeine and theobromine. It is
mildly diuretic and stimulant, and was
given for angina pains. The leaf is a
heart tonic in Colombia. Cocoa
butter is a popular cosmetic
emollient as it protects the
skin and is slow to go rancid.
• REMARK "Chocolatl" is
an Aztec word and it was the
Aztecs who developed cocoa
into a chocolate drink.

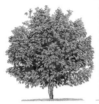

*cocoa
butter
pressed
from
seeds* •

up to
8m
(26ft)

*• ripens
to red-brown*

large, glossy leaf •

*fermented,
roasted seeds* •

Habitat Tropical lowlands; C. & S. America, W. Africa	Parts used

Family CUPRESSACEAE	Species *Thuja occidentalis*	Local name White Cedar

EASTERN ARBOR VITAE

This evergreen conifer has orange-brown bark, aromatic sprays
of yellow-green leaves, and upright cones on the shoot-tips.
• USES The foliage is used for bronchial, urinary, and
vaginal infections; the inner bark is given for delayed
menstruation; the twigs for rheumatism; and the anti-viral
and anti-fungal twig tincture for warts and
skin infections. The essential oil
is used similarly, but is toxic.
• REMARK *Thuja plicata*
leaves and twigs are
used to treat coughs
and rheumatism.

• flattened spray

△ THUJA OCCIDENTALIS

• small, upright cones

◁ THUJA PLICATA
The tall Western Red Cedar
has maroon bark, and flat
leaf sprays with a white
mark beneath.

up to
20m
(65ft)

THUJA
OCCIDENTALIS

*aromatic
leaf* •

Habitat Swamps & mountain slopes; E. Canada	Parts used

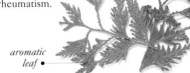

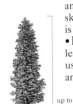

| Family TILIACEAE | Species *Tilia* species | Local name Linden |

LIME

Limes have very small fragrant flowers, but species can be difficult to identify as they hybridize freely.
• USES The flowers of the Common, Large-, and Small-leaved Limes are brewed for Linden tea, the classic digestive end to a continental meal, and a treatment for nervous tension, insomnia, and over-wrought children. It induces sweating which reduces colds, flu, and head-aches, and may lower blood pressure and help arteriosclerosis. Linden water is a skin tonic and is used in bath preparations to soothe rheumatic aches. The world's most valued honey is made from Lime blossom and is used in liqueurs and medicines. The inner bark treats kidney stones, gout, and coronary disease.
• REMARK The names "Lime", "Linden", and "Basswood" refer to the linen-like bass fibres below the bark, once used as cordage.

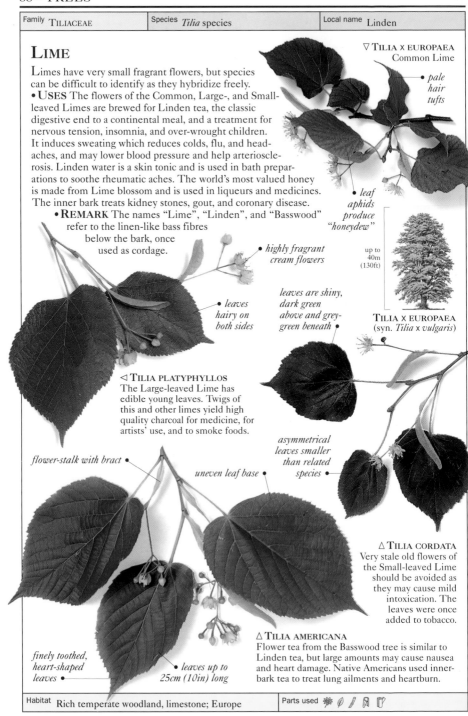

▽ **TILIA X EUROPAEA**
Common Lime

• *pale hair tufts*

• *leaf aphids produce "honeydew"*

• *highly fragrant cream flowers*

up to 40m (130ft)

TILIA X EUROPAEA
(syn. *Tilia* x *vulgaris*)

• *leaves hairy on both sides*

leaves are shiny, dark green above and grey-green beneath •

◁ **TILIA PLATYPHYLLOS**
The Large-leaved Lime has edible young leaves. Twigs of this and other limes yield high quality charcoal for medicine, for artists' use, and to smoke foods.

asymmetrical leaves smaller than related species •

flower-stalk with bract •

uneven leaf base •

△ **TILIA CORDATA**
Very stale old flowers of the Small-leaved Lime should be avoided as they may cause mild intoxication. The leaves were once added to tobacco.

△ **TILIA AMERICANA**
Flower tea from the Basswood tree is similar to Linden tea, but large amounts may cause nausea and heart damage. Native Americans used inner-bark tea to treat lung ailments and heartburn.

finely toothed, heart-shaped leaves •

• *leaves up to 25cm (10in) long*

| Habitat Rich temperate woodland, limestone; Europe | Parts used ✿ ⌀ ⫽ 🍃 🌿 |

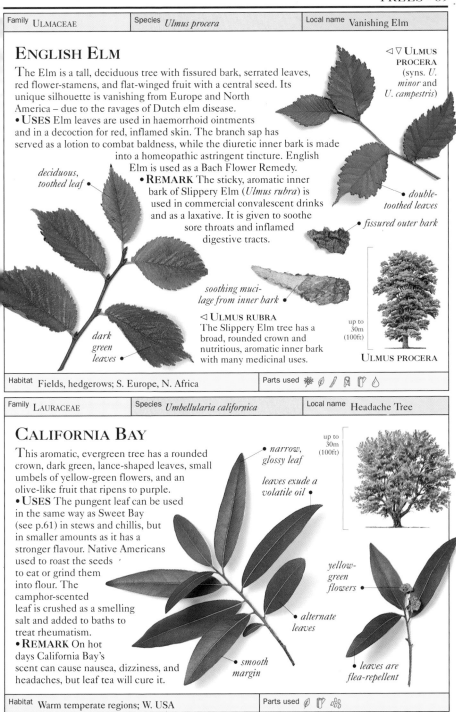

| Family ULMACEAE | Species *Ulmus procera* | Local name Vanishing Elm |

ENGLISH ELM

The Elm is a tall, deciduous tree with fissured bark, serrated leaves, red flower-stamens, and flat-winged fruit with a central seed. Its unique silhouette is vanishing from Europe and North America – due to the ravages of Dutch elm disease.
• **USES** Elm leaves are used in haemorrhoid ointments and in a decoction for red, inflamed skin. The branch sap has served as a lotion to combat baldness, while the diuretic inner bark is made into a homeopathic astringent tincture. English Elm is used as a Bach Flower Remedy.
• **REMARK** The sticky, aromatic inner bark of Slippery Elm (*Ulmus rubra*) is used in commercial convalescent drinks and as a laxative. It is given to soothe sore throats and inflamed digestive tracts.

◁ ▽ **ULMUS PROCERA** (syns. *U. minor* and *U. campestris*)

deciduous, toothed leaf •

• double-toothed leaves

• fissured outer bark

soothing muci-lage from inner bark •

◁ **ULMUS RUBRA**
The Slippery Elm tree has a broad, rounded crown and nutritious, aromatic inner bark with many medicinal uses.

dark green leaves •

up to 30m (100ft)

ULMUS PROCERA

| Habitat Fields, hedgerows; S. Europe, N. Africa | Parts used ❋ ∅ ∥ 🗚 🜂 ◊ |

| Family LAURACEAE | Species *Umbellularia californica* | Local name Headache Tree |

CALIFORNIA BAY

This aromatic, evergreen tree has a rounded crown, dark green, lance-shaped leaves, small umbels of yellow-green flowers, and an olive-like fruit that ripens to purple.
• **USES** The pungent leaf can be used in the same way as Sweet Bay (see p.61) in stews and chillis, but in smaller amounts as it has a stronger flavour. Native Americans used to roast the seeds to eat or grind them into flour. The camphor-scented leaf is crushed as a smelling salt and added to baths to treat rheumatism.
• **REMARK** On hot days California Bay's scent can cause nausea, dizziness, and headaches, but leaf tea will cure it.

• narrow, glossy leaf

leaves exude a volatile oil •

up to 30m (100ft)

yellow-green flowers •

• alternate leaves

• smooth margin

• leaves are flea-repellent

| Habitat Warm temperate regions; W. USA | Parts used ∅ 🗚 ⚘ |

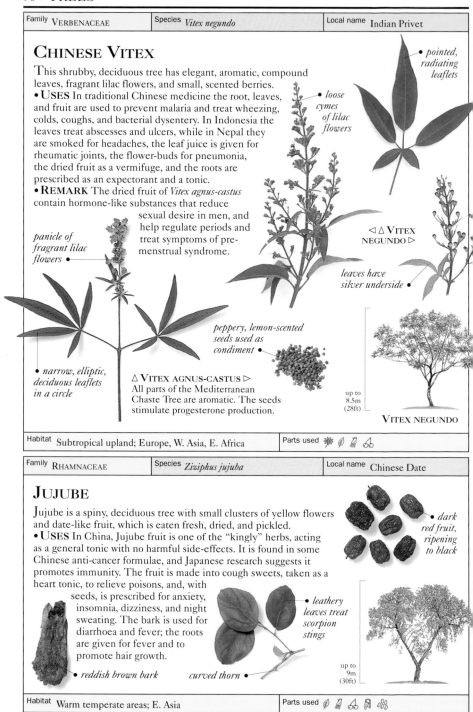

Family VERBENACEAE	Species *Vitex negundo*	Local name Indian Privet

CHINESE VITEX

This shrubby, deciduous tree has elegant, aromatic, compound leaves, fragrant lilac flowers, and small, scented berries.
• **USES** In traditional Chinese medicine the root, leaves, and fruit are used to prevent malaria and treat wheezing, colds, coughs, and bacterial dysentery. In Indonesia the leaves treat abscesses and ulcers, while in Nepal they are smoked for headaches, the leaf juice is given for rheumatic joints, the flower-buds for pneumonia, the dried fruit as a vermifuge, and the roots are prescribed as an expectorant and a tonic.
• **REMARK** The dried fruit of *Vitex agnus-castus* contain hormone-like substances that reduce sexual desire in men, and help regulate periods and treat symptoms of pre-menstrual syndrome.

pointed, radiating leaflets

loose cymes of lilac flowers

◁ △ **VITEX NEGUNDO** ▷

leaves have silver underside •

panicle of fragrant lilac flowers •

• narrow, elliptic, deciduous leaflets in a circle

peppery, lemon-scented seeds used as condiment •

△ **VITEX AGNUS-CASTUS** ▷
All parts of the Mediterranean Chaste Tree are aromatic. The seeds stimulate progesterone production.

up to 8.5m (28ft)

VITEX NEGUNDO

Habitat Subtropical upland; Europe, W. Asia, E. Africa	Parts used 🌸 🍃 🌿 🌾

Family RHAMNACEAE	Species *Ziziphus jujuba*	Local name Chinese Date

JUJUBE

Jujube is a spiny, deciduous tree with small clusters of yellow flowers and date-like fruit, which is eaten fresh, dried, and pickled.
• **USES** In China, Jujube fruit is one of the "kingly" herbs, acting as a general tonic with no harmful side-effects. It is found in some Chinese anti-cancer formulae, and Japanese research suggests it promotes immunity. The fruit is made into cough sweets, taken as a heart tonic, to relieve poisons, and, with seeds, is prescribed for anxiety, insomnia, dizziness, and night sweating. The bark is used for diarrhoea and fever; the roots are given for fever and to promote hair growth.

• dark red fruit, ripening to black

• leathery leaves treat scorpion stings

• reddish brown bark

curved thorn •

up to 9m (30ft)

Habitat Warm temperate areas; E. Asia	Parts used 🍃 🌿 🌾 🌱 🌰

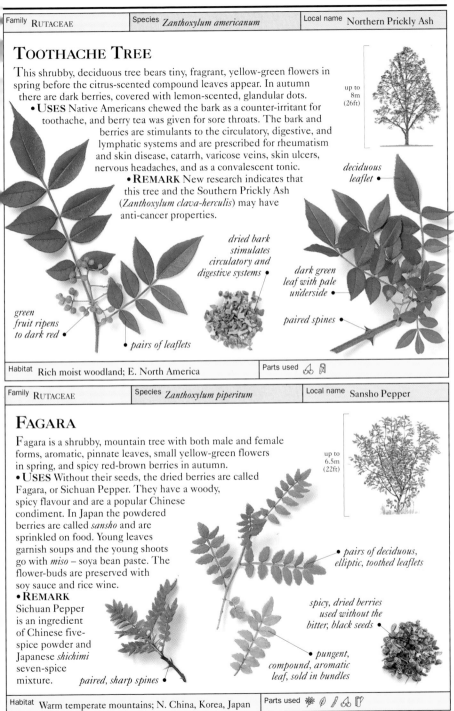

Family RUTACEAE	Species *Zanthoxylum americanum*	Local name Northern Prickly Ash

TOOTHACHE TREE

This shrubby, deciduous tree bears tiny, fragrant, yellow-green flowers in spring before the citrus-scented compound leaves appear. In autumn there are dark berries, covered with lemon-scented, glandular dots.

up to 8m (26ft)

• **USES** Native Americans chewed the bark as a counter-irritant for toothache, and berry tea was given for sore throats. The bark and berries are stimulants to the circulatory, digestive, and lymphatic systems and are prescribed for rheumatism and skin disease, catarrh, varicose veins, skin ulcers, nervous headaches, and as a convalescent tonic.

deciduous leaflet •

• **REMARK** New research indicates that this tree and the Southern Prickly Ash (*Zanthoxylum clava-herculis*) may have anti-cancer properties.

dried bark stimulates circulatory and digestive systems •

dark green leaf with pale underside •

green fruit ripens to dark red •

paired spines •

• pairs of leaflets

Habitat Rich moist woodland; E. North America	Parts used

Family RUTACEAE	Species *Zanthoxylum piperitum*	Local name Sansho Pepper

FAGARA

Fagara is a shrubby, mountain tree with both male and female forms, aromatic, pinnate leaves, small yellow-green flowers in spring, and spicy red-brown berries in autumn.

up to 6.5m (22ft)

• **USES** Without their seeds, the dried berries are called Fagara, or Sichuan Pepper. They have a woody, spicy flavour and are a popular Chinese condiment. In Japan the powdered berries are called *sansho* and are sprinkled on food. Young leaves garnish soups and the young shoots go with *miso* – soya bean paste. The flower-buds are preserved with soy sauce and rice wine.

• pairs of deciduous, elliptic, toothed leaflets

• **REMARK** Sichuan Pepper is an ingredient of Chinese five-spice powder and Japanese *shichimi* seven-spice mixture.

spicy, dried berries used without the bitter, black seeds •

paired, sharp spines •

• pungent, compound, aromatic leaf, sold in bundles

Habitat Warm temperate mountains; N. China, Korea, Japan	Parts used

SHRUBS

Family LEGUMINOSAE	Species *Acacia dealbata*	Local name Silver Wattle

MIMOSA

This evergreen shrub has blue-green to mid-green leaves, with fine, grey-white hairs and highly fragrant yellow inflorescences. Shrubs and trees in the genus *Acacia* are tolerant of dry conditions, where they help to restore fertility to the soil.
• **USES** Boiled young leaves, shoots, and seeds of *Acacia* are edible, and the roots can be tapped for water. Mimosa is sold in florists and grown in Natal (South Africa) for its bark-tannin and gum. The mimosa or cassie essential oil, used in perfumery, is distilled from the flowers of *A. farnesiana* and *A. baileyana*. *A. senegal* is the main source of Gum Arabic, used in sweets, inks, fabric printing, to thicken artists' paints, and to add shine to silk and crepes. The thorns of *A. cornigera* treat asthma, the root delays snakebite effects, and the bark is given for skin problems. *A. catechu* wood yields dye and catechu. The latter extract is chewed with betel-nuts and used as a disinfectant against throat inflammation.
• **REMARK** *Acacia* pods growing on trees in the savannah are irresistible food for elephants.

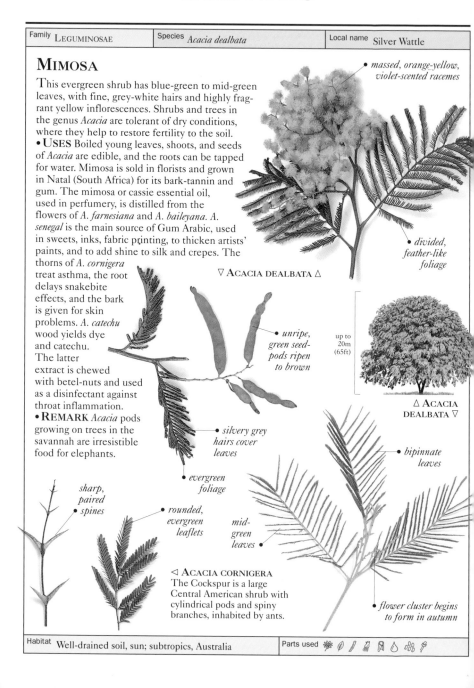

• *massed, orange-yellow, violet-scented racemes*

• *divided, feather-like foliage*

▽ ACACIA DEALBATA △

• *unripe, green seed-pods ripen to brown*

up to 20m (65ft)

△ ACACIA DEALBATA ▽

• *silvery grey hairs cover leaves*

• *bipinnate leaves*

evergreen foliage

sharp, paired spines

• *rounded, evergreen leaflets*

mid-green leaves •

◁ ACACIA CORNIGERA
The Cockspur is a large Central American shrub with cylindrical pods and spiny branches, inhabited by ants.

• *flower cluster begins to form in autumn*

Habitat Well-drained soil, sun; subtropics, Australia	Parts used ❋ ✐ ⫽ ⚭ ⎅ ◌ ⁂ ⚘

Family VERBENACEAE	Species *Aloysia triphylla*	Local name Limonetto

LEMON VERBENA

Lemon Verbena has strongly lemon-scented whorls of three or four leaves along its stems, and panicles of tiny, pale summer flowers.
• USES The leaves of *Aloysia triphylla* (syn. *Lippia citriodora*) are used to flavour drinks, fruit and sweet dishes, and to make herb tea. The tea is refreshing and mildly sedative; it soothes bronchial and nasal congestion and eases indigestion and nausea. The leaves yield a green colouring and an essential oil used in perfumes and bath lotions. A leaf infusion relieves puffy eyes and, as a floral vinegar, it softens the skin. Sprigs are used to scent pot-pourri.
• REMARK *Lippia dulcis* contains a sweetener 1,000 times sweeter than sucrose.

loose clusters of white and pale purple flowers •

long, pointed, rough-textured leaves •

up to 3m (10ft)

leaf scent retained for many years when dried •

Habitat Frost-free, well-drained areas; Argentina, Chile	Parts used

Family ROSACEAE	Species *Amelanchier alnifolia*	Local name Shadbush

SASKATOON BERRIES

This deciduous, thicket-forming shrub or small tree has racemes of small, fragrant white flowers followed by clusters of purple-black berries.
• USES The Saskatoon was the most important berry to the native peoples of western Canada, who ate it fresh, dried it for winter use, and used it to flavour stews and soup. Today the berries are eaten raw or cooked in pies, puddings, and preserves. The Cree tribe dried the whole plant for medicinal teas. The fruit was used to treat sore eyes, stomachache, and liver trouble, and yields black and purple dyes. The roots were used as a tobacco substitute.
• REMARK The berries were used by native Americans in *pemmican*, a pressed cake of meat, and fresh or dried fruit. They are now used mainly for emergency food rations.

thin layer of dark brown, finely furrowed bark •

strong, flexible wood •

up to 4m (13ft)

deciduous, alternate, rounded leaves on thin stalks •

purple-black berries •

• sweet berries eaten raw, cooked, and preserved

• upper leaf margins toothed

• matt green leaf

Habitat Wet woodland; W. Canada	Parts used

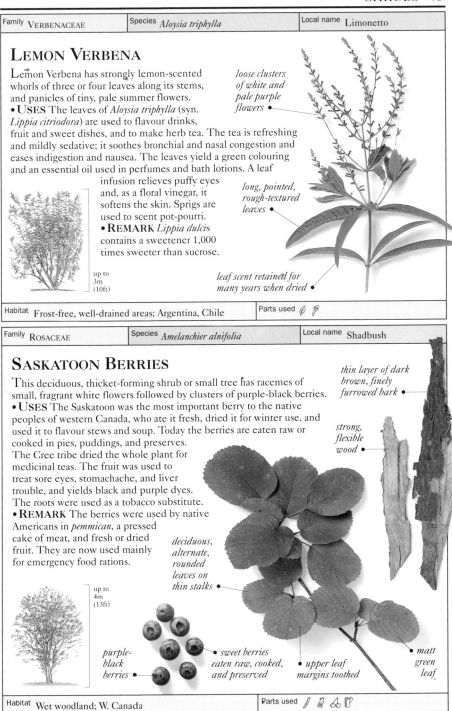

Family ERICACEAE	Species *Arctostaphylos uva-ursi*	Local name Bearberry

UVA-URSI

Uva-ursi is a low, mat-forming, evergreen shrub with long, trailing stems; tough, flexible twigs; hanging, urn-shaped, pinkish white spring flowers; and red autumn berries.

• USES The raw or dried berries make necklaces and rattles and are relied on as a bland survival food, improved by cooking. The stem and leaves are brewed by native Americans to treat headaches and to prevent and cure scurvy. They act as a diuretic and anti-bacterial treatment for cystitis and urinary tract disorders, and are applied externally for back sprain. The roots have been used as a dysentery cure. The leaves form a tobacco substitute, used in ceremonies of the Blackfoot tribe. The aerial parts yield yellow, green, and grey dyes.

• REMARK Persistent over-use may have toxic effects.

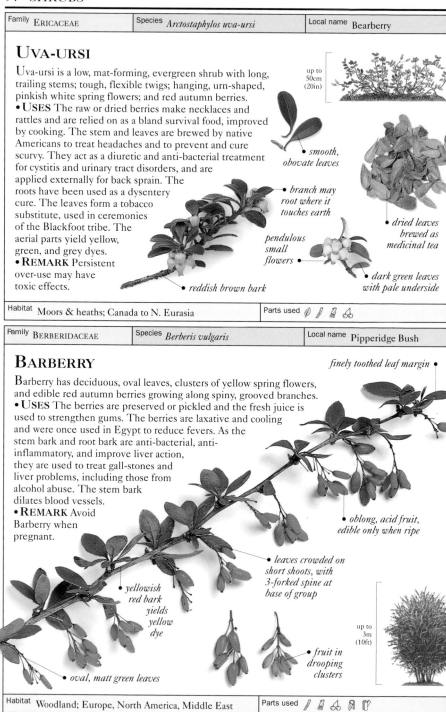

up to 50cm (20in)

smooth, obovate leaves

branch may root where it touches earth

dried leaves brewed as medicinal tea

pendulous small flowers

dark green leaves with pale underside

reddish brown bark

Habitat Moors & heaths; Canada to N. Eurasia	Parts used

Family BERBERIDACEAE	Species *Berberis vulgaris*	Local name Pipperidge Bush

BARBERRY

finely toothed leaf margin

Barberry has deciduous, oval leaves, clusters of yellow spring flowers, and edible red autumn berries growing along spiny, grooved branches.

• USES The berries are preserved or pickled and the fresh juice is used to strengthen gums. The berries are laxative and cooling and were once used in Egypt to reduce fevers. As the stem bark and root bark are anti-bacterial, anti-inflammatory, and improve liver action, they are used to treat gall-stones and liver problems, including those from alcohol abuse. The stem bark dilates blood vessels.

• REMARK Avoid Barberry when pregnant.

oblong, acid fruit, edible only when ripe

leaves crowded on short shoots, with 3-forked spine at base of group

yellowish red bark yields yellow dye

up to 3m (10ft)

fruit in drooping clusters

oval, matt green leaves

Habitat Woodland; Europe, North America, Middle East	Parts used

| Family BUXACEAE | Species *Buxus sempervirens* | Local name Boxwood |

BOX

Box is an evergreen shrub or small tree of variable form, with small, yellow-green flowers in spring, berries with black seeds, and leafy stems with a distinctive scent.
• USES Box leaves contain buxine and were once used to purify the blood, improve hair growth and horses' coats, and, with bark, were given to treat rheumatism and expel worms. They are now considered too toxic except in homeopathic doses. The wood is narcotic and sedative, and its distilled oil was given for toothache and piles. Leached leaves and wood yield an auburn hair dye and the bark is used in perfumery.
• REMARK Animals can die from eating Box leaves. The hard wood is used to make some scientific instruments, flutes, and combs.

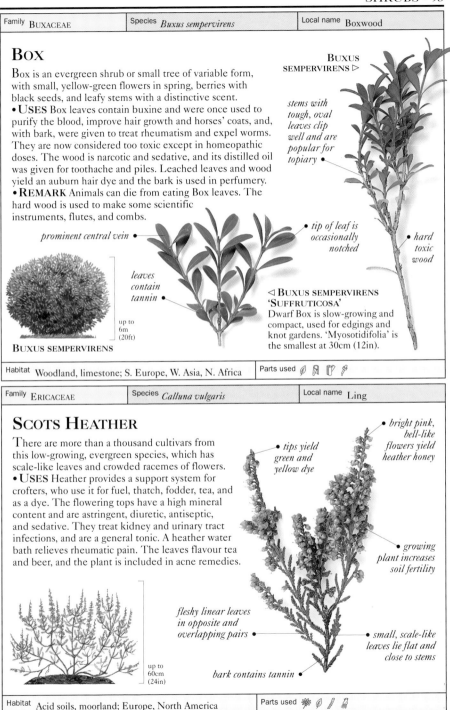

BUXUS
SEMPERVIRENS ▷

stems with tough, oval leaves clip well and are popular for topiary •

prominent central vein •

leaves contain tannin •

tip of leaf is occasionally notched •

• *hard toxic wood*

up to
6m
(20ft)

BUXUS SEMPERVIRENS

◁ BUXUS SEMPERVIRENS
'SUFFRUTICOSA'
Dwarf Box is slow-growing and compact, used for edgings and knot gardens. 'Myosotidifolia' is the smallest at 30cm (12in).

| Habitat Woodland, limestone; S. Europe, W. Asia, N. Africa | Parts used 🌿 🍃 🍂 |

| Family ERICACEAE | Species *Calluna vulgaris* | Local name Ling |

SCOTS HEATHER

There are more than a thousand cultivars from this low-growing, evergreen species, which has scale-like leaves and crowded racemes of flowers.
• USES Heather provides a support system for crofters, who use it for fuel, thatch, fodder, tea, and as a dye. The flowering tops have a high mineral content and are astringent, diuretic, antiseptic, and sedative. They treat kidney and urinary tract infections, and are a general tonic. A heather water bath relieves rheumatic pain. The leaves flavour tea and beer, and the plant is included in acne remedies.

• *bright pink, bell-like flowers yield heather honey*

• *tips yield green and yellow dye*

• *growing plant increases soil fertility*

fleshy linear leaves in opposite and overlapping pairs •

• *small, scale-like leaves lie flat and close to stems*

up to
60cm
(24in)

bark contains tannin •

| Habitat Acid soils, moorland; Europe, North America | Parts used 🌸 🌿 🍃 🍂 |

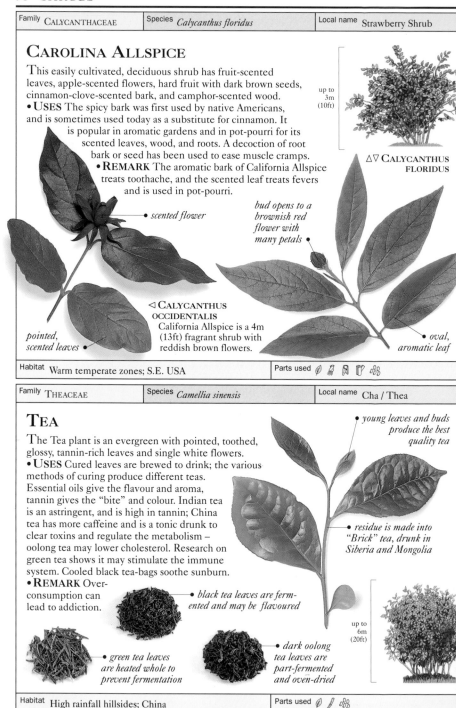

Family CALYCANTHACEAE	Species *Calycanthus floridus*	Local name Strawberry Shrub

CAROLINA ALLSPICE

This easily cultivated, deciduous shrub has fruit-scented leaves, apple-scented flowers, hard fruit with dark brown seeds, cinnamon-clove-scented bark, and camphor-scented wood.
• USES The spicy bark was first used by native Americans, and is sometimes used today as a substitute for cinnamon. It is popular in aromatic gardens and in pot-pourri for its scented leaves, wood, and roots. A decoction of root bark or seed has been used to ease muscle cramps.
• REMARK The aromatic bark of California Allspice treats toothache, and the scented leaf treats fevers and is used in pot-pourri.

up to 3m (10ft)

△▽ CALYCANTHUS FLORIDUS

• *scented flower*

bud opens to a brownish red flower with many petals •

◁ CALYCANTHUS OCCIDENTALIS
California Allspice is a 4m (13ft) fragrant shrub with reddish brown flowers.

pointed, scented leaves •

• *oval, aromatic leaf*

Habitat Warm temperate zones; S.E. USA	Parts used

Family THEACEAE	Species *Camellia sinensis*	Local name Cha / Thea

TEA

The Tea plant is an evergreen with pointed, toothed, glossy, tannin-rich leaves and single white flowers.
• USES Cured leaves are brewed to drink; the various methods of curing produce different teas. Essential oils give the flavour and aroma, tannin gives the "bite" and colour. Indian tea is an astringent, and is high in tannin; China tea has more caffeine and is a tonic drunk to clear toxins and regulate the metabolism – oolong tea may lower cholesterol. Research on green tea shows it may stimulate the immune system. Cooled black tea-bags soothe sunburn.
• REMARK Over-consumption can lead to addiction.

• *young leaves and buds produce the best quality tea*

• *residue is made into "Brick" tea, drunk in Siberia and Mongolia*

• *black tea leaves are fermented and may be flavoured*

up to 6m (20ft)

• *green tea leaves are heated whole to prevent fermentation*

• *dark oolong tea leaves are part-fermented and oven-dried*

Habitat High rainfall hillsides; China	Parts used

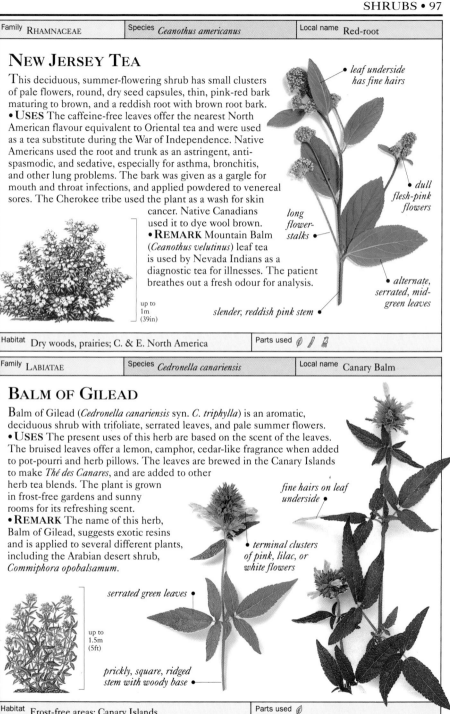

Family RHAMNACEAE	Species *Ceanothus americanus*	Local name Red-root

New Jersey Tea

This deciduous, summer-flowering shrub has small clusters of pale flowers, round, dry seed capsules, thin, pink-red bark maturing to brown, and a reddish root with brown root bark.
• USES The caffeine-free leaves offer the nearest North American flavour equivalent to Oriental tea and were used as a tea substitute during the War of Independence. Native Americans used the root and trunk as an astringent, anti-spasmodic, and sedative, especially for asthma, bronchitis, and other lung problems. The bark was given as a gargle for mouth and throat infections, and applied powdered to venereal sores. The Cherokee tribe used the plant as a wash for skin cancer. Native Canadians used it to dye wool brown.
• REMARK Mountain Balm (*Ceanothus velutinus*) leaf tea is used by Nevada Indians as a diagnostic tea for illnesses. The patient breathes out a fresh odour for analysis.

leaf underside has fine hairs

dull flesh-pink flowers

long flower-stalks

alternate, serrated, mid-green leaves

up to 1m (39in)

slender, reddish pink stem

Habitat Dry woods, prairies; C. & E. North America	Parts used

Family LABIATAE	Species *Cedronella canariensis*	Local name Canary Balm

Balm of Gilead

Balm of Gilead (*Cedronella canariensis* syn. *C. triphylla*) is an aromatic, deciduous shrub with trifoliate, serrated leaves, and pale summer flowers.
• USES The present uses of this herb are based on the scent of the leaves. The bruised leaves offer a lemon, camphor, cedar-like fragrance when added to pot-pourri and herb pillows. The leaves are brewed in the Canary Islands to make *Thé des Canares*, and are added to other herb tea blends. The plant is grown in frost-free gardens and sunny rooms for its refreshing scent.
• REMARK The name of this herb, Balm of Gilead, suggests exotic resins and is applied to several different plants, including the Arabian desert shrub, *Commiphora opobalsamum*.

fine hairs on leaf underside

terminal clusters of pink, lilac, or white flowers

serrated green leaves

up to 1.5m (5ft)

prickly, square, ridged stem with woody base

Habitat Frost-free areas; Canary Islands	Parts used

Family COMPOSITAE	Species *Chrysothamnus nauseosus*	Local name Grey Rabbitbrush

RABBITBRUSH

Rabbitbrush is an low, rounded, aromatic
bush with soft, feathery foliage, clusters of
yellow tubular florets, each with a calyx of
soft bristles, and dry seed capsules.
• **USES** Various native American tribes
once used it medicinally, inhaling smoke
from a smouldering plant for colds. They
brewed a flower or twig infusion to treat
coughs, colds, and tuberculosis; used leaves
and stems in a skin wash for smallpox; and a
root decoction for
menstrual pain,
colds, and flu. A salve
of the branches and leaves helps
keep flies away from horses, and
the flowers yield yellow and orange dyes.
• **REMARK** The tribal practice of chewing gum
from the knots on plant stems led the US
government to consider Rabbitbrush as a
source of rubber during the First World War.

• *hair-like, grey-green foliage*

• *linear leaves placed alternately*

plant can be propagated from seed or cuttings

multi-branched
• *stem*

• *white- or grey-felted stems contain a rubbery resin when mature*

up to
2m
(6½ft)

Habitat Gravelly arid areas; W. North America	Parts used 🌼 ✐ ∥ ♨ ◊

Family CISTACEAE	Species *Cistus ladanifer*	Local name Ladanum

LABDANUM

This twiggy evergreen has large, white flowers with a
crimson spot on each petal. During the intense heat of
summer, glandular hairs on the leaves and stem exude a
sticky, aromatic resin that becomes opaque in the cold,
giving the plant an unreal, leaden appearance.
• **USES** The resin, called labdanum, was once collected
on the fleece of browsing goats, but now the leafy twigs are
usually gathered and boiled, and the resin skimmed off the
water surface. It is distilled to produce a heavy fragrance used
as a perfume fixative, in soaps, cosmetics, and
deodorants. It can be used as a substitute for amber-
gris from whales, and has insecticidal properties.
• **REMARK** *Cistus creticus* (syn. *C. incanus*), with
rose-purple flowers, is also a prolific source of
labdanum, which is used locally to treat bronchitis.

aromatic dark green leaves •

• *leaf feels gummy*

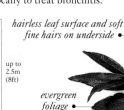

hairless leaf surface and soft fine hairs on underside •

up to
2.5m
(8ft)

evergreen foliage •

• *summer heat causes leaf and stem to exude a balsamic resin called labdanum*

• *leaves in opposite pairs*

Habitat Rocky scrubland; Mediterranean	Parts used ✐ ∥ ◊

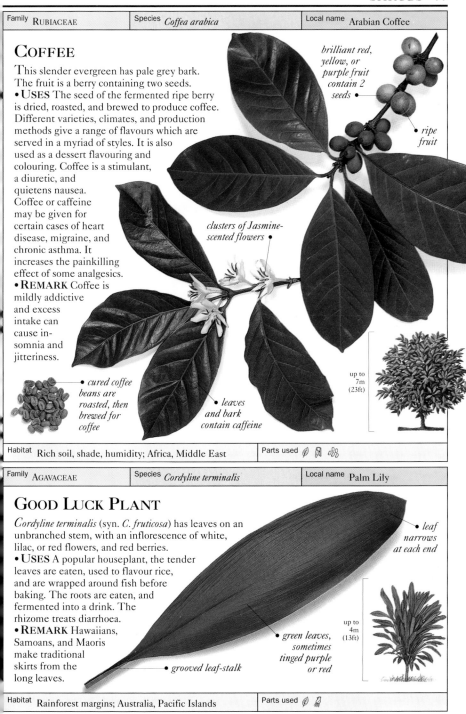

| Family RUBIACEAE | Species *Coffea arabica* | Local name Arabian Coffee |

COFFEE

This slender evergreen has pale grey bark.
The fruit is a berry containing two seeds.
• **USES** The seed of the fermented ripe berry
is dried, roasted, and brewed to produce coffee.
Different varieties, climates, and production
methods give a range of flavours which are
served in a myriad of styles. It is also
used as a dessert flavouring and
colouring. Coffee is a stimulant,
a diuretic, and
quietens nausea.
Coffee or caffeine
may be given for
certain cases of heart
disease, migraine, and
chronic asthma. It
increases the painkilling
effect of some analgesics.
• **REMARK** Coffee is
mildly addictive
and excess
intake can
cause in-
somnia and
jitteriness.

*brilliant red,
yellow, or
purple fruit
contain 2
seeds •*

*• ripe
fruit*

*clusters of Jasmine-
scented flowers •*

*• cured coffee
beans are
roasted, then
brewed for
coffee*

*• leaves
and bark
contain caffeine*

up to
7m
(23ft)

| Habitat Rich soil, shade, humidity; Africa, Middle East | Parts used |

| Family AGAVACEAE | Species *Cordyline terminalis* | Local name Palm Lily |

GOOD LUCK PLANT

Cordyline terminalis (syn. *C. fruticosa*) has leaves on an
unbranched stem, with an inflorescence of white,
lilac, or red flowers, and red berries.
• **USES** A popular houseplant, the tender
leaves are eaten, used to flavour rice,
and are wrapped around fish before
baking. The roots are eaten, and
fermented into a drink. The
rhizome treats diarrhoea.
• **REMARK** Hawaiians,
Samoans, and Maoris
make traditional
skirts from the
long leaves.

*• leaf
narrows
at each end*

up to
4m
(13ft)

*• green leaves,
sometimes
tinged purple
or red*

• grooved leaf-stalk

| Habitat Rainforest margins; Australia, Pacific Islands | Parts used |

Family CORYLACEAE	Species *Corylus avellana*	Local name Cobnut

HAZEL

Hazel is a deciduous, suckering shrub with pendulous male catkins in spring and clusters of nuts in autumn.
• **USES** Hazelnuts are eaten raw and used in confectionery, cakes, and liqueurs. The edible nut oil is extracted and used in cooking, perfumery, massage oils, soaps, and lubricants. The nuts are ground into a fine flour for face masks. The leaves have served as a tobacco substitute.
• **REMARK** Hazel branches are the traditional material for water divining.

rounded, toothed leaves

short leaf-stalk

shelled nuts are cream under the papery brown skin

bud-like female flowers

yellow-brown male catkins

nuts contain sulphur and magnesium

up to 10m (33ft)

Habitat Woodland, hedgerows; Europe, W. Asia, N. Africa	Parts used

Family ROSACEAE	Species *Crataegus* species	Local name May Blossom

HAWTHORN

This deciduous, thorny shrub has serrated, lobed leaves, dense, white flower clusters in late spring, and red false fruit (haws).
• **USES** The leaves, flowers, and haws are a cardiac and circulation tonic, treating heart weakness caused by kidney disease, thickening tissue, artery spasm, and irregular heartbeat. Hawthorn dilates the heart's blood vessels and improves pumping, which controls both high and low blood pressure. Japanese research has confirmed improvement in cardiac function.
• **REMARK** During the First World War, young Hawthorn leaves were used as substitutes for tea and tobacco, and the seeds were ground in place of coffee.

up to 10m (33ft)

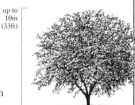

▽△ CRATAEGUS LAEVIGATA
(syn. *Crataegus oxycanthoides*)

• *dried ripe haws*

△▷ CRATAEGUS MONOGYNA
English Hawthorn has deeply lobed leaves and single-seeded haws.

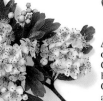

△ CRATAEGUS CUNEATA
Chinese Hawthorn haws are now used in China to treat stomach and ovarian cancer.

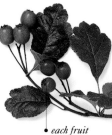

• *each fruit has 2 seeds*

Habitat Woodland, hedgerows; Europe, N. Africa, India	Parts used

Family EUPHORBIACEAE	Species *Croton tiglium*	Local name Purging Croton

CROTON

Croton has malodorous, dark green leaves, inconspicuous flower racemes, and a brown seed capsule with three hard black seeds.
• **USES** The seed oil is a dangerous, violent purgative now only used for extreme blockages or externally as a counter-irritant. In China tiny amounts of processed seed are used to treat epilepsy, malaria, and chest congestion. In Malaysia whole seeds are used to stun fish. The tumour-promoting properties of the oil are being used to investigate how cancerous cells develop from normal ones.
• **REMARK** Sweetbark (*Croton eleuteria*) is a decorative shrub with a metallic appearance, fragrant white flowers, and aromatic tonic bark which burns with a musky scent. It has mild narcotic properties and is given for malaria, nausea, and headaches.

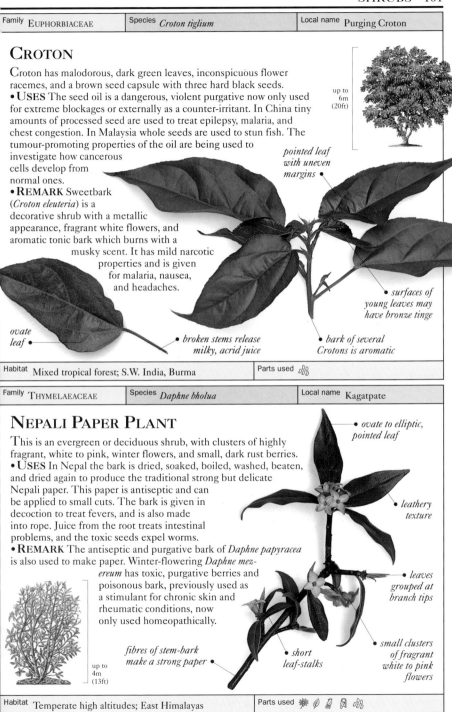

up to
6m
(20ft)

*pointed leaf
with uneven
margins*

*surfaces of
young leaves may
have bronze tinge*

*ovate
leaf*

*broken stems release
milky, acrid juice*

*bark of several
Crotons is aromatic*

Habitat Mixed tropical forest; S.W. India, Burma	Parts used

Family THYMELAEACEAE	Species *Daphne bholua*	Local name Kagatpate

NEPALI PAPER PLANT

This is an evergreen or deciduous shrub, with clusters of highly fragrant, white to pink, winter flowers, and small, dark rust berries.
• **USES** In Nepal the bark is dried, soaked, boiled, washed, beaten, and dried again to produce the traditional strong but delicate Nepali paper. This paper is antiseptic and can be applied to small cuts. The bark is given in decoction to treat fevers, and is also made into rope. Juice from the root treats intestinal problems, and the toxic seeds expel worms.
• **REMARK** The antiseptic and purgative bark of *Daphne papyracea* is also used to make paper. Winter-flowering *Daphne mezereum* has toxic, purgative berries and poisonous bark, previously used as a stimulant for chronic skin and rheumatic conditions, now only used homeopathically.

*ovate to elliptic,
pointed leaf*

*leathery
texture*

*leaves
grouped at
branch tips*

*fibres of stem-bark
make a strong paper*

up to
4m
(13ft)

*short
leaf-stalks*

*small clusters
of fragrant
white to pink
flowers*

Habitat Temperate high altitudes; East Himalayas	Parts used

Family ARALIACEAE	Species *Eleutherococcus sieboldianus*	Local name Free Pips

HEDGING ELEUTHEROCOCCUS

This deciduous shrub has arching stems, umbels of green-white, early summer flowers, and clusters of black fruit.
• USES This elegant hedging plant, tolerant of urban pollution, may have medicinal properties, but so far research has centred on the similar-looking shrub Siberian Ginseng (*Eleutherococcus senticosus*), whose roots and leaves share the medicinal attributes of Panax Ginseng and are cheaper and less heating (stimulating). Russian research on astronauts and athletes shows it increases stamina, strengthens resistance, and reduces stress.

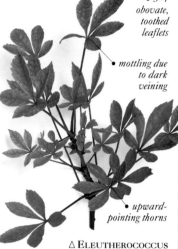

• *3–7 obovate, toothed leaflets*

• *mottling due to dark veining*

• REMARK Siberian Ginseng was given to reduce radiation sickness after the 1986 nuclear disaster at Chernobyl.

up to 3m (10ft)

▽ ELEUTHEROCOCCUS SENTICOSUS
Siberian Ginseng is a hardy shrub.

ELEUTHEROCOCCUS SIEBOLDIANUS

• *powdered root*

• *upward-pointing thorns*

△ ELEUTHEROCOCCUS SIEBOLDIANUS

Habitat Well-drained, poor soil, sun; E. China, Japan	Parts used

Family EPHEDRACEAE	Species *Ephedra sinica*	Local name Ma Huang

EPHEDRA

Ephedra is a primitive shrub with long, jointed, cylindrical stems, scale-like leaves, and male cones.
• USES Several species, notably *Ephedra sinica*, are the source of the drug ephedrine, used for asthma, hay fever, and allergies until the side-effect of very high blood pressure was recognized. But the whole herb contains counteracting alkaloids which balance this. It has been used successfully for 5,000 years in China for the above, and for rheumatism and coughs, and by modern herbalists with no apparent side-effects.
• REMARK *E. gerardiana* and *E. americana* are diuretic and purify the system.

female "flowers" •

△ E. AMERICANA

• *downward arch*

• *whorled branchlets*

△ EPHEDRA GERARDIANA

△ EPHEDRA SINICA
The dried stems contain alkaloids.

up to 75cm (30in)

EPHEDRA SINICA

Habitat Semi-arid, rocky hills; China	Parts used

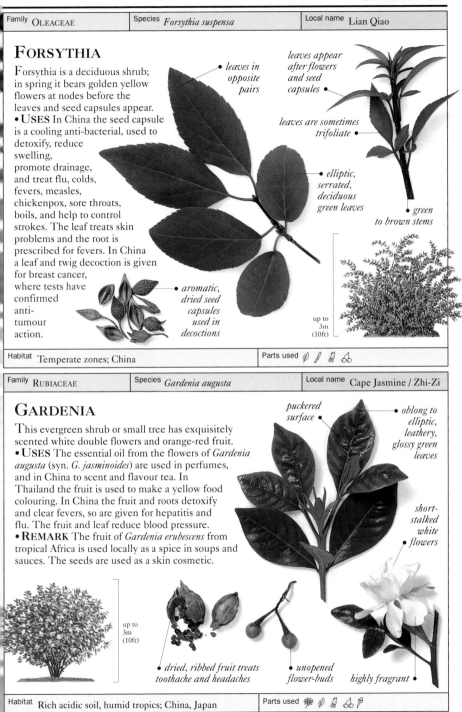

Family OLEACEAE	Species *Forsythia suspensa*	Local name Lian Qiao

FORSYTHIA

Forsythia is a deciduous shrub; in spring it bears golden yellow flowers at nodes before the leaves and seed capsules appear.
• **USES** In China the seed capsule is a cooling anti-bacterial, used to detoxify, reduce swelling, promote drainage, and treat flu, colds, fevers, measles, chickenpox, sore throats, boils, and help to control strokes. The leaf treats skin problems and the root is prescribed for fevers. In China a leaf and twig decoction is given for breast cancer, where tests have confirmed anti-tumour action.

leaves in opposite pairs

leaves appear after flowers and seed capsules

leaves are sometimes trifoliate

elliptic, serrated, deciduous green leaves

green to brown stems

aromatic, dried seed capsules used in decoctions

up to 3m (10ft)

Habitat Temperate zones; China	Parts used

Family RUBIACEAE	Species *Gardenia augusta*	Local name Cape Jasmine / Zhi-Zi

GARDENIA

This evergreen shrub or small tree has exquisitely scented white double flowers and orange-red fruit.
• **USES** The essential oil from the flowers of *Gardenia augusta* (syn. *G. jasminoides*) are used in perfumes, and in China to scent and flavour tea. In Thailand the fruit is used to make a yellow food colouring. In China the fruit and roots detoxify and clear fevers, so are given for hepatitis and flu. The fruit and leaf reduce blood pressure.
• **REMARK** The fruit of *Gardenia erubescens* from tropical Africa is used locally as a spice in soups and sauces. The seeds are used as a skin cosmetic.

puckered surface

oblong to elliptic, leathery, glossy green leaves

short-stalked white flowers

up to 3m (10ft)

dried, ribbed fruit treats toothache and headaches

unopened flower-buds

highly fragrant

Habitat Rich acidic soil, humid tropics; China, Japan	Parts used

Family ERICACEAE	Species *Gaultheria procumbens*	Local name Checkerberry

WINTERGREEN

This creeping shrub flowers in summer and bears aromatic scarlet pseudo-berries from autumn into spring.
• **USES** Wintergreen Oil, with its rich, refreshing scent, is distilled from the leaves after 24 hours of maceration to flavour sweets and toothpaste. The oil, present in the leaves and fruit, contains methyl salicylate, related to aspirin. Easily absorbed through the skin, the oil is astringent, diuretic, and stimulant, and is used externally for muscular aches, especially in foot balms and treatments for rheumatism. In aromatherapy the oil is used with others to reduce cellulite. The leaves are brewed for Mountain Tea and are used by the Inuit of Labrador, Canada, to treat paralysis, headaches, aching muscles, and sore throats. They eat raw berries, which can be added to jams.
• **REMARK** Wintergreen Oil can irritate the skin, and should be taken internally only under close medical supervision.

aromatic, evergreen leaves grouped at the end of stiff shoots

slightly toothed leaves

red leaf-stalks on short, erect shoots

flowers open white to pale pink

bell-shaped flowers usually appear singly from base of leaves

pale stems

up to 15cm (6in)

Habitat Woodland, acid, sandy moorland; North America	Parts used

Family LEGUMINOSAE	Species *Genista tinctoria*	Local name Dyer's Broom

DYER'S GREENWEED

Dyer's Greenweed is a variable deciduous shrub with golden flowers and small fruit-pods with four to ten seeds.
• **USES** The flowering tops are used as a yellow dye and are added to woad-dyed blue cloth to turn it Kendal green. The plant was once used for its diuretic, purgative, and weak cardio-active properties and to treat rheumatism. Common Broom has flexible branches, ideal for brooms. The narcotic flowering tops first excite then stupefy the system, and the whole herb was used to treat tumours.
• **REMARK** A flowering sprig of broom was a heraldic battle device of Henry II of England, who is said to have taken the family name Plantagenet from this medieval "planta genista".

flowers grouped at ends of branches

pea-like, 2-lipped, yellow summer flowers

small, bright green leaves

△ GENISTA TINCTORIA ▷

rich yellow, fragrant flowers

flowers on slender stalks

green fruit-pod ripens nearly black

up to 2m (6½ft)

1–2 flowers from each leaf-joint

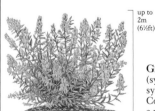

GENISTA TINCTORIA

GENISTA SCOPARIUS ▷
(syn. *Cytisus scoparius* and syn. *Sarothamnus scoparius*)
Common or Scotch Broom is a many-branched erect shrub with simple or trifoliate leaves.

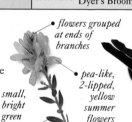

ripe pods explode

Habitat Northern temperate areas; Europe to S.W. Siberia	Parts used

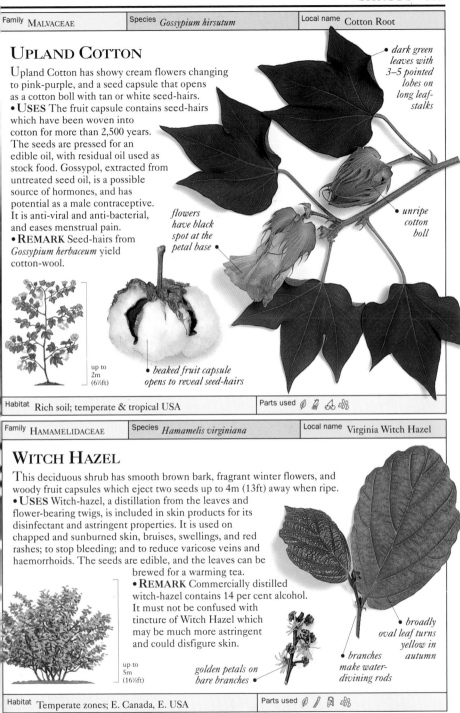

Family MALVACEAE	Species *Gossypium hirsutum*	Local name Cotton Root

UPLAND COTTON

Upland Cotton has showy cream flowers changing to pink-purple, and a seed capsule that opens as a cotton boll with tan or white seed-hairs.
• USES The fruit capsule contains seed-hairs which have been woven into cotton for more than 2,500 years. The seeds are pressed for an edible oil, with residual oil used as stock food. Gossypol, extracted from untreated seed oil, is a possible source of hormones, and has potential as a male contraceptive. It is anti-viral and anti-bacterial, and eases menstrual pain.
• REMARK Seed-hairs from *Gossypium herbaceum* yield cotton-wool.

• dark green leaves with 3–5 pointed lobes on long leaf-stalks

flowers have black spot at the petal base •

• *unripe cotton boll*

up to 2m (6½ft)

• *beaked fruit capsule opens to reveal seed-hairs*

Habitat Rich soil; temperate & tropical USA	Parts used

Family HAMAMELIDACEAE	Species *Hamamelis virginiana*	Local name Virginia Witch Hazel

WITCH HAZEL

This deciduous shrub has smooth brown bark, fragrant winter flowers, and woody fruit capsules which eject two seeds up to 4m (13ft) away when ripe.
• USES Witch-hazel, a distillation from the leaves and flower-bearing twigs, is included in skin products for its disinfectant and astringent properties. It is used on chapped and sunburned skin, bruises, swellings, and red rashes; to stop bleeding; and to reduce varicose veins and haemorrhoids. The seeds are edible, and the leaves can be brewed for a warming tea.
• REMARK Commercially distilled witch-hazel contains 14 per cent alcohol. It must not be confused with tincture of Witch Hazel which may be much more astringent and could disfigure skin.

• *broadly oval leaf turns yellow in autumn*

up to 5m (16½ft)

golden petals on bare branches •

• *branches make water-divining rods*

Habitat Temperate zones; E. Canada, E. USA	Parts used

Family COMPOSITAE	Species *Helichrysum italicum*	Local name Everlasting

CURRY PLANT

clusters of tiny mustard-yellow flowers used in pot-pourri •

Curry Plant is a subshrub with intensely silver foliage, golden flowers, and shining, white, cylindrical fruit.
• USES Unlike two other plants of the same name, the Curry Plant's name does result from its curry-like smell, but it is not part of curry blends. The leaf gives a mild curry flavour to soups or casseroles, but should be removed from the dish before eating as it can upset stomachs.
• REMARK A form of *Helichrysum italicum* yields the essential oil *Immortelle*, used in aromatherapy for bacterial and fungal infections, lethargy, and depression.

linear silver leaves have a strong curry scent •

small, linear, silver leaf with mild curry scent •

up to 50cm (20in)

H. ITALICUM VAR. NANA ▷
The Dwarf Curry Plant grows to 25cm (10in).

woolly stem •

HELICHRYSUM ITALICUM

△ **H. ITALICUM (SUBSP. SEROTINUM)** (syn. *H. angustifolium*)

Habitat Sunny, sheltered positions; S.W. Europe	Parts used ※ ∅

Family BORAGINACEAE	Species *Heliotropium arborescens*	Local name Cherry Pie

HELIOTROPE

Heliotrope is a much-branched shrub, with a curved inflorescence of purple or white flowers, and small, elliptic fruit with four nutlets.
• USES A flower powder is used to scent soaps and talcum powder, and an oil is extracted for perfumes. The fresh plant was taken by the Incas of Peru to reduce fevers. A homeopathic tincture treats the hoarseness of "clergyman's sore throat".
• REMARK The name, from the Greek *helios* (sun) and *trope* (to turn), is from an old belief that the flowers turn with the sun as it crosses the sky.

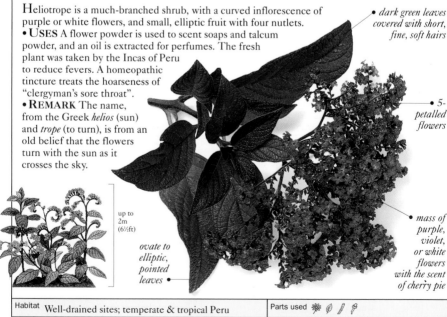

• dark green leaves covered with short, fine, soft hairs

• 5-petalled flowers

up to 2m (6½ft)

ovate to elliptic, pointed leaves •

• mass of purple, violet, or white flowers with the scent of cherry pie

Habitat Well-drained sites; temperate & tropical Peru	Parts used ※ ∅ ∥ ⸙

Family MALVACEAE	Species *Hibiscus sabdariffa*	Local name Lemonade Bush

ROSELLE

This annual shrub has yellow-petalled flowers which drop off leaving protective sepals; these swell into a succulent "fruit".
• USES The "fruit" give a burgundy colour and acid flavour to jellies, sauces, wines, and herb teas. The young leaves are cooked, the fermented juice of young "fruit" is added to rum, and the ripe "fruit" is made into jam. The "fruit" is astringent and is used to dress wounds and treat coughs. The dried petals treat fevers and tapeworm. The inner stem bark yields a strong, jute-like fibre.
• REMARK The flowers of Choublac (*Hibiscus rosa-sinensis*) yield a red food colouring, a tea, and a shoe black. Chinese women used the petal juice to blacken eyebrows. In South East Asia the bark, root, leaf, and flowers have medicinal uses.

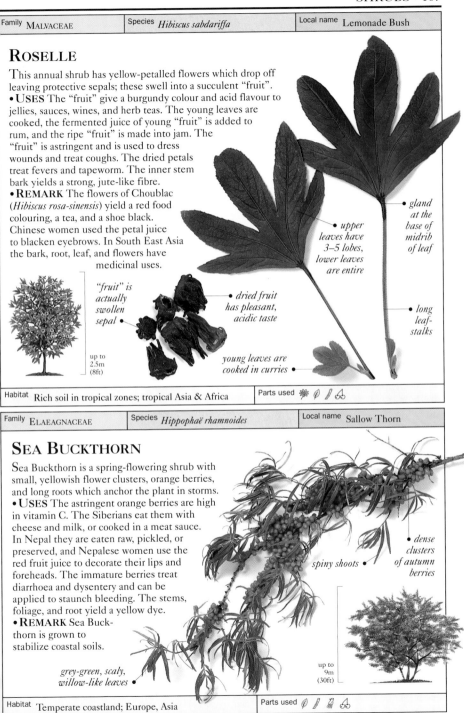

gland at the base of midrib of leaf

upper leaves have 3–5 lobes, lower leaves are entire

long leaf-stalks

"fruit" is actually swollen sepal

dried fruit has pleasant, acidic taste

young leaves are cooked in curries

up to 2.5m (8ft)

Habitat Rich soil in tropical zones; tropical Asia & Africa	Parts used ❋ 🌸 / 🌿

Family ELAEAGNACEAE	Species *Hippophaë rhamnoides*	Local name Sallow Thorn

SEA BUCKTHORN

Sea Buckthorn is a spring-flowering shrub with small, yellowish flower clusters, orange berries, and long roots which anchor the plant in storms.
• USES The astringent orange berries are high in vitamin C. The Siberians eat them with cheese and milk, or cooked in a meat sauce. In Nepal they are eaten raw, pickled, or preserved, and Nepalese women use the red fruit juice to decorate their lips and foreheads. The immature berries treat diarrhoea and dysentery and can be applied to staunch bleeding. The stems, foliage, and root yield a yellow dye.
• REMARK Sea Buck-thorn is grown to stabilize coastal soils.

dense clusters of autumn berries

spiny shoots

grey-green, scaly, willow-like leaves

up to 9m (30ft)

Habitat Temperate coastland; Europe, Asia	Parts used 🌸 / 🌿

Family LABIATAE	Species *Hyssopus officinalis*	Local name Issopo Celestino

HYSSOP

Hyssop is a semi-evergreen shrub or subshrub with aromatic leaves and spikes of blue, two-lipped, late-summer flowers.
• USES The sharp-flavoured leaf is added to liqueurs, adds bite to sweet and savoury dishes, and aids the digestion of fatty meat. Once used for purifying temples and cleansing lepers, the leaves contain an antiseptic, anti-viral oil. A mould that produces penicillin grows on the leaves. An infusion is taken as a sedative expectorant for flu, bronchitis, and catarrh. A leaf poultice treats bruises and wounds. The antiseptic, anti-viral, but hazardous essential oil is used in perfumes and to treat cold sores, disperse bruises, and heal scars. Hyssop is added to pot-pourri and laundry rinses.
• REMARK Hyssop is used in companion planting to distract cabbage butterflies and planted near vines to increase their yield. It should be avoided when pregnant and by those with high blood pressure.

up to
1.5m
(5ft)

HYSSOPUS OFFICINALIS

• *flower clusters borne in whorls in leaf-axils*

• *pungent-flavoured leaves*

WHITE FORM ▽

leaves and flowering tops yield essential oil •

flowers are enjoyed by bees and butterflies •

• *pink flowers*

• *branching stems turn woody at base in second year*

• *rich blue, 2-lipped flowers*

◁ **BLUE FORM**

◁ **PINK FORM**

◁ **PURPLE FORM**

• *narrow, pointed, aromatic leaves*

stems are green in first year •

leaves in opposite pairs •

pungent-flavoured leaves •

blue and purple flowers •

peppery stem useful for barbeque skewers •

HYSSOPUS OFFICINALIS 'NETHERFIELD' ▷
A new form with green and gold leaves and white flowers.

dense growth •

◁ **HYSSOPUS OFFICINALIS SUBSP. ARISTATUS**
Rock Hyssop is a compact plant and a useful hedging herb.

Habitat Well-drained, sunny sites; S. Europe	Parts used ❋ ∅ ℘

Family AQUIFOLIACEAE	Species *Ilex vomitoria*	Local name Yaupon / Emetic Holly

BLACK DRINK PLANT

This evergreen shrub has white flowers and scarlet fruit.
• USES The narcotic leaves are used ceremonially by native
Americans. They are brewed for a stimulant emetic called
Black Drink, taken by warriors for purification before war
councils. The berries also cause vomiting and have been
used as emergency treatment for poisoning. The leaves of
several *Ilex* species yield caffeine drinks used locally as tea.
Ilex guayusa is the source of *guayusa*, an Amazon stimulant tea.
I. paraguariensis gives *Yerba Maté*, popular in South America, and a
tonic, laxative, diuretic, and muscle relaxant which reduces
appetite and is said to increase intellectual vigour.
• REMARK English Holly
(*I. aquifolium*) does not yield
a stimulant tea. Infused
leaves treat colds and coughs.

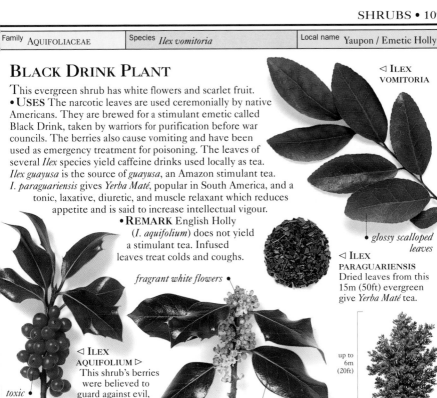

◁ ILEX
VOMITORIA

*glossy scalloped
leaves*

◁ ILEX
PARAGUARIENSIS
Dried leaves from this
15m (50ft) evergreen
give *Yerba Maté* tea.

fragrant white flowers •

◁ ILEX
AQUIFOLIUM ▷
This shrub's berries
were believed to
guard against evil,
becoming part of
Christmas
festivities.

toxic •
berries

up to
6m
(20ft)

• *leaves usually spined
but may be spine-free*

ILEX VOMITORIA

Habitat Moist, well-drained soils; S.E. USA, Mexico	Parts used 🍃 ⚘

Family LEGUMINOSAE	Species *Indigofera tinctoria*	Local name Nil-awari

INDIGO

This deciduous subshrub has pinnate leaves
and racemes of purplish summer flowers.
• USES Fermented stems and leaves are the
source of a rich blue dye, valued for 4,000
years. In India the leaves are used to deepen
the blackness of hair. In China the roots and
leaves treat depression, swollen
glands, and heat rash. The
leaves show anti-cancer activity.
• REMARK *Indigofera arrecta* and
I. sumatrana have the highest dye
content and have become the main
commercially grown crops.

• *pairs of
oval,
pointed
leaflets*

up to
2m
(6½ft)

*leaves and stems produce
famous blue dye* •

Habitat Tropics, subtropics; S.E. Asia	Parts used 🍃 ⚘ 🌿

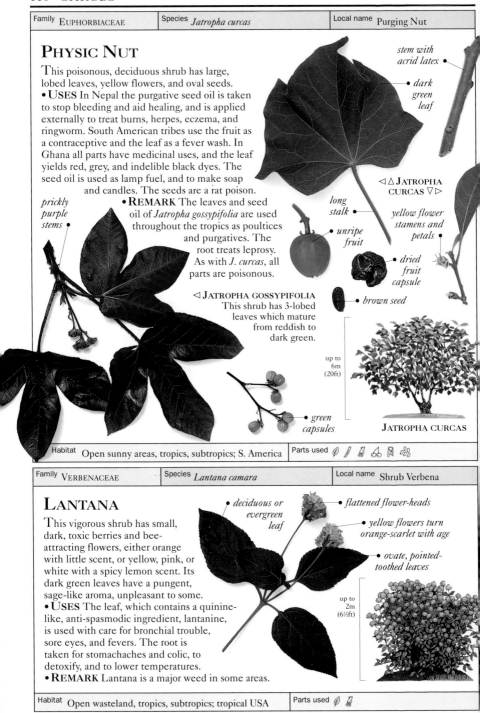

Family EUPHORBIACEAE	Species *Jatropha curcas*	Local name Purging Nut

PHYSIC NUT

This poisonous, deciduous shrub has large, lobed leaves, yellow flowers, and oval seeds.
• **USES** In Nepal the purgative seed oil is taken to stop bleeding and aid healing, and is applied externally to treat burns, herpes, eczema, and ringworm. South American tribes use the fruit as a contraceptive and the leaf as a fever wash. In Ghana all parts have medicinal uses, and the leaf yields red, grey, and indelible black dyes. The seed oil is used as lamp fuel, and to make soap and candles. The seeds are a rat poison.
• **REMARK** The leaves and seed oil of *Jatropha gossypifolia* are used throughout the tropics as poultices and purgatives. The root treats leprosy. As with *J. curcas*, all parts are poisonous.

stem with acrid latex

dark green leaf

◁ △ **JATROPHA CURCAS** ▽ ▷

yellow flower stamens and petals

long stalk

unripe fruit

dried fruit capsule

brown seed

prickly purple stems

◁ **JATROPHA GOSSYPIFOLIA**
This shrub has 3-lobed leaves which mature from reddish to dark green.

up to 6m (20ft)

green capsules

JATROPHA CURCAS

Habitat Open sunny areas, tropics, subtropics; S. America	Parts used

Family VERBENACEAE	Species *Lantana camara*	Local name Shrub Verbena

LANTANA

This vigorous shrub has small, dark, toxic berries and bee-attracting flowers, either orange with little scent, or yellow, pink, or white with a spicy lemon scent. Its dark green leaves have a pungent, sage-like aroma, unpleasant to some.
• **USES** The leaf, which contains a quinine-like, anti-spasmodic ingredient, lantanine, is used with care for bronchial trouble, sore eyes, and fevers. The root is taken for stomachaches and colic, to detoxify, and to lower temperatures.
• **REMARK** Lantana is a major weed in some areas.

deciduous or evergreen leaf

flattened flower-heads

yellow flowers turn orange-scarlet with age

ovate, pointed-toothed leaves

up to 2m (6½ft)

Habitat Open wasteland, tropics, subtropics; tropical USA	Parts used

Family LYTHRACEAE	Species *Lawsonia inerma*	Local name Mignonette Tree

HENNA

Henna is an open shrub with heavily scented, small cream flowers and blue-black fruit.
• USES Henna leaves yield the famous red dye used as body paint, and to stain hair, nails, cloth, and sometimes the manes of white Arab horses. The cooling, astringent leaves soothe fevers, headaches, stings, aching joints, and skin irritations. The leaves are also deodorizers, carried under the arm by Nubians, and recommended in Apina's medieval herbals to treat "evil-smelling feet". The bark, leaves, and fruit are used in folk medicine. The flowers' scented oil, *Mehndi*, is an Indian and African perfume, and is used in Arab religious festivals.
• REMARK The flower scent was known as "camphire" in the Bible, and was the source of Cleopatra's famous seductive perfume, *cyprinum*, used to soak the sails of her barge before her first meeting with Antony.

• *panicle of small, powerfully scented, cream flowers*

• *fruit capsule contains thick, triangular seeds*

• *leaves in opposite pairs*

• *narrow, obovate to oblong, pointed leaves*

up to 6m (20ft)

• *leaves yield the henna dye*

Habitat Well-drained soil, sun; N. Africa, S.W. Asia	Parts used ✳ 🌰 📗 ⚖ 🏺 ⚗ 🥄

Family LAURACEAE	Species *Lindera benzoin*	Local name Benjamin Bush

SPICE BUSH

This deciduous, aromatic shrub releases a spicy fragrance from bruised branches, and has clusters of pale, yellow-green flowers on bare spring branches, with olive-sized, red autumn fruit.
• USES Dried ground fruit are used as a substitute for Allspice, while fresh leaves and bark can be made into an aromatic tea, popular during the American War of Independence. The bark and twigs are given for coughs, colds, and dysentery, and to reduce fevers. The plant yields three scented oils: a spicy-camphor type from the fruit, a lavender-like oil from the leaves, and a wintergreen-scented oil from the bark and twigs.
• REMARK The Chinese species *Lindera strychnifolia* has aromatic leaves and sausage-like roots, used medicinally. The leaves are used externally, and the roots decocted; both reduce the pain, inflammation, and congestion from gastric problems, headaches, strokes, rheumatic legs and back, hernias, and menstrual problems.

obovate leaves •

▷ LINDERA BENZOIN

• *dried, sliced roots*

up to 4m (13ft)

LINDERA BENZOIN

△ LINDERA STRYCHNIFOLIA
This 10m (33ft) evergreen has rusty-haired branches, yellowish flowers, and black berries.

• *bark and twigs yield a wintergreen-scented oil*

Habitat Rich woodland; E. North America	Parts used 🌰 ✒ ⚖ 🏺 ⚗

Family LABIATAE	Species *Lavandula* species	Local name Various

LAVENDER

There are 28 species of these aromatic, evergreen, shrubby perennials, all with small, linear leaves and spikes of fragrant, usually purple or blue, two-lipped flowers.

• USES Aromatic oil glands cover all aerial parts of the plants but are most concentrated in the flowers. The flowers flavour jams, vinegar, sweets, cream, and Provençal stews, and are crystallized for decoration. Dried flowers add long-lasting fragrance to sachets and pot-pourri. Flower water is a useful skin toner to speed cell renewal and is an antiseptic for acne. Flower tea treats anxiety, headaches, flatulence, nausea, dizziness, and halitosis. Flower sprigs, particularly those of Spike Lavender (*Lavandula latifolia*), are a fly repellent. The essential oil is a highly valued perfume and healer. It is antiseptic, mildly sedative, and painkilling. It is applied to insect bites, and treats burns, sore throats, and headaches. It is added to baths as a relaxant. It treats rheumatic aches, insomnia, depression, high blood pressure, lymphatic congestion, poor digestion, and menstrual problems.

• REMARK The best quality essential oil comes from *L. stoechas* and *L. angustifolia*.

LAVANDULA
ANGUSTIFOLIA ▷
English Lavender may
grow to 75cm (30in) tall.

• *soft pink flowers*

• *silver-grey leaves*

• *spikes of purplish blue, scented flowers in summer*

△ LAVANDULA
ANGUSTIFOLIA
'LODDEN PINK'
This plant grows
to 45cm (17½in).

△ LAVANDULA
ANGUSTIFOLIA
'HIDCOTE'
A slow-growing
cultivar that may
reach 40cm (16in).

rich, purple-blue flowers •

long flower-spikes •

purple flowers •

• *narrow, grey-green, fragrant leaves*

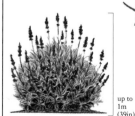

LAVANDULA
ANGUSTIFOLIA

up to
1m
(39in)

LAVANDULA △
ANGUSTIFOLIA
'VERA'
The leaves of Dutch
Lavender are more
silver and compact
than *L. angustifolia*.

LAVANDULA △
ANGUSTIFOLIA
'FOLGATE'
This 45cm (18in)
compact Lavender
has narrow, grey-
green leaves.

LAVANDULA △
ANGUSTIFOLIA
'TWICKEL PURPLE'
A bushy and compact
plant with green
leaves, sometimes
flushed purple.

Habitat Sunny sites, warm temperate regions; Mediterranean	Parts used ✳ ⊘ ∥ ⸜

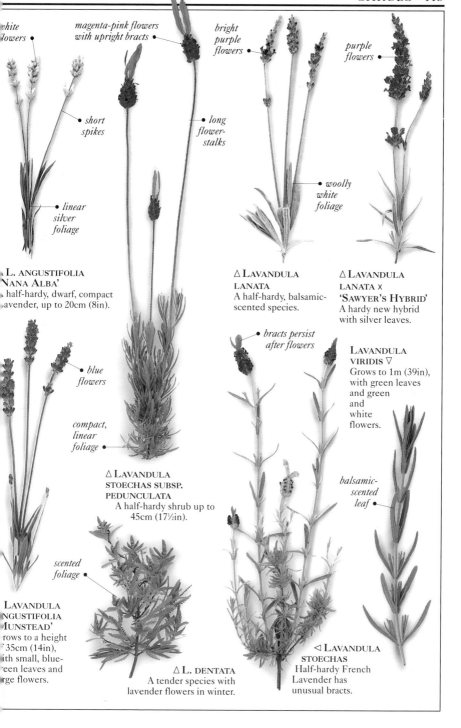

white flowers •

magenta-pink flowers with upright bracts •

bright purple flowers •

purple flowers •

• short spikes

• long flower-stalks

• woolly white foliage

• linear silver foliage

L. ANGUSTIFOLIA NANA ALBA'
A half-hardy, dwarf, compact lavender, up to 20cm (8in).

△ **LAVANDULA LANATA**
A half-hardy, balsamic-scented species.

△ **LAVANDULA LANATA x 'SAWYER'S HYBRID'**
A hardy new hybrid with silver leaves.

• blue flowers

• bracts persist after flowers

LAVANDULA VIRIDIS ▽
Grows to 1m (39in), with green leaves and green and white flowers.

compact, linear foliage •

△ **LAVANDULA STOECHAS SUBSP. PEDUNCULATA**
A half-hardy shrub up to 45cm (17½in).

balsamic-scented leaf •

scented foliage •

LAVANDULA ANGUSTIFOLIA 'HUNSTEAD'
Grows to a height of 35cm (14in), with small, blue-green leaves and large flowers.

△ **L. DENTATA**
A tender species with lavender flowers in winter.

◁ **LAVANDULA STOECHAS**
Half-hardy French Lavender has unusual bracts.

Family SOLANACEAE	Species *Lycium chinense*	Local name Matrimony Vine

WOLFBERRY

This is a deciduous, summer-flowering shrub with bright green leaves on arching stems, purple flowers, and long-lasting, vermilion to scarlet berries that appear in autumn and early winter.
• USES The berries, root bark, and, occasionally, leaves are used in Chinese medicine to lift the spirits and tone the liver, kidneys, and blood. Wolfberry is used to treat pneumonia in children, diabetes, tuberculosis, and dimmed vision as a result of malnutrition. It is taken with other herbs to slow the ageing process by improving muscle growth and preventing premature grey hair, facial skin roughness, and pigmentation.
• REMARK Wolfberries are often included in Chinese medicinal meals, in a recipe for tonic soup, *congee* (rice porridge), and a spirit drink.

ripening orange-red fruit

dried scarlet wolfberries are a Chinese tonic, Ji Zi

alternate leaves

long, narrow leaves, slightly wider below the middle

up to 4m (13ft)

flowers with pointed, light purple, sometimes yellow, petals

Habitat Temperate zones; E. Asia	Parts used

Family BERBERIDACEAE	Species *Mahonia aquifolium*	Local name Mountain Grape

OREGON GRAPE

The evergreen *Mahonia aquifolium* (syn. *Berberis aquifolium*) has grey-brown bark, dark green leaves that turn purple-red in autumn, fragrant flowers, and mauve-black berries.
• USES The root and underground suckers are used by herbalists for their blood-cleansing properties to treat skin disorders, such as eczema, acne, psoriasis, and cold sores. They act as a digestive and liver tonic, and are given to improve the appetite, suppress nausea, and reduce rheumatic inflammation. The root yields a yellow dye. Avoid during pregnancy.
• REMARK *M. japonica* leaves have shown anti-cancer activity in tests.

spiny-toothed leaves

up to 2m (6½ft)

underground suckers are used to cleanse blood

tight clusters of golden flowers

smooth bark

Habitat Open temperate areas; N.W. America, W. Canada	Parts used

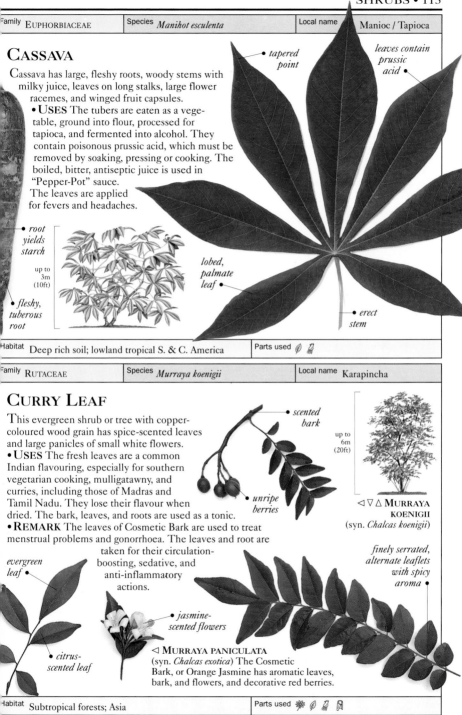

| Family EUPHORBIACEAE | Species *Manihot esculenta* | Local name | Manioc / Tapioca |

CASSAVA

Cassava has large, fleshy roots, woody stems with milky juice, leaves on long stalks, large flower racemes, and winged fruit capsules.
- **USES** The tubers are eaten as a vegetable, ground into flour, processed for tapioca, and fermented into alcohol. They contain poisonous prussic acid, which must be removed by soaking, pressing or cooking. The boiled, bitter, antiseptic juice is used in "Pepper-Pot" sauce.
The leaves are applied for fevers and headaches.

• *tapered point*

leaves contain prussic acid •

• *root yields starch*

up to 3m (10ft)

• *fleshy, tuberous root*

lobed, palmate leaf •

• *erect stem*

| Habitat Deep rich soil; lowland tropical S. & C. America | Parts used |

| Family RUTACEAE | Species *Murraya koenigii* | Local name Karapincha |

CURRY LEAF

This evergreen shrub or tree with copper-coloured wood grain has spice-scented leaves and large panicles of small white flowers.
- **USES** The fresh leaves are a common Indian flavouring, especially for southern vegetarian cooking, mulligatawny, and curries, including those of Madras and Tamil Nadu. They lose their flavour when dried. The bark, leaves, and roots are used as a tonic.
- **REMARK** The leaves of Cosmetic Bark are used to treat menstrual problems and gonorrhoea. The leaves and root are taken for their circulation-boosting, sedative, and anti-inflammatory actions.

• *scented bark*

up to 6m (20ft)

• *unripe berries*

◁ ▽ △ **MURRAYA KOENIGII**
(syn. *Chalcas koenigii*)

finely serrated, alternate leaflets with spicy aroma •

evergreen leaf •

• *jasmine-scented flowers*

• *citrus-scented leaf*

◁ **MURRAYA PANICULATA**
(syn. *Chalcas exotica*) The Cosmetic Bark, or Orange Jasmine has aromatic leaves, bark, and flowers, and decorative red berries.

| Habitat Subtropical forests; Asia | Parts used |

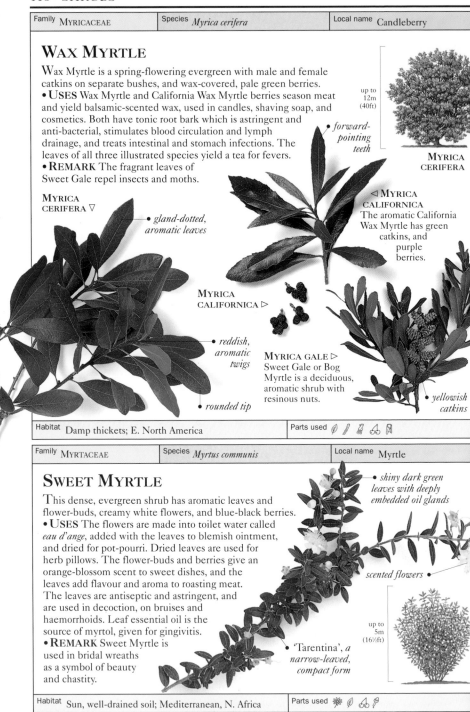

Family MYRICACEAE	Species *Myrica cerifera*	Local name Candleberry

WAX MYRTLE

Wax Myrtle is a spring-flowering evergreen with male and female catkins on separate bushes, and wax-covered, pale green berries.
• **USES** Wax Myrtle and California Wax Myrtle berries season meat and yield balsamic-scented wax, used in candles, shaving soap, and cosmetics. Both have tonic root bark which is astringent and anti-bacterial, stimulates blood circulation and lymph drainage, and treats intestinal and stomach infections. The leaves of all three illustrated species yield a tea for fevers.
• **REMARK** The fragrant leaves of Sweet Gale repel insects and moths.

up to
12m
(40ft)

• *forward-pointing teeth*

MYRICA CERIFERA

MYRICA CERIFERA ▽

• *gland-dotted, aromatic leaves*

◁ **MYRICA CALIFORNICA**
The aromatic California Wax Myrtle has green catkins, and purple berries.

MYRICA CALIFORNICA ▷

• *reddish, aromatic twigs*

MYRICA GALE ▷
Sweet Gale or Bog Myrtle is a deciduous, aromatic shrub with resinous nuts.

• *yellowish catkins*

• *rounded tip*

Habitat Damp thickets; E. North America	Parts used ✐ ⬭ ⚘ △ 🍃

Family MYRTACEAE	Species *Myrtus communis*	Local name Myrtle

SWEET MYRTLE

This dense, evergreen shrub has aromatic leaves and flower-buds, creamy white flowers, and blue-black berries.
• **USES** The flowers are made into toilet water called *eau d'ange*, added with the leaves to blemish ointment, and dried for pot-pourri. Dried leaves are used for herb pillows. The flower-buds and berries give an orange-blossom scent to sweet dishes, and the leaves add flavour and aroma to roasting meat. The leaves are antiseptic and astringent, and are used in decoction, on bruises and haemorrhoids. Leaf essential oil is the source of myrtol, given for gingivitis.
• **REMARK** Sweet Myrtle is used in bridal wreaths as a symbol of beauty and chastity.

• *shiny dark green leaves with deeply embedded oil glands*

scented flowers •

up to
5m
(16½ft)

• *'Tarentina', a narrow-leaved, compact form*

Habitat Sun, well-drained soil; Mediterranean, N. Africa	Parts used ✻ ✐ ⚘ 🍃

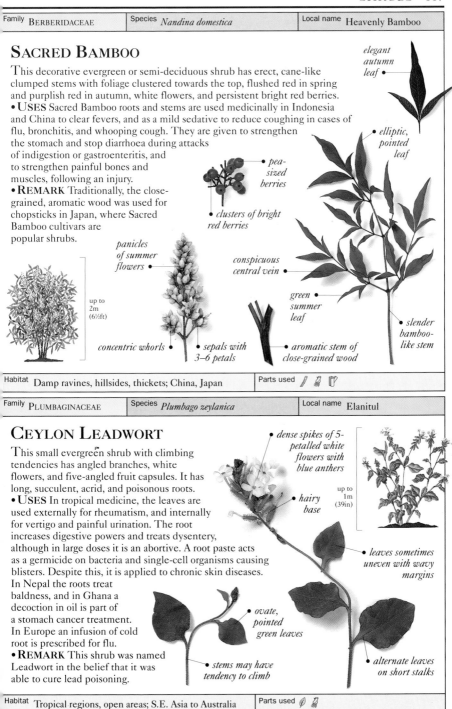

Family BERBERIDACEAE	Species *Nandina domestica*	Local name Heavenly Bamboo

SACRED BAMBOO

This decorative evergreen or semi-deciduous shrub has erect, cane-like clumped stems with foliage clustered towards the top, flushed red in spring and purplish red in autumn, white flowers, and persistent bright red berries.
• USES Sacred Bamboo roots and stems are used medicinally in Indonesia and China to clear fevers, and as a mild sedative to reduce coughing in cases of flu, bronchitis, and whooping cough. They are given to strengthen the stomach and stop diarrhoea during attacks of indigestion or gastroenteritis, and to strengthen painful bones and muscles, following an injury.
• REMARK Traditionally, the close-grained, aromatic wood was used for chopsticks in Japan, where Sacred Bamboo cultivars are popular shrubs.

elegant autumn leaf

elliptic, pointed leaf

pea-sized berries

clusters of bright red berries

panicles of summer flowers

conspicuous central vein

green summer leaf

up to 2m (6½ft)

concentric whorls

sepals with 3–6 petals

aromatic stem of close-grained wood

slender bamboo-like stem

Habitat Damp ravines, hillsides, thickets; China, Japan	Parts used

Family PLUMBAGINACEAE	Species *Plumbago zeylanica*	Local name Elanitul

CEYLON LEADWORT

This small evergreen shrub with climbing tendencies has angled branches, white flowers, and five-angled fruit capsules. It has long, succulent, acrid, and poisonous roots.
• USES In tropical medicine, the leaves are used externally for rheumatism, and internally for vertigo and painful urination. The root increases digestive powers and treats dysentery, although in large doses it is an abortive. A root paste acts as a germicide on bacteria and single-cell organisms causing blisters. Despite this, it is applied to chronic skin diseases. In Nepal the roots treat baldness, and in Ghana a decoction in oil is part of a stomach cancer treatment. In Europe an infusion of cold root is prescribed for flu.
• REMARK This shrub was named Leadwort in the belief that it was able to cure lead poisoning.

dense spikes of 5-petalled white flowers with blue anthers

hairy base

up to 1m (39in)

leaves sometimes uneven with wavy margins

ovate, pointed green leaves

stems may have tendency to climb

alternate leaves on short stalks

Habitat Tropical regions, open areas; S.E. Asia to Australia	Parts used

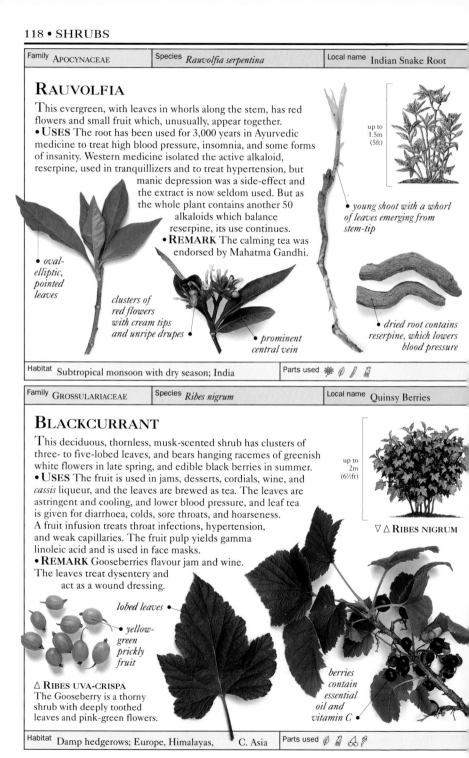

Family APOCYNACEAE	Species *Rauvolfia serpentina*	Local name Indian Snake Root

RAUVOLFIA

This evergreen, with leaves in whorls along the stem, has red flowers and small fruit which, unusually, appear together.
• **USES** The root has been used for 3,000 years in Ayurvedic medicine to treat high blood pressure, insomnia, and some forms of insanity. Western medicine isolated the active alkaloid, reserpine, used in tranquillizers and to treat hypertension, but manic depression was a side-effect and the extract is now seldom used. But as the whole plant contains another 50 alkaloids which balance reserpine, its use continues.
• **REMARK** The calming tea was endorsed by Mahatma Gandhi.

up to 1.5m (5ft)

• young shoot with a whorl of leaves emerging from stem-tip

• oval-elliptic, pointed leaves

clusters of red flowers with cream tips and unripe drupes •

• prominent central vein

• dried root contains reserpine, which lowers blood pressure

Habitat Subtropical monsoon with dry season; India	Parts used ✱ 🌿 🍃 🪵

Family GROSSULARIACEAE	Species *Ribes nigrum*	Local name Quinsy Berries

BLACKCURRANT

This deciduous, thornless, musk-scented shrub has clusters of three- to five-lobed leaves, and bears hanging racemes of greenish white flowers in late spring, and edible black berries in summer.
• **USES** The fruit is used in jams, desserts, cordials, wine, and *cassis* liqueur, and the leaves are brewed as tea. The leaves are astringent and cooling, and lower blood pressure, and leaf tea is given for diarrhoea, colds, sore throats, and hoarseness. A fruit infusion treats throat infections, hypertension, and weak capillaries. The fruit pulp yields gamma linoleic acid and is used in face masks.
• **REMARK** Gooseberries flavour jam and wine. The leaves treat dysentery and act as a wound dressing.

up to 2m (6½ft)

▽ △ **RIBES NIGRUM**

lobed leaves •

• yellow-green prickly fruit

△ **RIBES UVA-CRISPA**
The Gooseberry is a thorny shrub with deeply toothed leaves and pink-green flowers.

berries contain essential oil and vitamin C •

Habitat Damp hedgerows; Europe, Himalayas, C. Asia	Parts used 🌿 🪵 🍃🌸

Family ANACARDIACEAE	Species *Rhus typhina*	Local name Indian Lemonade

STAG HORN SUMACH

The narrow leaflets of this deciduous shrub turn vermilion in autumn, and dense flower panicles produce acid-flavoured berries.
• **USES** Romans in Britain used the flowers to colour rice. The sour berries feature extensively in Middle Eastern cooking, although Sicilian Sumach berries are preferred. Juice from the soaked seeds or dried berries are used in salad dressings, yoghurt, sauces, and marinades. The powdered berries flavour fish and meat.
• **REMARK**
Plants of the *Toxicodendron* genus such as Poison Ivy, also called Sumachs, are highly poisonous.

up to 10m (33ft)

cluster of brick-red berries used to make "Indian Lemonade" in the USA •

RHUS TYPHINA

• *dried berries soaked to make a drink*

◁ ▽ **RHUS GLABRA**
Smooth Sumach or the Vinegar Tree is a 3m (10ft) North American tree or shrub with sour culinary berries.

△ **RHUS TYPHINA**

RHUS COPALLINA ▽
The fruit of the deciduous Mountain Sumach flavour a drink, and the roots treat dysentery.

• *ripe red berries*

• *pinnate leaves*

unripe berries •

cracked, seedless berries •

• *brown seeds from centre of berries*

dried berries •

red autumn leaves used for tanning and dyeing •

◁ △ **RHUS CORIORIA**
The Sicilian Sumach produces the best flavoured berries, which are soaked for a fruity-sour, culinary juice.

• *red-tinged twigs*

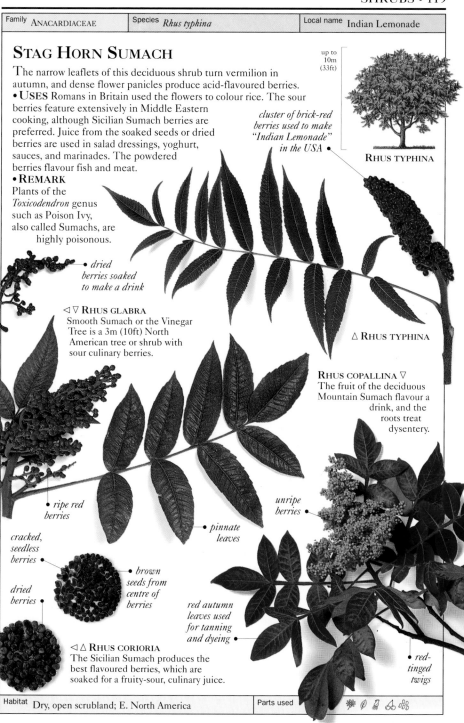

Habitat Dry, open scrubland; E. North America	Parts used

Family ROSACEAE	Species *Rosa* species	Local name Various

ROSE

Roses are mainly deciduous with prickly stems, compound leaves of up to nine leaflets, fragrant summer flowers, and autumn hips.
• USES The Rose has aromatic, cosmetic, medicinal, culinary, and craft uses. Fresh petals and rose-water flavour sweet and savoury dishes, and are crystallized for decoration. Rose-water revives tired skin and eyes. Dried petals retain their scent and are the basis of pot-pourri. Dog Rose (*Rosa canina*) is the major source of hips for jam, syrup, tea, and wine. Leaf tea has a mild laxative effect, and is applied as a wound poultice. Rose oil, from Damask, Bourbon, and other Rose species, is used in most good perfumes. Associated with pure love and femininity, it is valued by aromatherapists for its rejuvenating qualities.
• REMARK Oil from Rosa Mosqueta, the Amazon rose (*Rosa rubirinova*), is used in surgery to speed up healing and is noteworthy in the growing Amazon cosmetic industry.

up to 5.5m (18ft)

ROSA CANINA

white or pink flowers with 5 petals

solitary or grouped flowers with green sepals

scented flower

dried petals add scent and colour to pot-pourri and sachets

mid-green toothed leaflets

◁ △ ROSA CANINA ▽

vigorous arching or climbing stems with strong, downward-hooked prickles

fragrant petals feature in Turkish delight and Arab and Indian dishes

5–7 elliptic, serrated leaflets

vermilion hips

fragrant petals with bitter base removed are used for flavouring

smooth, pointed leaves

stiff bristles

◁ ROSA DAMASCENA 'TRIGINTIPETALA'
The Damask Rose is among the most fragrant and is grown for attar of roses.

dried hips

△▽ ROSA CANINA

when fresh, hips are rich in vitamins, C, B, E, and K

normally 5–7 serrated leaflets

deciduous grey-green leaves

flower-bud can be dried whole for pot-pourri and posies

hips contain irritant hairs which must be strained from hip tea

Habitat Temperate & subtropical zones; China	Parts used ❋ ∅ ⚭ ♀

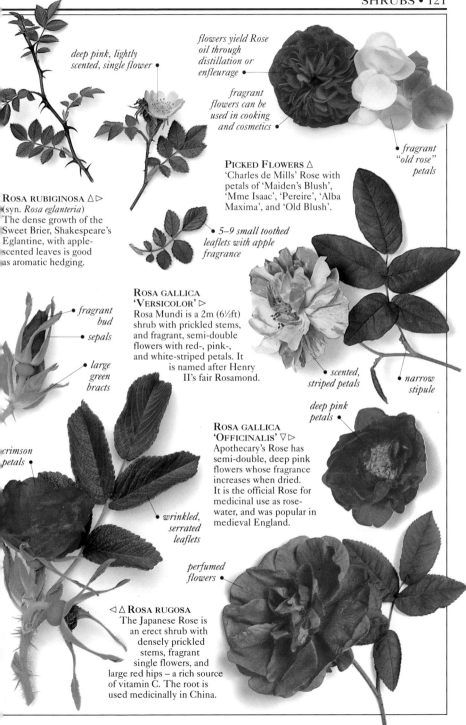

deep pink, lightly scented, single flower •

flowers yield Rose oil through distillation or enfleurage •

fragrant flowers can be used in cooking and cosmetics •

• fragrant "old rose" petals

ROSA RUBIGINOSA △▷
(syn. *Rosa eglanteria*)
The dense growth of the
Sweet Brier, Shakespeare's
Eglantine, with apple-
scented leaves is good
as aromatic hedging.

PICKED FLOWERS △
'Charles de Mills' Rose with
petals of 'Maiden's Blush',
'Mme Isaac', 'Pereire', 'Alba
Maxima', and 'Old Blush'.

• 5–9 small toothed
leaflets with apple
fragrance

• fragrant bud

• sepals

• large green bracts

ROSA GALLICA
'VERSICOLOR' ▷
Rosa Mundi is a 2m (6½ft)
shrub with prickled stems,
and fragrant, semi-double
flowers with red-, pink-,
and white-striped petals. It
is named after Henry
II's fair Rosamond.

• scented, striped petals

• narrow stipule

deep pink petals •

crimson petals •

ROSA GALLICA
'OFFICINALIS' ▽▷
Apothecary's Rose has
semi-double, deep pink
flowers whose fragrance
increases when dried.
It is the official Rose for
medicinal use as rose-
water, and was popular in
medieval England.

• wrinkled,
serrated
leaflets

perfumed flowers •

◁△ **ROSA RUGOSA**
The Japanese Rose is
an erect shrub with
densely prickled
stems, fragrant
single flowers, and
large red hips – a rich source
of vitamin C. The root is
used medicinally in China.

Family LABIATAE	Species *Rosmarinus officinalis*	Local name Sea Dew

ROSEMARY

Rosemary is a dense, evergreen, aromatic shrub with resinous, needle-like leaves, and soft, blue, pollen-rich spring flowers loved by bees.
• USES Rosemary leaves are an ancient savoury herb, especially popular in Italian dishes, and with shellfish, pork, and lamb. The antiseptic, anti-oxidant leaves help preserve food, aid digestion of fat, and are included in several slimming compounds. The flowers can be used fresh as a garnish or crystallized as decoration. Distilled flower water makes a soothing eye wash. The leaves are used in eau-de-Cologne, dark hair conditioning rinses, and dandruff shampoos.
Rosemary stimulates circulation and eases aching joints by increasing blood supply.
• REMARK The distilled oil of the flowering tops is invigorating, anti-bacterial, and anti-fungal. It stimulates the central nervous system and blood circulation, relieving muscular pain.

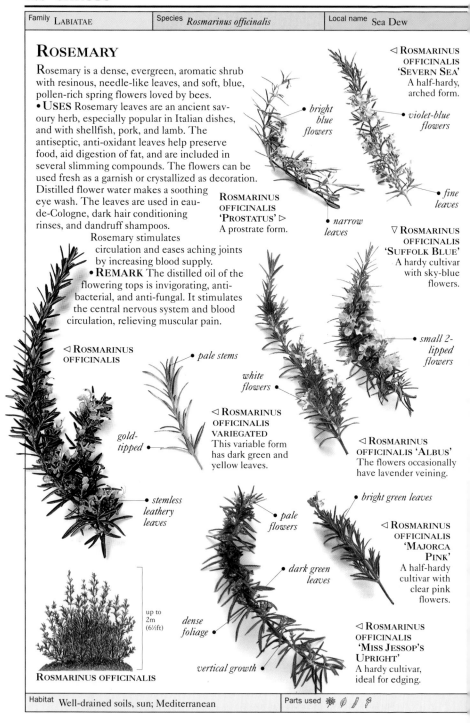

◁ ROSEMARINUS
OFFICINALIS
'SEVERN SEA'
A half-hardy,
arched form.

*violet-blue
flowers*

*bright
blue
flowers*

ROSMARINUS
OFFICINALIS
'PROSTATUS' ▷
A prostrate form.

*narrow
leaves*

*fine
leaves*

▽ ROSMARINUS
OFFICINALIS
'SUFFOLK BLUE'
A hardy cultivar
with sky-blue
flowers.

*small 2-
lipped
flowers*

◁ ROSMARINUS
OFFICINALIS

pale stems

*white
flowers*

*gold-
tipped*

◁ ROSMARINUS
OFFICINALIS
VARIEGATED
This variable form
has dark green and
yellow leaves.

◁ ROSMARINUS
OFFICINALIS 'ALBUS'
The flowers occasionally
have lavender veining.

bright green leaves

*stemless
leathery
leaves*

*pale
flowers*

*dark green
leaves*

◁ ROSMARINUS
OFFICINALIS
'MAJORCA
PINK'
A half-hardy
cultivar with
clear pink
flowers.

up to
2m
(6½ft)

*dense
foliage*

vertical growth

ROSMARINUS OFFICINALIS

◁ ROSMARINUS
OFFICINALIS
'MISS JESSOP'S
UPRIGHT'
A hardy cultivar,
ideal for edging.

Habitat Well-drained soils, sun; Mediterranean	Parts used 🌸 🖊 ⎗ 🍂

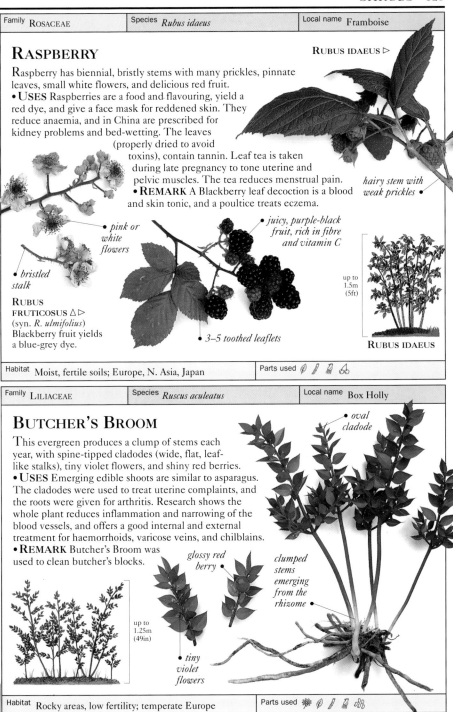

Family ROSACEAE	Species *Rubus idaeus*	Local name Framboise

RASPBERRY

RUBUS IDAEUS ▷

Raspberry has biennial, bristly stems with many prickles, pinnate leaves, small white flowers, and delicious red fruit.
• USES Raspberries are a food and flavouring, yield a red dye, and give a face mask for reddened skin. They reduce anaemia, and in China are prescribed for kidney problems and bed-wetting. The leaves (properly dried to avoid toxins), contain tannin. Leaf tea is taken during late pregnancy to tone uterine and pelvic muscles. The tea reduces menstrual pain.
• REMARK A Blackberry leaf decoction is a blood and skin tonic, and a poultice treats eczema.

hairy stem with weak prickles •

• *pink or white flowers*

• *juicy, purple-black fruit, rich in fibre and vitamin C*

• *bristled stalk*

RUBUS FRUTICOSUS △▷
(syn. *R. ulmifolius*)
Blackberry fruit yields a blue-grey dye.

• *3–5 toothed leaflets*

up to 1.5m (5ft)

RUBUS IDAEUS

Habitat Moist, fertile soils; Europe, N. Asia, Japan	Parts used

Family LILIACEAE	Species *Ruscus aculeatus*	Local name Box Holly

BUTCHER'S BROOM

• *oval cladode*

This evergreen produces a clump of stems each year, with spine-tipped cladodes (wide, flat, leaf-like stalks), tiny violet flowers, and shiny red berries.
• USES Emerging edible shoots are similar to asparagus. The cladodes were used to treat uterine complaints, and the roots were given for arthritis. Research shows the whole plant reduces inflammation and narrowing of the blood vessels, and offers a good internal and external treatment for haemorrhoids, varicose veins, and chilblains.
• REMARK Butcher's Broom was used to clean butcher's blocks.

glossy red berry •

clumped stems emerging from the rhizome •

up to 1.25m (49in)

• *tiny violet flowers*

Habitat Rocky areas, low fertility; temperate Europe	Parts used

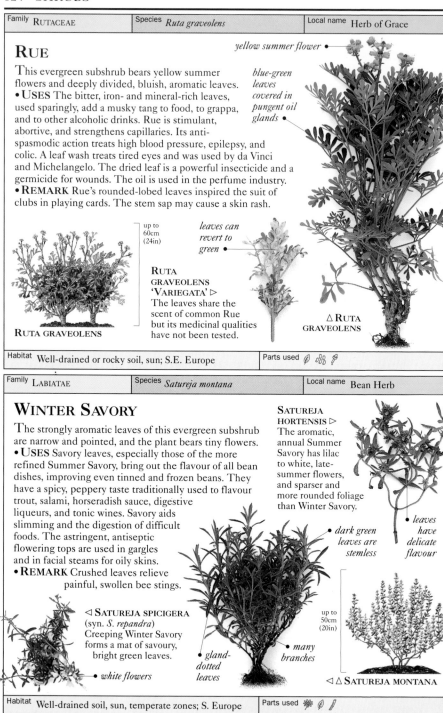

Family RUTACEAE	Species *Ruta graveolens*	Local name Herb of Grace

RUE

yellow summer flower •

This evergreen subshrub bears yellow summer flowers and deeply divided, bluish, aromatic leaves.
• USES The bitter, iron- and mineral-rich leaves, used sparingly, add a musky tang to food, to grappa, and to other alcoholic drinks. Rue is stimulant, abortive, and strengthens capillaries. Its anti-spasmodic action treats high blood pressure, epilepsy, and colic. A leaf wash treats tired eyes and was used by da Vinci and Michelangelo. The dried leaf is a powerful insecticide and a germicide for wounds. The oil is used in the perfume industry.
• REMARK Rue's rounded-lobed leaves inspired the suit of clubs in playing cards. The stem sap may cause a skin rash.

blue-green leaves covered in pungent oil glands •

up to 60cm (24in)

leaves can revert to green •

RUTA GRAVEOLENS 'VARIEGATA' ▷
The leaves share the scent of common Rue but its medicinal qualities have not been tested.

RUTA GRAVEOLENS

△ RUTA GRAVEOLENS

Habitat Well-drained or rocky soil, sun; S.E. Europe	Parts used

Family LABIATAE	Species *Satureja montana*	Local name Bean Herb

WINTER SAVORY

The strongly aromatic leaves of this evergreen subshrub are narrow and pointed, and the plant bears tiny flowers.
• USES Savory leaves, especially those of the more refined Summer Savory, bring out the flavour of all bean dishes, improving even tinned and frozen beans. They have a spicy, peppery taste traditionally used to flavour trout, salami, horseradish sauce, digestive liqueurs, and tonic wines. Savory aids slimming and the digestion of difficult foods. The astringent, antiseptic flowering tops are used in gargles and in facial steams for oily skins.
• REMARK Crushed leaves relieve painful, swollen bee stings.

SATUREJA HORTENSIS ▷
The aromatic, annual Summer Savory has lilac to white, late-summer flowers, and sparser and more rounded foliage than Winter Savory.

• leaves have delicate flavour

• dark green leaves are stemless

◁ SATUREJA SPICIGERA
(syn. *S. repandra*)
Creeping Winter Savory forms a mat of savoury, bright green leaves.

up to 50cm (20in)

• many branches

• gland-dotted leaves

• white flowers

◁ △ SATUREJA MONTANA

Habitat Well-drained soil, sun, temperate zones; S. Europe	Parts used

Family COMPOSITAE	Species *Santolina chamaecyparissus*	Local name Cotton Lavender

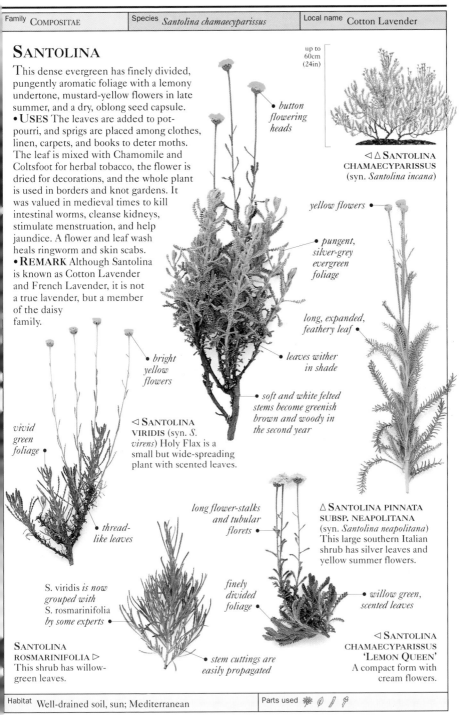

SANTOLINA

This dense evergreen has finely divided, pungently aromatic foliage with a lemony undertone, mustard-yellow flowers in late summer, and a dry, oblong seed capsule.
• USES The leaves are added to potpourri, and sprigs are placed among clothes, linen, carpets, and books to deter moths. The leaf is mixed with Chamomile and Coltsfoot for herbal tobacco, the flower is dried for decorations, and the whole plant is used in borders and knot gardens. It was valued in medieval times to kill intestinal worms, cleanse kidneys, stimulate menstruation, and help jaundice. A flower and leaf wash heals ringworm and skin scabs.
• REMARK Although Santolina is known as Cotton Lavender and French Lavender, it is not a true lavender, but a member of the daisy family.

up to 60cm (24in)

• *button flowering heads*

◁ △ SANTOLINA CHAMAECYPARISSUS (syn. *Santolina incana*)

yellow flowers •

• *pungent, silver-grey evergreen foliage*

• *long, expanded, feathery leaf*

• *leaves wither in shade*

• *soft and white felted stems become greenish brown and woody in the second year*

• *bright yellow flowers*

vivid green foliage •

◁ SANTOLINA VIRIDIS (syn. *S. virens*) Holy Flax is a small but wide-spreading plant with scented leaves.

long flower-stalks and tubular florets •

△ SANTOLINA PINNATA SUBSP. NEAPOLITANA (syn. *Santolina neapolitana*) This large southern Italian shrub has silver leaves and yellow summer flowers.

• *thread-like leaves*

S. viridis *is now grouped with* S. rosmarinifolia *by some experts* •

finely divided foliage •

• *willow green, scented leaves*

SANTOLINA ROSMARINIFOLIA ▷ This shrub has willow-green leaves.

• *stem cuttings are easily propagated*

◁ SANTOLINA CHAMAECYPARISSUS 'LEMON QUEEN' A compact form with cream flowers.

Habitat Well-drained soil, sun; Mediterranean	Parts used ❀ ∅ ∥ ♀

Family LABIATAE	Species *Salvia elegans*	Local name House Plant Sage

PINEAPPLE SAGE

This half-hardy Sage has red-edged, oval leaves and red stems with racemes of scarlet winter flowers.
• **USES** The pineapple-scented leaf enhances poultry, pork, and cheeses. Young leaves are fried in batter and served with cream. They scent pot-pourri and can be burned to produce a deo-dorizing smoke to counter household smells. Sage leaves do the same.
• **REMARK** *Salvia lavandulifolia* is used as an astringent cleanser. *S. hispanica* seeds yield a tonic drink and an oil used in artists' paints.

◁ **SALVIA ELEGANS**
(syn. *Salvia rutilans*)

up to 90cm (35in)

blue-green to grey leaves

scented leaf

◁ **SALVIA LAVANDULIFOLIA**
Narrow Leaf Sage has pointed, balsamic-scented leaves and violet-blue flowers.

SALVIA ELEGANS

Habitat Fertile, well-drained soil, sun; Mexico, Guatemala	Parts used

Family LABIATAE	Species *Salvia miltiorrhiza*	Local name Hung Ken

RED-ROOTED SAGE

This medicinal perennial has unusual, lobed green leaves, the middle lobe being the largest. It has long leaf-stalks, and spikes of purple-blue flowers in summer. The fresh roots are scarlet and rounded.
• **USES** In Chinese medicine a decoction of the roots treats irregular menstruation, uterine bleeding, and abdominal pain caused by stagnant blood. It invigorates the blood in cases of hepatitis or liver ulcers, helps to heal bruises, and treats inflamed breasts, bones, or kidneys. It is taken for nervous exhaustion and insomnia.

dried flower bracts

up to 60cm (24in)

serrated edge

dried root

3–5 lobed leaves

Habitat Sunny hillsides, stream edges; China	Parts used

Family LABIATAE	Species *Salvia sclarea*	Local name Clear Eye

CLARY SAGE

Hardy biennial Clary Sage has tall inflorescences with persistent, coloured bracts and large pungent leaves.
• **USES** Distilled flower- and leaf-water soothes tired eyes, while a soaked seed mucilage dislodges foreign bodies. The leaf essential oil is used for flavouring, perfume, and cosmetics. In aromatherapy it is a powerful relaxant for stress, fatigue, digestive and menstrual problems, and asthma.
• **REMARK** If applied when consuming alcohol it can cause nausea or nightmares.

purple and white flowers

up to 1m (39in)

bracts range from rose to lilac, mauve, and peach

pointed, ovate leaf

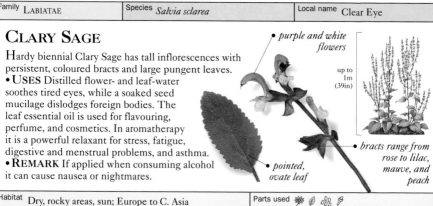

Habitat Dry, rocky areas, sun; Europe to C. Asia	Parts used

Family LABIATAE	Species *Salvia officinalis*	Local name Garden Sage

SAGE

Sage is an aromatic evergreen with grey-green, textured leaves, and mauve-blue flowers in summer.

• USES Sage leaf has a strong taste which increases when dried. Used sparingly to flavour and aid the digestion of fatty meats, it is popular in poultry stuffing and combines well with strongly flavoured foods. The flowers are tossed in salads and brewed for a light, balsamic tea, while the leaf tea is an antiseptic nerve and blood tonic. Sage contains hormone precursors that help irregular menstruation and menopause symptoms.

• REMARK Avoid large doses during pregnancy.

up to
80cm
(32in)

◁ △ SALVIA OFFICINALIS

• *flowers are most common in mauve-blue, but may be white or pink*

oval, pointed aromatic leaves •

SALVIA OFFICINALIS 'ICTERINA' ▷
Gold Variegated Sage has mottled green and gold leaves with a mild flavour.

• *purple leaf*

• *finely serrated edge*

SALVIA OFFICINALIS 'PROSTRATUS' ▽
Half-hardy Prostrate Sage has balsamic-scented leaves.

• *leaves yield powerful, toxic Sage Oil*

SALVIA OFFICINALIS 'PURPURASCENS' △
Purple Sage is a hardy cultivar. A leaf tea treats sore throats.

variegation on flower, bracts, and leaf •

leaf colour lasts all year •

square stems •

△ SALVIA OFFICINALIS

minutely bumpy surface •

SALVIA OFFICINALIS 'PURPURESCENS VARIEGATA' ▷
This variegated cultivar has white, peach, rose, and purple marks.

leaves can trigger epileptic fits •

• *wide, serrated leaves*

• *red stem*

leaf rub whitens teeth •

rose-coloured stems •

SALVIA OFFICINALIS 'TRICOLOR' ▷
This half-hardy cultivar has mild-flavoured green leaves with pink and white margins.

square-sectioned stem •

◁ SALVIA OFFICINALIS 'BROAD-LEAF'
This useful cultivar seldom flowers in cooler climates.

Habitat Dry, well-drained soil; Mediterranean, N. Africa	Parts used 🌸 🍃 🌱

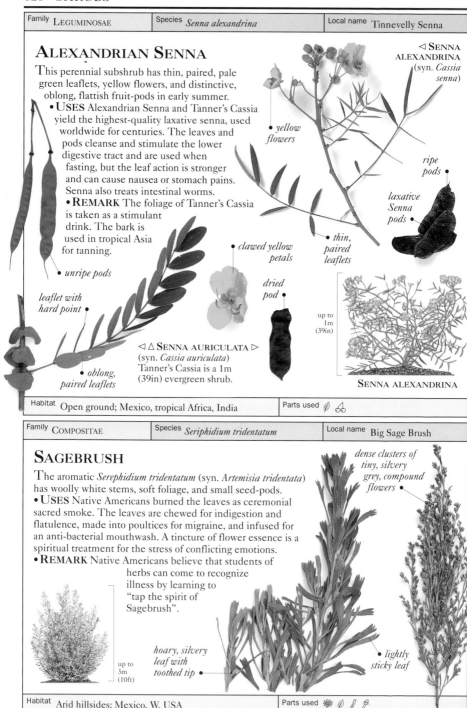

Family LEGUMINOSAE	Species *Senna alexandrina*	Local name Tinnevelly Senna

ALEXANDRIAN SENNA

This perennial subshrub has thin, paired, pale green leaflets, yellow flowers, and distinctive, oblong, flattish fruit-pods in early summer.

• **USES** Alexandrian Senna and Tanner's Cassia yield the highest-quality laxative senna, used worldwide for centuries. The leaves and pods cleanse and stimulate the lower digestive tract and are used when fasting, but the leaf action is stronger and can cause nausea or stomach pains. Senna also treats intestinal worms.

• **REMARK** The foliage of Tanner's Cassia is taken as a stimulant drink. The bark is used in tropical Asia for tanning.

◁ **SENNA ALEXANDRINA** (syn. *Cassia senna*)

yellow flowers

ripe pods

laxative Senna pods

thin, paired leaflets

clawed yellow petals

dried pod

unripe pods

leaflet with hard point

◁ △ **SENNA AURICULATA** ▷ (syn. *Cassia auriculata*) Tanner's Cassia is a 1m (39in) evergreen shrub.

oblong, paired leaflets

up to 1m (39in)

SENNA ALEXANDRINA

Habitat Open ground; Mexico, tropical Africa, India	Parts used 🌿 ✂

Family COMPOSITAE	Species *Seriphidium tridentatum*	Local name Big Sage Brush

SAGEBRUSH

The aromatic *Serephidium tridentatum* (syn. *Artemisia tridentata*) has woolly white stems, soft foliage, and small seed-pods.

• **USES** Native Americans burned the leaves as ceremonial sacred smoke. The leaves are chewed for indigestion and flatulence, made into poultices for migraine, and infused for an anti-bacterial mouthwash. A tincture of flower essence is a spiritual treatment for the stress of conflicting emotions.

• **REMARK** Native Americans believe that students of herbs can come to recognize illness by learning to "tap the spirit of Sagebrush".

dense clusters of tiny, silvery grey, compound flowers

up to 3m (10ft)

hoary, silvery leaf with toothed tip

lightly sticky leaf

Habitat Arid hillsides; Mexico, W. USA	Parts used 🌼 🌿 ⫰ 🥄

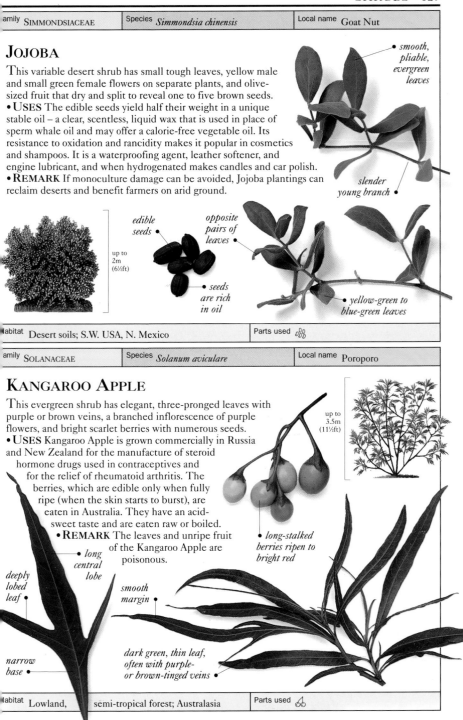

Family	SIMMONDSIACEAE	Species	*Simmondsia chinensis*	Local name	Goat Nut

JOJOBA

This variable desert shrub has small tough leaves, yellow male and small green female flowers on separate plants, and olive-sized fruit that dry and split to reveal one to five brown seeds.
• **USES** The edible seeds yield half their weight in a unique stable oil – a clear, scentless, liquid wax that is used in place of sperm whale oil and may offer a calorie-free vegetable oil. Its resistance to oxidation and rancidity makes it popular in cosmetics and shampoos. It is a waterproofing agent, leather softener, and engine lubricant, and when hydrogenated makes candles and car polish.
• **REMARK** If monoculture damage can be avoided, Jojoba plantings can reclaim deserts and benefit farmers on arid ground.

smooth, pliable, evergreen leaves

slender young branch

edible seeds

opposite pairs of leaves

up to 2m (6½ft)

seeds are rich in oil

yellow-green to blue-green leaves

Habitat	Desert soils; S.W. USA, N. Mexico	Parts used

Family	SOLANACEAE	Species	*Solanum aviculare*	Local name	Poroporo

KANGAROO APPLE

This evergreen shrub has elegant, three-pronged leaves with purple or brown veins, a branched inflorescence of purple flowers, and bright scarlet berries with numerous seeds.
• **USES** Kangaroo Apple is grown commercially in Russia and New Zealand for the manufacture of steroid hormone drugs used in contraceptives and for the relief of rheumatoid arthritis. The berries, which are edible only when fully ripe (when the skin starts to burst), are eaten in Australia. They have an acid-sweet taste and are eaten raw or boiled.
• **REMARK** The leaves and unripe fruit of the Kangaroo Apple are poisonous.

up to 3.5m (11½ft)

long central lobe

deeply lobed leaf

narrow base

smooth margin

long-stalked berries ripen to bright red

dark green, thin leaf, often with purple- or brown-tinged veins

Habitat	Lowland, semi-tropical forest; Australasia	Parts used

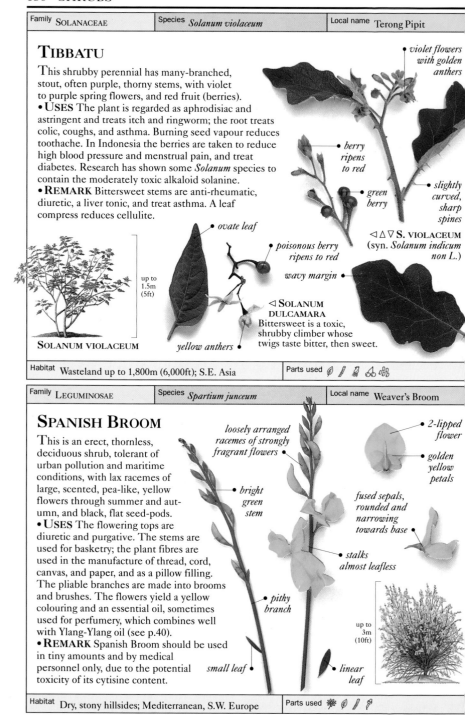

Family SOLANACEAE	Species *Solanum violaceum*	Local name Terong Pipit

TIBBATU

This shrubby perennial has many-branched, stout, often purple, thorny stems, with violet to purple spring flowers, and red fruit (berries).
• **USES** The plant is regarded as aphrodisiac and astringent and treats itch and ringworm; the root treats colic, coughs, and asthma. Burning seed vapour reduces toothache. In Indonesia the berries are taken to reduce high blood pressure and menstrual pain, and treat diabetes. Research has shown some *Solanum* species to contain the moderately toxic alkaloid solanine.
• **REMARK** Bittersweet stems are anti-rheumatic, diuretic, a liver tonic, and treat asthma. A leaf compress reduces cellulite.

violet flowers with golden anthers

berry ripens to red

green berry

slightly curved, sharp spines

△ △ ▽ **S. VIOLACEUM** (syn. *Solanum indicum non L.*)

ovate leaf

poisonous berry ripens to red

wavy margin

up to 1.5m (5ft)

SOLANUM VIOLACEUM

yellow anthers

◁ **SOLANUM DULCAMARA** Bittersweet is a toxic, shrubby climber whose twigs taste bitter, then sweet.

Habitat Wasteland up to 1,800m (6,000ft); S.E. Asia	Parts used

Family LEGUMINOSAE	Species *Spartium junceum*	Local name Weaver's Broom

SPANISH BROOM

This is an erect, thornless, deciduous shrub, tolerant of urban pollution and maritime conditions, with lax racemes of large, scented, pea-like, yellow flowers through summer and autumn, and black, flat seed-pods.
• **USES** The flowering tops are diuretic and purgative. The stems are used for basketry; the plant fibres are used in the manufacture of thread, cord, canvas, and paper, and as a pillow filling. The pliable branches are made into brooms and brushes. The flowers yield a yellow colouring and an essential oil, sometimes used for perfumery, which combines well with Ylang-Ylang oil (see p.40).
• **REMARK** Spanish Broom should be used in tiny amounts and by medical personnel only, due to the potential toxicity of its cytisine content.

loosely arranged racemes of strongly fragrant flowers

2-lipped flower

golden yellow petals

bright green stem

fused sepals, rounded and narrowing towards base

stalks almost leafless

pithy branch

up to 3m (10ft)

small leaf

linear leaf

Habitat Dry, stony hillsides; Mediterranean, S.W. Europe	Parts used

Family LOGANIACEAE	Species *Strychnos nux-vomica*	Local name Nux-vomica

STRYCHNINE

This shrub or tree has oval leaves and clusters
of greenish white flowers, followed by yellow,
tennis-ball fruit with greyish disc seeds.
• USES The bark, root, and seed coat contain
poisonous strychnine and brucine, once
used to stimulate nerves, but now
used only in homeopathy. In Nepal
the treated seeds are given as a
digestive tonic, and for rabies,
menstrual problems, and paralysis.
• REMARK In India the Clearing
Nut (*Strychnos potatorum*) is put in water jars,
causing any impurities in the water to sink to
the bottom. The
Amazon climber
S. toxifera, was part
of the curare arrow
poison and is now a life-
saving muscle relaxant
in surgical operations.

smooth shiny leaves in opposite pairs

bark treats cholera in India

up to 20m (65ft)

fine hairs give satin sheen •

ash-grey seed

leaves used as poultice

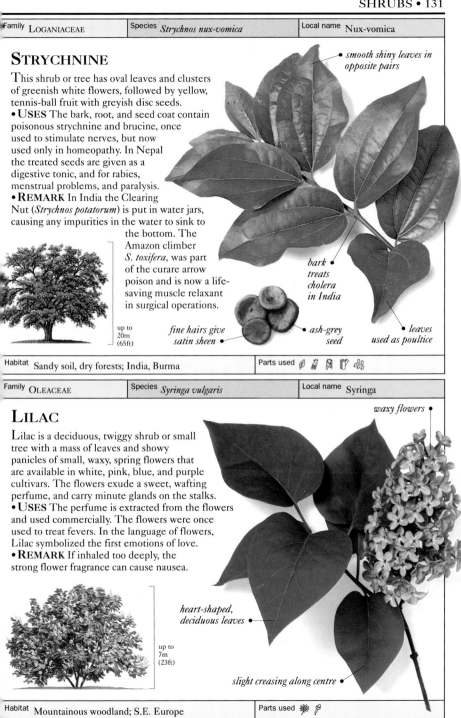

Habitat Sandy soil, dry forests; India, Burma	Parts used

Family OLEACEAE	Species *Syringa vulgaris*	Local name Syringa

LILAC

Lilac is a deciduous, twiggy shrub or small
tree with a mass of leaves and showy
panicles of small, waxy, spring flowers that
are available in white, pink, blue, and purple
cultivars. The flowers exude a sweet, wafting
perfume, and carry minute glands on the stalks.
• USES The perfume is extracted from the flowers
and used commercially. The flowers were once
used to treat fevers. In the language of flowers,
Lilac symbolized the first emotions of love.
• REMARK If inhaled too deeply, the
strong flower fragrance can cause nausea.

waxy flowers •

heart-shaped, deciduous leaves •

up to 7m (23ft)

slight creasing along centre •

Habitat Mountainous woodland; S.E. Europe	Parts used

Family LABIATAE	Species *Thymus serpyllum*	Local name Mother of Thyme

CREEPING WILD THYME

This mat-forming, creeping, aromatic shrub has oval leaves and pink or mauve flowering heads.
• USES Wild Thyme can be used as Common Thyme in flavouring. Both have medicinal uses, especially to reduce indigestion and flatulence, although Wild Thyme also has a sedative action. Thyme honey is a sweetener for expectorant herb teas and is used externally to heal sore skin. Antiseptic, expectorant, and calming, Wild Thyme tea treats hangovers, cough spasms, flu, and sore throats.
• REMARK *Thymus praecox* is almost identical to *T. serpyllum*, but with a purple calyx.

up to 10cm (4in)

• *mildly scented leaves*

◁ △ THYMUS SERPYLLUM

• *mat-forming, creeping roots*

cochineal flowers •

THYMUS SERPYLLUM 'COCCINEUS' ▷
This has small, faintly scented, dark green leaves and crimson flowers.

THYMUS X CITRIODORUS 'AUREUS' ▷
Golden Lemon Creeping Thyme has golden leaves.

• *lemon-scented leaves*

bright gold summer leaves •

◁ THYMUS SERPYLLUM 'AUREUS'
Golden Creeping Thyme has golden leaves that fade without strong sun, and rose-purple flowers.

wiry • *branches*

dense clusters •

◁ THYMUS DOERFLERI
This species has mauve flowers and narrow, grey, clustered leaves, closer than Woolly Thyme.

• *pinky brown stem*

T. PSEUDOLANUGINOSUS ▽
Woolly Thyme has hairy grey leaves and pale pink flowers.

• *pine-scented leaves*

THYMUS HERBA-BARONA ▷
The Caraway Thyme has heavily caraway-scented, dark green leaves on lax stems, which are used to flavour "barons" of beef.

THYMUS SERPYLLUM △ 'LEMON CURD'
This creeper has sweet-acid, lemon-scented, green leaves and pink flowers.

◁ THYMUS CAESPITITIUS (syn. *T. azoricus*)
This forms a hummock-like mat with tiny leaf clusters.

profuse flowers •

gold-splashed leaves •

• *rose flowers*

bright green leaf •

pink flowers •

THYMUS SERPYLLUM 'CITRIODORUS' ▷
This is a hardy creeper with lemon-scented leaves.

◁ THYMUS X CITRIODORUS 'DOONE VALLEY'
This sturdy creeper has strongly lemon-scented leaves.

△ THYMUS SERPYLLUM 'SNOWDRIFT'
This creeper is faintly scented.

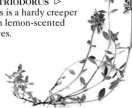

Habitat Light, well-drained, alkaline soil, full sun; N. Europe	Parts used ❀ 🌿 ✒ ✿

Family LABIATAE	Species *Thymus vulgaris*	Local name Garden Thyme

COMMON THYME

Thyme is a much-branching subshrub with woody stems; numerous small, pointed, mid-green, and strongly aromatic leaves; and lilac summer flowers.

• **USES** Culinary Thyme aids the digestion of fatty foods, and is part of *bouquet garni* and Benedictine liqueur. It is ideal for the long, slow cooking of stews and soups. Lemon Thyme (*Thymus* x *citriodorus*) is delicious with chicken and fresh fruit dishes. Thyme oil is distilled from the leaves and flowering tops and is stimulant and antiseptic. It is a nerve-tonic used externally to treat depression, colds, muscular pain, and respiratory problems. The oil is added to spot lotions, soaps, and mouthwashes.

• **REMARK** Research has confirmed it strengthens the immune system.

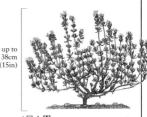

up to 38cm (15in)

◁ ▽ △ THYMUS VULGARIS

• leaf flavour blends with other herbs

small, 2-lipped, pale lilac flowers •

young plant leaves have best flavour •

• dense mat of greyish brown roots

◁ THYMUS X CITRIODORUS 'FRAGRANTISSIMUS'
This 38cm (15in) shrub has pale lilac flowers and sweet, fruity, blue-grey leaves.

THYMUS PULEGIOIDES ▽
Broad-leaf Thyme is a hardy, bushy shrub with mauve-pink flowers.

• leaves have robust flavour

leaves larger and rounder than Common Thyme •

bright green leaves •

▽ THYMUS X CITRIODORUS
This is a lemon-scented shrub with pale lilac flowers.

• antiseptic leaves are a natural preservative

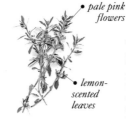

• leaves have subtle flavouring

• tiny pointed leaves

△ THYMUS NITIDUS
(syn. *Thymus richardii*)
This petite shrub has narrow bright green leaves and pale purple flowers.

• pale pink flowers

• lemon-scented leaves

△ THYMUS X CITRIODORUS 'SILVER QUEEN'
This variegated shrub has cream to silver leaves and rose-pink terminal leaf-buds in winter.

THYMUS VULGARIS 'SILVER POSIE' ▽
This shrub has silver variegated leaves with mild Common Thyme flavour.

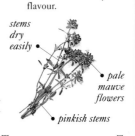

stems dry easily •

• pale mauve flowers

• pinkish stems

THYMUS ODORATISSIMUS ▽
(syn. *T. pallasianus*)
This herb has long, loose, lax branches of sweet, citrus-like leaves, and pink flowers with purple calyx.

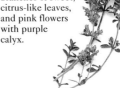

Habitat Light, well-drained soil, sun; W. Mediterranean	Parts used 🌿 ⬭ ⫽ 🗡

Family ERICACEAE	Species *Vaccinium oxycoccos*	Local name Small Cranberry

EUROPEAN CRANBERRY

This dwarf, prostrate evergreen has wiry stems, four-petalled, light purple flowers, green leaves tinged blue beneath, and dark red berries which remain on the plant throughout winter.
• USES Cranberries are eaten raw, jellied, and dried, ground with flour, and accompany poultry. The refreshing juice is drunk to treat cystitis.
• REMARK New research shows that Bilberry berries help with vein problems, increasing capillary strength and reducing permeability. They also replenish "retina purple", helping to correct visual fatigue. A leaf decoction lowers blood sugar levels. A leaf tea treats diarrhoea, vomiting, and nerves and is an antiseptic gargle for sore throats.

slim flexible stems

◁ VACCINIUM OXYCOCCUS

edible berry

ripe berries

VACCINIUM VITIS-IDAEA ▷
Cowberry is an evergreen with edible berries and leaves.

VACCINIUM MACROCARPON ▷
This cranberry is grown commercially in the USA.

serrated leaf

medicinal dried leaves

up to 30cm (12in)

VACCINIUM OXYCOCCUS

ripe berry

◁ VACCINIUM MYRTILLUS ▷
Bilberry is a deciduous shrub of Europe and N. Asia with greenish flowers and pleasantly acid berries.

Habitat Boggy heaths; N. Eurasia, North America	Parts used

Family APOCYNACEAE	Species *Vinca major*	Local name Sorcerer's Violet

GREATER PERIWINKLE

This spreading evergreen subshrub has glossy, oval leaves and purple-blue, tubular flowers from spring to summer.
• USES The leaves are tonic and astringent, and reduce internal and menstrual bleeding. They are given for ulcers and sore throats, and to reduce blood pressure. They also treat piles, nose-bleeds, and small wounds.
• REMARK Research has isolated an alkaloid, vincamine, which benefits cerebral blood flow. Lesser Periwinkle provides a medicinal wine and a homeopathic tincture.

up to 30cm (12in)

▽△ VINCA MAJOR

flower tube spreads into 5 flat lobes

flat lobes

◁ VINCA MINOR
Lesser Periwinkle is an evergreen with blue, pink, white, or wine-coloured flowers.

margin of minute hairs

pointed, oval leaf

flower is laxative

◁ VINCA MINOR 'PLENA'
This is a decorative, double-flowered form which provides ground cover.

prostrate rooting stems

Habitat Any soil, sun, shade; France, Italy, former Yugoslavia	Parts used

Family CAPRIFOLIACEAE	Species *Viburnum opulus*	Local name Guelder Rose

CRAMPBARK

This deciduous, thicket-forming
shrub has attractive, creamy flower-
heads, maple-like leaves that turn
burgundy in autumn, and red berries.
• USES The poisonous fresh berries are
edible when cooked and are used in a tart
jelly or a distilled spirit. The stem bark is
sedative and anti-spasmodic, reducing muscle
cramps and intestinal spasm. Native Americans
used stem bark to treat mumps. The berries yield a dye.
• REMARK *Viburnum prunifolium* bark is used similarly. The
leaf, stem, and bark of *V. edule* and *V.*
trilobum are given by the Alberta Cree
tribe for many illnesses, especially
high fever and pain relief.

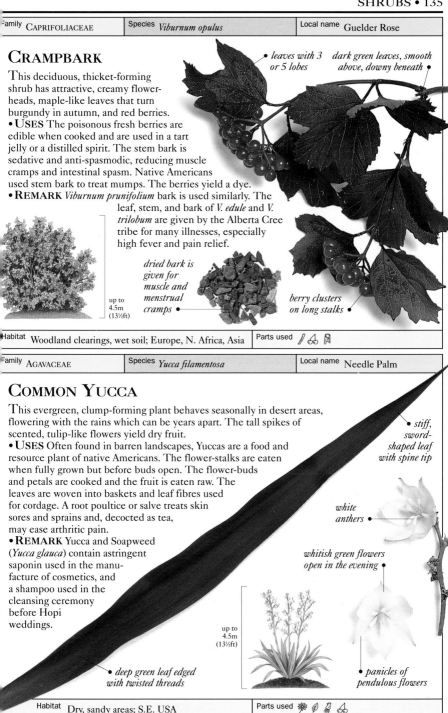

*leaves with 3
or 5 lobes*

*dark green leaves, smooth
above, downy beneath*

*dried bark is
given for
muscle and
menstrual
cramps* •

up to
4.5m
(13½ft)

*berry clusters
on long stalks* •

Habitat Woodland clearings, wet soil; Europe, N. Africa, Asia	Parts used

Family AGAVACEAE	Species *Yucca filamentosa*	Local name Needle Palm

COMMON YUCCA

This evergreen, clump-forming plant behaves seasonally in desert areas,
flowering with the rains which can be years apart. The tall spikes of
scented, tulip-like flowers yield dry fruit.
• USES Often found in barren landscapes, Yuccas are a food and
resource plant of native Americans. The flower-stalks are eaten
when fully grown but before buds open. The flower-buds
and petals are cooked and the fruit is eaten raw. The
leaves are woven into baskets and leaf fibres used
for cordage. A root poultice or salve treats skin
sores and sprains and, decocted as tea,
may ease arthritic pain.
• REMARK Yucca and Soapweed
(*Yucca glauca*) contain astringent
saponin used in the manu-
facture of cosmetics, and
a shampoo used in the
cleansing ceremony
before Hopi
weddings.

• *stiff,
sword-
shaped leaf
with spine tip*

*white
anthers* •

*whitish green flowers
open in the evening* •

up to
4.5m
(13½ft)

• *deep green leaf edged
with twisted threads*

• *panicles of
pendulous flowers*

Habitat Dry, sandy areas; S.E. USA	Parts used

HERBACEOUS PERENNIALS

Family COMPOSITAE	Species *Achillea millefolium*	Local name Milfoil

YARROW

Yarrow has a creeping rhizome; erect, downy stems; soft, pungent, finely divided leaves; and dense, flat, white or pink-tinged flower-heads from summer to autumn.
• **USES** The peppery leaf is finely chopped into salads and, with the flowers, used to flavour liqueurs. The flowering tops are a digestive and cleansing tonic, a diuretic, and reduce high blood pressure. Fresh leaves arrest bleeding and are applied as a poultice to wounds or placed on shaving cuts. Flowers treat eczema and catarrh from allergies. Flower essential oil treats colds, flu, and inflamed joints. Native Americans used a root decoction to strengthen muscles.
• **REMARK** Over-use can make the skin sensitive to sunlight and it should be taken in small doses. Avoid during pregnancy.

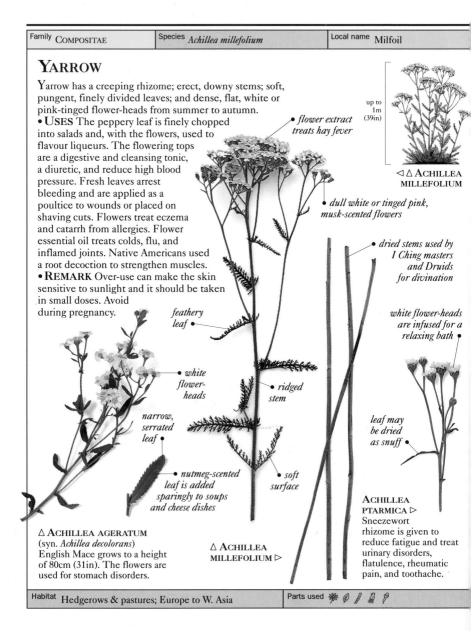

up to 1m (39in)

• *flower extract treats hay fever*

◁ △ **ACHILLEA MILLEFOLIUM**

• *dull white or tinged pink, musk-scented flowers*

• *dried stems used by I Ching masters and Druids for divination*

white flower-heads are infused for a relaxing bath •

feathery leaf •

• *white flower-heads*

• *ridged stem*

narrow, serrated leaf •

leaf may be dried as snuff •

• *nutmeg-scented leaf is added sparingly to soups and cheese dishes*

• *soft surface*

ACHILLEA PTARMICA ▷
Sneezewort rhizome is given to reduce fatigue and treat urinary disorders, flatulence, rheumatic pain, and toothache.

△ **ACHILLEA AGERATUM** (syn. *Achillea decolorans*) English Mace grows to a height of 80cm (31in). The flowers are used for stomach disorders.

△ **ACHILLEA MILLEFOLIUM** ▷

Habitat Hedgerows & pastures; Europe to W. Asia	Parts used ❋ ∅ ⫽ ⧨ ⚘

| Family RANUNCULACEAE | Species *Aconitum napellus* | Local name Aconite / Wolf's Bane |

MONKSHOOD

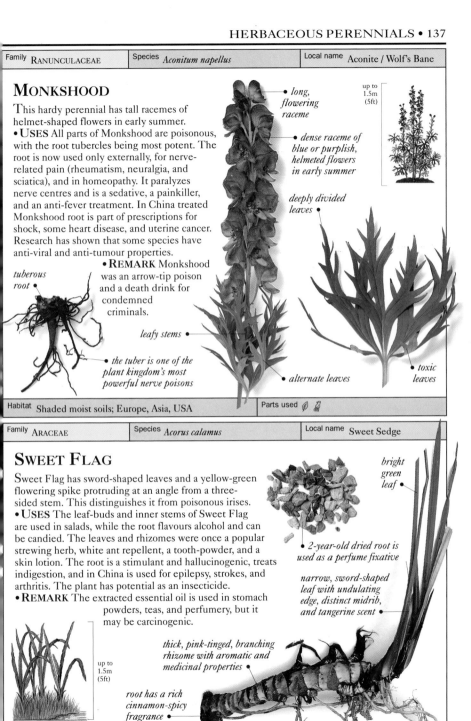

This hardy perennial has tall racemes of helmet-shaped flowers in early summer.
• **USES** All parts of Monkshood are poisonous, with the root tubercles being most potent. The root is now used only externally, for nerve-related pain (rheumatism, neuralgia, and sciatica), and in homeopathy. It paralyzes nerve centres and is a sedative, a painkiller, and an anti-fever treatment. In China treated Monkshood root is part of prescriptions for shock, some heart disease, and uterine cancer. Research has shown that some species have anti-viral and anti-tumour properties.
• **REMARK** Monkshood was an arrow-tip poison and a death drink for condemned criminals.

long, flowering raceme

dense raceme of blue or purplish, helmeted flowers in early summer

up to 1.5m (5ft)

deeply divided leaves

tuberous root

leafy stems

the tuber is one of the plant kingdom's most powerful nerve poisons

alternate leaves

toxic leaves

| Habitat Shaded moist soils; Europe, Asia, USA | Parts used |

| Family ARACEAE | Species *Acorus calamus* | Local name Sweet Sedge |

SWEET FLAG

Sweet Flag has sword-shaped leaves and a yellow-green flowering spike protruding at an angle from a three-sided stem. This distinguishes it from poisonous irises.
• **USES** The leaf-buds and inner stems of Sweet Flag are used in salads, while the root flavours alcohol and can be candied. The leaves and rhizomes were once a popular strewing herb, white ant repellent, a tooth-powder, and a skin lotion. The root is a stimulant and hallucinogenic, treats indigestion, and in China is used for epilepsy, strokes, and arthritis. The plant has potential as an insecticide.
• **REMARK** The extracted essential oil is used in stomach powders, teas, and perfumery, but it may be carcinogenic.

bright green leaf

2-year-old dried root is used as a perfume fixative

narrow, sword-shaped leaf with undulating edge, distinct midrib, and tangerine scent

up to 1.5m (5ft)

thick, pink-tinged, branching rhizome with aromatic and medicinal properties

root has a rich cinnamon-spicy fragrance

| Habitat Near fresh water; Asia, E. USA | Parts used |

Family RANUNCULACEAE	Species *Adonis vernalis*	Local name Spring Adonis

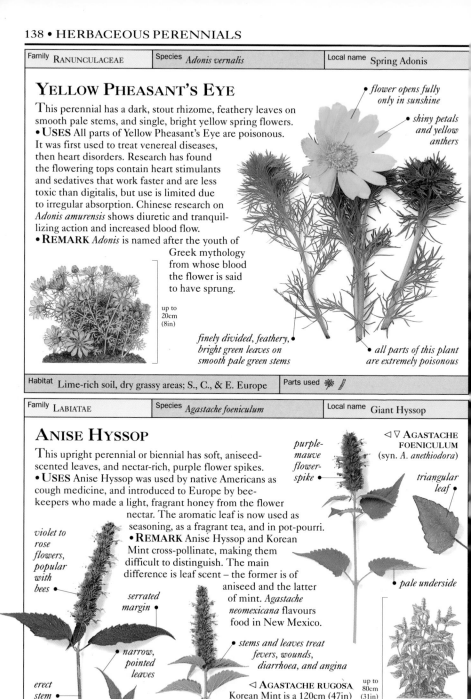

YELLOW PHEASANT'S EYE

This perennial has a dark, stout rhizome, feathery leaves on smooth pale stems, and single, bright yellow spring flowers.
• USES All parts of Yellow Pheasant's Eye are poisonous. It was first used to treat venereal diseases, then heart disorders. Research has found the flowering tops contain heart stimulants and sedatives that work faster and are less toxic than digitalis, but use is limited due to irregular absorption. Chinese research on *Adonis amurensis* shows diuretic and tranquillizing action and increased blood flow.
• REMARK *Adonis* is named after the youth of Greek mythology from whose blood the flower is said to have sprung.

flower opens fully only in sunshine

shiny petals and yellow anthers

up to 20cm (8in)

finely divided, feathery, bright green leaves on smooth pale green stems

all parts of this plant are extremely poisonous

Habitat Lime-rich soil, dry grassy areas; S., C., & E. Europe	Parts used ✳ ∥

Family LABIATAE	Species *Agastache foeniculum*	Local name Giant Hyssop

ANISE HYSSOP

This upright perennial or biennial has soft, aniseed-scented leaves, and nectar-rich, purple flower spikes.
• USES Anise Hyssop was used by native Americans as cough medicine, and introduced to Europe by bee-keepers who made a light, fragrant honey from the flower nectar. The aromatic leaf is now used as seasoning, as a fragrant tea, and in pot-pourri.
• REMARK Anise Hyssop and Korean Mint cross-pollinate, making them difficult to distinguish. The main difference is leaf scent – the former is of aniseed and the latter of mint. *Agastache neomexicana* flavours food in New Mexico.

purple-mauve flower-spike

◁▽ AGASTACHE FOENICULUM (syn. *A. anethiodora*)

triangular leaf

violet to rose flowers, popular with bees

pale underside

serrated margin

narrow, pointed leaves

stems and leaves treat fevers, wounds, diarrhoea, and angina

erect stem

◁ AGASTACHE RUGOSA Korean Mint is a 120cm (47in) scented perennial or biennial, used in Chinese medicine.

up to 80cm (31in)

AGASTACHE FOENICULUM

Habitat Moist woodland, high plains; North America	Parts used ✳ ∅ ∥

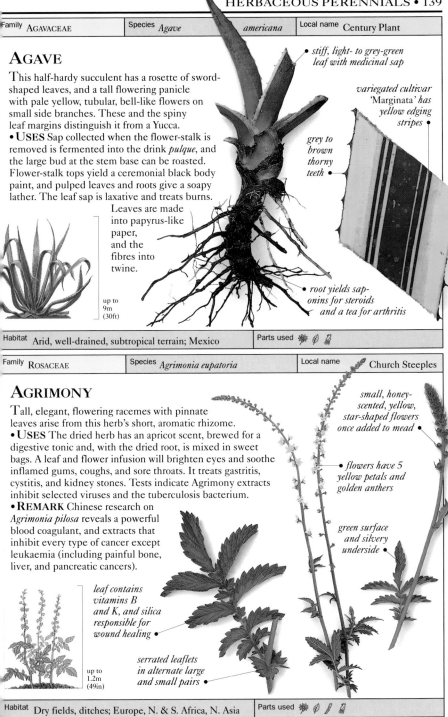

| Family AGAVACEAE | Species *Agave* | *americana* | Local name Century Plant |

AGAVE

This half-hardy succulent has a rosette of sword-shaped leaves, and a tall flowering panicle with pale yellow, tubular, bell-like flowers on small side branches. These and the spiny leaf margins distinguish it from a Yucca.
• USES Sap collected when the flower-stalk is removed is fermented into the drink *pulque*, and the large bud at the stem base can be roasted. Flower-stalk tops yield a ceremonial black body paint, and pulped leaves and roots give a soapy lather. The leaf sap is laxative and treats burns. Leaves are made into papyrus-like paper, and the fibres into twine.

stiff, light- to grey-green leaf with medicinal sap

variegated cultivar 'Marginata' has yellow edging stripes •

grey to brown thorny teeth •

• root yields sap-onins for steroids and a tea for arthritis

up to 9m (30ft)

| Habitat Arid, well-drained, subtropical terrain; Mexico | Parts used |

| Family ROSACEAE | Species *Agrimonia eupatoria* | Local name Church Steeples |

AGRIMONY

Tall, elegant, flowering racemes with pinnate leaves arise from this herb's short, aromatic rhizome.
• USES The dried herb has an apricot scent, brewed for a digestive tonic and, with the dried root, is mixed in sweet bags. A leaf and flower infusion will brighten eyes and soothe inflamed gums, coughs, and sore throats. It treats gastritis, cystitis, and kidney stones. Tests indicate Agrimony extracts inhibit selected viruses and the tuberculosis bacterium.
• REMARK Chinese research on *Agrimonia pilosa* reveals a powerful blood coagulant, and extracts that inhibit every type of cancer except leukaemia (including painful bone, liver, and pancreatic cancers).

small, honey-scented, yellow, star-shaped flowers once added to mead •

• flowers have 5 yellow petals and golden anthers

green surface and silvery underside •

leaf contains vitamins B and K, and silica responsible for wound healing •

serrated leaflets in alternate large and small pairs •

up to 1.2m (49in)

| Habitat Dry fields, ditches; Europe, N. & S. Africa, N. Asia | Parts used |

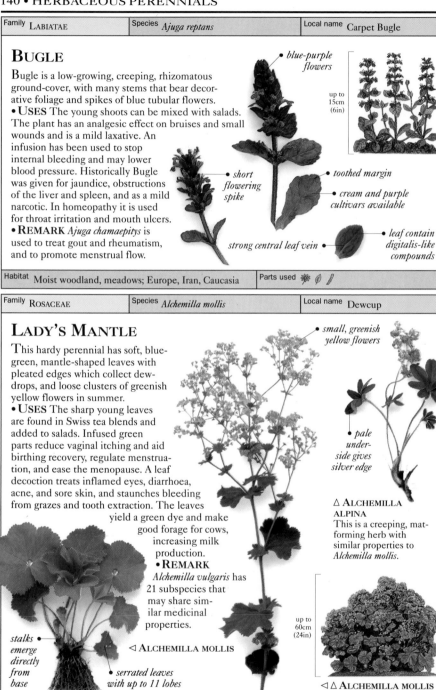

| Family LABIATAE | Species *Ajuga reptans* | Local name Carpet Bugle |

BUGLE

Bugle is a low-growing, creeping, rhizomatous ground-cover, with many stems that bear decorative foliage and spikes of blue tubular flowers.
• USES The young shoots can be mixed with salads. The plant has an analgesic effect on bruises and small wounds and is a mild laxative. An infusion has been used to stop internal bleeding and may lower blood pressure. Historically Bugle was given for jaundice, obstructions of the liver and spleen, and as a mild narcotic. In homeopathy it is used for throat irritation and mouth ulcers.
• REMARK *Ajuga chamaepitys* is used to treat gout and rheumatism, and to promote menstrual flow.

blue-purple flowers

up to 15cm (6in)

short flowering spike

toothed margin

cream and purple cultivars available

strong central leaf vein

leaf contain digitalis-like compounds

| Habitat Moist woodland, meadows; Europe, Iran, Caucasia | Parts used ✳ ◕ ⫽ |

| Family ROSACEAE | Species *Alchemilla mollis* | Local name Dewcup |

LADY'S MANTLE

This hardy perennial has soft, blue-green, mantle-shaped leaves with pleated edges which collect dew-drops, and loose clusters of greenish yellow flowers in summer.
• USES The sharp young leaves are found in Swiss tea blends and added to salads. Infused green parts reduce vaginal itching and aid birthing recovery, regulate menstruation, and ease the menopause. A leaf decoction treats inflamed eyes, diarrhoea, acne, and sore skin, and staunches bleeding from grazes and tooth extraction. The leaves yield a green dye and make good forage for cows, increasing milk production.
• REMARK *Alchemilla vulgaris* has 21 subspecies that may share similar medicinal properties.

small, greenish yellow flowers

pale underside gives silver edge

△ ALCHEMILLA ALPINA
This is a creeping, mat-forming herb with similar properties to *Alchemilla mollis*.

◁ ALCHEMILLA MOLLIS

up to 60cm (24in)

stalks emerge directly from base

serrated leaves with up to 11 lobes

◁ △ ALCHEMILLA MOLLIS

| Habitat Meadows in temperate climates; E. Europe | Parts used ◕ ⫽ |

Family LILIACEAE	Species *Aloe vera*	Local name Barbados Aloe

ALOE VERA

This evergreen, stemless perennial forms a dense rosette of leaves with irregular white marks, and a spike of yellow flowers.

• USES The plant has remarkable qualities. Two parts are used: the clear, gel-like central leaf pulp, and the yellow-green juice from the green part of the leaf. The gel is used in creams to soothe, heal, and moisturize the skin, and in shampoos for dry, itchy scalps. It cools the skin, protects it from airborne infections and fungi, and reduces scarring. It speeds cell regeneration, and so treats radiation burns, coral wounds, and dermatitis. It can be scraped from split leaves for first-aid treatment of small burns, cuts, chapped skin, sunburn, eczema, and Poison Ivy rash. Compounds in the leaf juice are added to sun creams for protection against UV rays, and have shown anti-cancer activity.

• REMARK *Aloe perryi* was famed for its rich, violet dye.

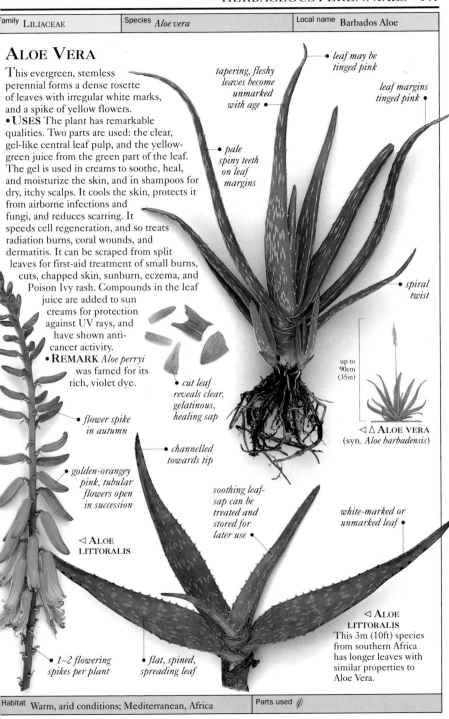

tapering, fleshy leaves become unmarked with age

leaf may be tinged pink

leaf margins tinged pink

pale spiny teeth on leaf margins

spiral twist

cut leaf reveals clear, gelatinous, healing sap

channelled towards tip

up to 90cm (35in)

◁△ ALOE VERA
(syn. *Aloe barbadensis*)

flower spike in autumn

golden-orangey pink, tubular flowers open in succession

◁ ALOE LITTORALIS

soothing leaf-sap can be treated and stored for later use

white-marked or unmarked leaf

◁ ALOE LITTORALIS
This 3m (10ft) species from southern Africa has longer leaves with similar properties to Aloe Vera.

1–2 flowering spikes per plant

flat, spined, spreading leaf

Habitat Warm, arid conditions; Mediterranean, Africa	Parts used 🖉

| Family LILIACEAE | Species *Allium sativum* | Local name Poor Man's Treacle |

GARLIC

Garlic has a clustered bulb made up of several bulblets (cloves) enclosed in a papery tunic. It has a single stem with long, thin leaves and an umbel of edible flowers, of which some are replaced by sterile bulbils.
• USES The cloves add flavour to savoury dishes, especially in hot countries where the plants develop the best flavour. Garlic purifies the blood, helps control acne, and reduces blood pressure, cholesterol, and clotting. Tests confirm antibiotic activity against samples of candida, cholera, staphylococcus, salmonella, dysentery, and typhus; and a mild anti-fungal action. Garlic clears catarrh, thus providing treatment for colds, bronchitis, pulmonary tuberculosis, and whooping cough. New tests suggest it has a role in treating lead poisoning, some carcinomas, and diabetes.
• REMARK The *Allium* species form one of the most popular and widely used flavouring groups. All *Alliums* contain iron and vitamins and are mildly antibiotic.

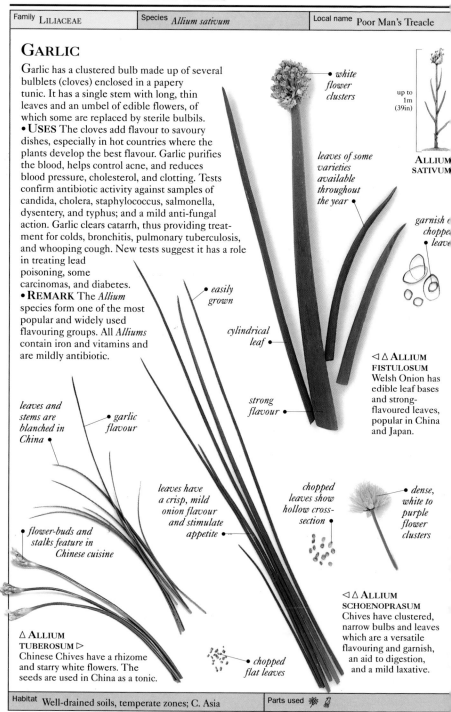

up to 1m (39in)

ALLIUM SATIVUM

• white flower clusters

leaves of some varieties available throughout the year •

garnish of chopped leaves •

⊲ △ ALLIUM FISTULOSUM
Welsh Onion has edible leaf bases and strong-flavoured leaves, popular in China and Japan.

• easily grown

cylindrical leaf •

strong flavour •

leaves and stems are blanched in China •

• garlic flavour

leaves have a crisp, mild onion flavour and stimulate appetite •

chopped leaves show hollow cross-section •

• dense, white to purple flower clusters

• flower-buds and stalks feature in Chinese cuisine

⊲ △ ALLIUM SCHOENOPRASUM
Chives have clustered, narrow bulbs and leaves which are a versatile flavouring and garnish, an aid to digestion, and a mild laxative.

△ ALLIUM TUBEROSUM ⊳
Chinese Chives have a rhizome and starry white flowers. The seeds are used in China as a tonic.

• chopped flat leaves

| Habitat Well-drained soils, temperate zones; C. Asia | Parts used |

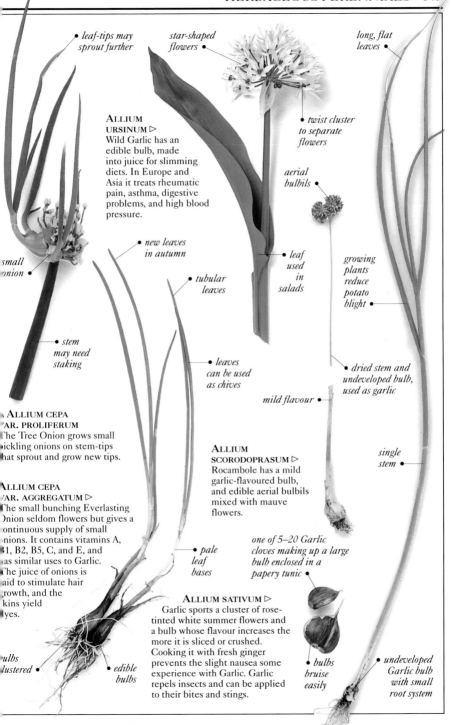

leaf-tips may sprout further •

star-shaped flowers •

long, flat leaves •

ALLIUM URSINUM ▷
Wild Garlic has an edible bulb, made into juice for slimming diets. In Europe and Asia it treats rheumatic pain, asthma, digestive problems, and high blood pressure.

• twist cluster to separate flowers

aerial bulbils •

small onion •

• new leaves in autumn

• leaf used in salads

growing plants reduce potato blight •

• tubular leaves

• stem may need staking

• leaves can be used as chives

mild flavour •

• dried stem and undeveloped bulb, used as garlic

ALLIUM CEPA VAR. PROLIFERUM
The Tree Onion grows small pickling onions on stem-tips that sprout and grow new tips.

ALLIUM SCORODOPRASUM ▷
Rocambole has a mild garlic-flavoured bulb, and edible aerial bulbils mixed with mauve flowers.

single stem •

ALLIUM CEPA VAR. AGGREGATUM ▷
The small bunching Everlasting Onion seldom flowers but gives a continuous supply of small onions. It contains vitamins A, B1, B2, B5, C, and E, and has similar uses to Garlic. The juice of onions is said to stimulate hair growth, and the skins yield dyes.

• pale leaf bases

one of 5–20 Garlic cloves making up a large bulb enclosed in a papery tunic •

ALLIUM SATIVUM ▷
Garlic sports a cluster of rose-tinted white summer flowers and a bulb whose flavour increases the more it is sliced or crushed. Cooking it with fresh ginger prevents the slight nausea some experience with Garlic. Garlic repels insects and can be applied to their bites and stings.

bulbs clustered •

• edible bulbs

• bulbs bruise easily

• undeveloped Garlic bulb with small root system

Family ZINGIBERACEAE	Species *Alpinia galanga*	Local name Siamese Ginger

GREATER GALANGAL

Galangal has dark green, sword-shaped leaves, white flowers with pink veins, round red seed-capsules, and an aromatic rhizome.
• USES The rhizome has a spicy, ginger-like flavour used in South East Asian soups and curries. The young shoots and flowers are eaten raw, and the flowers can be boiled or pickled. In Asia the fresh rhizome treats bronchitis, measles, gastritis, cholera, and scaly skin diseases, and is used in a snuff for catarrh. The seed is given for digestive problems. The rhizome yields an essential oil, *Essence d'Amali*, used in perfumery.
• REMARK Lesser Galangal (*Alpinia officinarum*) rhizome flavours tea, curries, pickles, and Russian *Nastoika* liqueur. It treats indigestion and ulcers.

ALPINIA OFFICINARUM ▽
(syn. *Languas officinarum*)

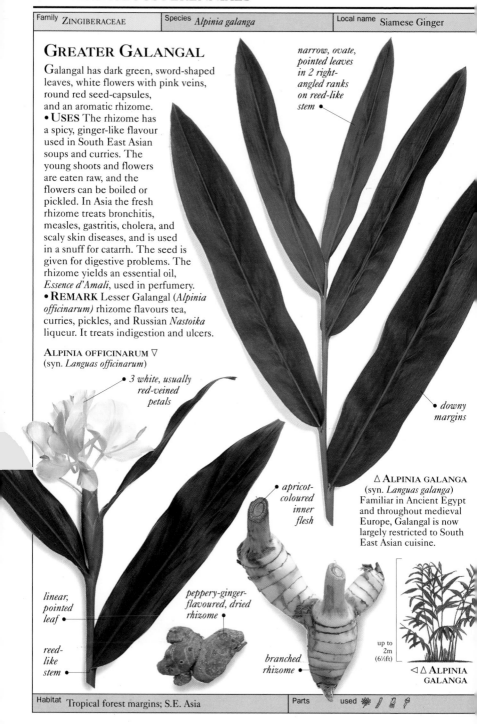

narrow, ovate, pointed leaves in 2 right-angled ranks on reed-like stem •

• *3 white, usually red-veined petals*

• *downy margins*

• *apricot-coloured inner flesh*

△ ALPINIA GALANGA
(syn. *Languas galanga*)
Familiar in Ancient Egypt and throughout medieval Europe, Galangal is now largely restricted to South East Asian cuisine.

linear, pointed leaf •

peppery-ginger-flavoured, dried rhizome •

reed-like stem •

branched rhizome •

up to 2m (6¼ft)

◁ △ ALPINIA GALANGA

Habitat Tropical forest margins; S.E. Asia	Parts used ❋ 〽 〽 ⬚

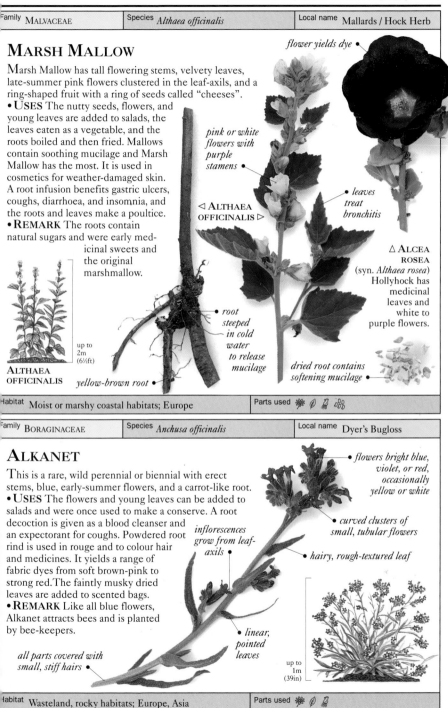

| Family MALVACEAE | Species *Althaea officinalis* | Local name Mallards / Hock Herb |

MARSH MALLOW

Marsh Mallow has tall flowering stems, velvety leaves, late-summer pink flowers clustered in the leaf-axils, and a ring-shaped fruit with a ring of seeds called "cheeses".
• **USES** The nutty seeds, flowers, and young leaves are added to salads, the leaves eaten as a vegetable, and the roots boiled and then fried. Mallows contain soothing mucilage and Marsh Mallow has the most. It is used in cosmetics for weather-damaged skin. A root infusion benefits gastric ulcers, coughs, diarrhoea, and insomnia, and the roots and leaves make a poultice.
• **REMARK** The roots contain natural sugars and were early medicinal sweets and the original marshmallow.

flower yields dye •

pink or white flowers with purple stamens •

◁ **ALTHAEA OFFICINALIS** ▷

• leaves treat bronchitis

△ **ALCEA ROSEA** (syn. *Althaea rosea*) Hollyhock has medicinal leaves and white to purple flowers.

up to 2m (6½ft)

ALTHAEA OFFICINALIS

yellow-brown root •

• root steeped in cold water to release mucilage

dried root contains softening mucilage •

| Habitat Moist or marshy coastal habitats; Europe | Parts used 🌸 🌿 🥕 🌰 |

| Family BORAGINACEAE | Species *Anchusa officinalis* | Local name Dyer's Bugloss |

ALKANET

This is a rare, wild perennial or biennial with erect stems, blue, early-summer flowers, and a carrot-like root.
• **USES** The flowers and young leaves can be added to salads and were once used to make a conserve. A root decoction is given as a blood cleanser and an expectorant for coughs. Powdered root rind is used in rouge and to colour hair and medicines. It yields a range of fabric dyes from soft brown-pink to strong red. The faintly musky dried leaves are added to scented bags.
• **REMARK** Like all blue flowers, Alkanet attracts bees and is planted by bee-keepers.

• flowers bright blue, violet, or red, occasionally yellow or white

• curved clusters of small, tubular flowers

inflorescences grow from leaf-axils •

• hairy, rough-textured leaf

• linear, pointed leaves

up to 1m (39in)

all parts covered with small, stiff hairs •

| Habitat Wasteland, rocky habitats; Europe, Asia | Parts used 🌸 🌿 🥕 |

Family BROMELIACEAE	Species *Ananas comosus*	Local name Annasi / Nana

PINEAPPLE

Unlike tree-perching bromeliads, Pineapple is planted in the ground. It has a dense rosette of leaves allowing it to make maximum use of rainwater, and a conical spike of violet-red flowers with yellow bracts.
• USES A popular tropical fruit, it has a high sugar content and is rich in vitamins A, B, and C. The flesh is eaten raw, cooked, battered, jellied, candied, juiced, or made into alcohol, including *Vin d'Ananas*. New shoots are added to curries, waste is made into vinegar or fed to livestock, and the flesh is used in face masks as the enzymes digest dead skin. The fruit helps menstrual, urinary, and digestive problems, beri-beri, worms, and nervous exhaustion. Plant enzymes reduce swelling, intensify antibiotics, and break down the fibrin protein which causes heart attacks and strokes.
• REMARK In Sri Lanka it is taken by smokers to clear the lungs, but it can aggravate skin rashes.

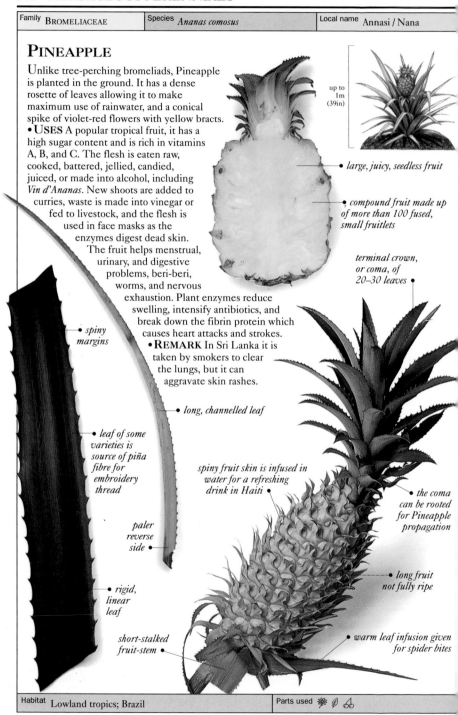

up to 1m (39in)

• *large, juicy, seedless fruit*

• *compound fruit made up of more than 100 fused, small fruitlets*

terminal crown, or coma, of 20–30 leaves •

spiny margins

• *long, channelled leaf*

• *leaf of some varieties is source of piña fibre for embroidery thread*

spiny fruit skin is infused in water for a refreshing drink in Haiti •

paler reverse side •

• *rigid, linear leaf*

short-stalked fruit-stem •

• *the coma can be rooted for Pineapple propagation*

• *long fruit not fully ripe*

• *warm leaf infusion given for spider bites*

Habitat Lowland tropics; Brazil	Parts used

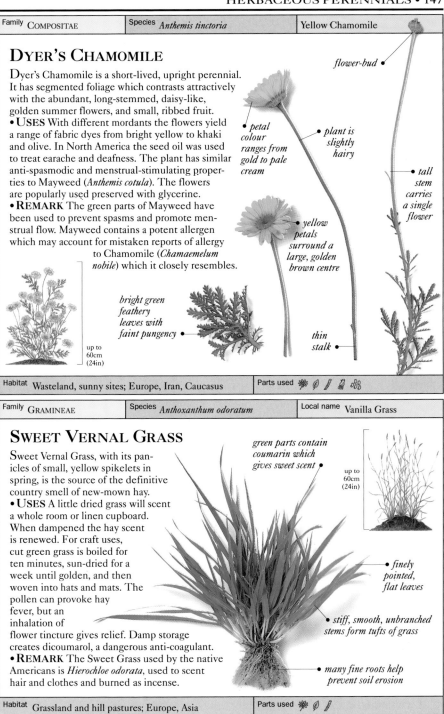

| Family COMPOSITAE | Species *Anthemis tinctoria* | Yellow Chamomile |

DYER'S CHAMOMILE

Dyer's Chamomile is a short-lived, upright perennial. It has segmented foliage which contrasts attractively with the abundant, long-stemmed, daisy-like, golden summer flowers, and small, ribbed fruit.

• USES With different mordants the flowers yield a range of fabric dyes from bright yellow to khaki and olive. In North America the seed oil was used to treat earache and deafness. The plant has similar anti-spasmodic and menstrual-stimulating proper-ties to Mayweed (*Anthemis cotula*). The flowers are popularly used preserved with glycerine.

• REMARK The green parts of Mayweed have been used to prevent spasms and promote men-strual flow. Mayweed contains a potent allergen which may account for mistaken reports of allergy to Chamomile (*Chamaemelum nobile*) which it closely resembles.

flower-bud

petal colour ranges from gold to pale cream

plant is slightly hairy

tall stem carries a single flower

yellow petals surround a large, golden brown centre

bright green feathery leaves with faint pungency

up to 60cm (24in)

thin stalk

| Habitat Wasteland, sunny sites; Europe, Iran, Caucasus | Parts used |

| Family GRAMINEAE | Species *Anthoxanthum odoratum* | Local name Vanilla Grass |

SWEET VERNAL GRASS

Sweet Vernal Grass, with its pan-icles of small, yellow spikelets in spring, is the source of the definitive country smell of new-mown hay.

• USES A little dried grass will scent a whole room or linen cupboard. When dampened the hay scent is renewed. For craft uses, cut green grass is boiled for ten minutes, sun-dried for a week until golden, and then woven into hats and mats. The pollen can provoke hay fever, but an inhalation of flower tincture gives relief. Damp storage creates dicoumarol, a dangerous anti-coagulant.

• REMARK The Sweet Grass used by the native Americans is *Hierochloe odorata*, used to scent hair and clothes and burned as incense.

green parts contain coumarin which gives sweet scent

up to 60cm (24in)

finely pointed, flat leaves

stiff, smooth, unbranched stems form tufts of grass

many fine roots help prevent soil erosion

| Habitat Grassland and hill pastures; Europe, Asia | Parts used |

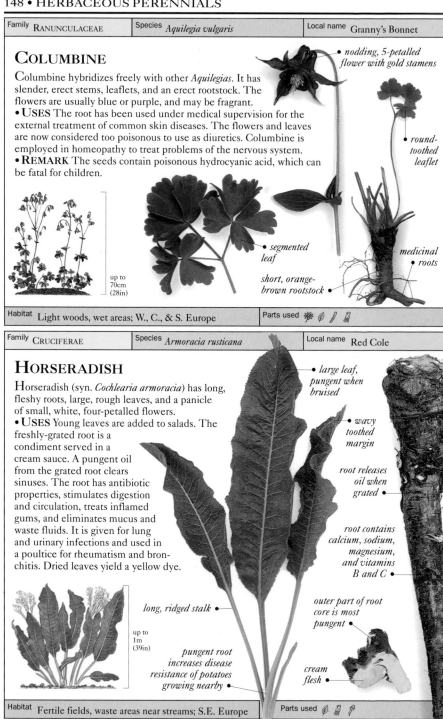

| Family RANUNCULACEAE | Species *Aquilegia vulgaris* | Local name Granny's Bonnet |

COLUMBINE

Columbine hybridizes freely with other *Aquilegias*. It has slender, erect stems, leaflets, and an erect rootstock. The flowers are usually blue or purple, and may be fragrant.
• USES The root has been used under medical supervision for the external treatment of common skin diseases. The flowers and leaves are now considered too poisonous to use as diuretics. Columbine is employed in homeopathy to treat problems of the nervous system.
• REMARK The seeds contain poisonous hydrocyanic acid, which can be fatal for children.

• nodding, 5-petalled flower with gold stamens

• round-toothed leaflet

• segmented leaf

short, orange-brown rootstock •

medicinal • roots

up to 70cm (28in)

| Habitat Light woods, wet areas; W., C., & S. Europe | Parts used |

| Family CRUCIFERAE | Species *Armoracia rusticana* | Local name Red Cole |

HORSERADISH

Horseradish (syn. *Cochlearia armoracia*) has long, fleshy roots, large, rough leaves, and a panicle of small, white, four-petalled flowers.
• USES Young leaves are added to salads. The freshly-grated root is a condiment served in a cream sauce. A pungent oil from the grated root clears sinuses. The root has antibiotic properties, stimulates digestion and circulation, treats inflamed gums, and eliminates mucus and waste fluids. It is given for lung and urinary infections and used in a poultice for rheumatism and bronchitis. Dried leaves yield a yellow dye.

• large leaf, pungent when bruised

• wavy toothed margin

root releases oil when grated •

root contains calcium, sodium, magnesium, and vitamins B and C •

outer part of root core is most pungent •

long, ridged stalk •

up to 1m (39in)

pungent root increases disease resistance of potatoes growing nearby •

cream flesh •

| Habitat Fertile fields, waste areas near streams; S.E. Europe | Parts used |

Family COMPOSITAE	Species *Arnica montana*	Local name Leopard's Bane

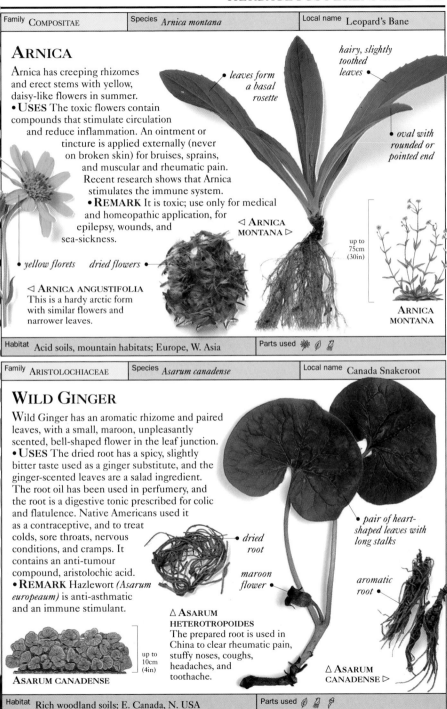

ARNICA

Arnica has creeping rhizomes and erect stems with yellow, daisy-like flowers in summer.
• **USES** The toxic flowers contain compounds that stimulate circulation and reduce inflammation. An ointment or tincture is applied externally (never on broken skin) for bruises, sprains, and muscular and rheumatic pain. Recent research shows that Arnica stimulates the immune system.
• **REMARK** It is toxic; use only for medical and homeopathic application, for epilepsy, wounds, and sea-sickness.

leaves form a basal rosette

hairy, slightly toothed leaves •

• oval with rounded or pointed end

◁ **ARNICA MONTANA** ▷

up to 75cm (30in)

yellow florets   *dried flowers •*

◁ **ARNICA ANGUSTIFOLIA**
This is a hardy arctic form with similar flowers and narrower leaves.

ARNICA MONTANA

Habitat Acid soils, mountain habitats; Europe, W. Asia	Parts used

Family ARISTOLOCHIACEAE	Species *Asarum canadense*	Local name Canada Snakeroot

WILD GINGER

Wild Ginger has an aromatic rhizome and paired leaves, with a small, maroon, unpleasantly scented, bell-shaped flower in the leaf junction.
• **USES** The dried root has a spicy, slightly bitter taste used as a ginger substitute, and the ginger-scented leaves are a salad ingredient. The root oil has been used in perfumery, and the root is a digestive tonic prescribed for colic and flatulence. Native Americans used it as a contraceptive, and to treat colds, sore throats, nervous conditions, and cramps. It contains an anti-tumour compound, aristolochic acid.
• **REMARK** Hazlewort (*Asarum europeaum*) is anti-asthmatic and an immune stimulant.

• dried root

maroon flower •

• pair of heart-shaped leaves with long stalks

aromatic root •

△ **ASARUM HETEROTROPOIDES**
The prepared root is used in China to clear rheumatic pain, stuffy noses, coughs, headaches, and toothache.

up to 10cm (4in)

ASARUM CANADENSE

△ **ASARUM CANADENSE** ▷

Habitat Rich woodland soils; E. Canada, N. USA	Parts used

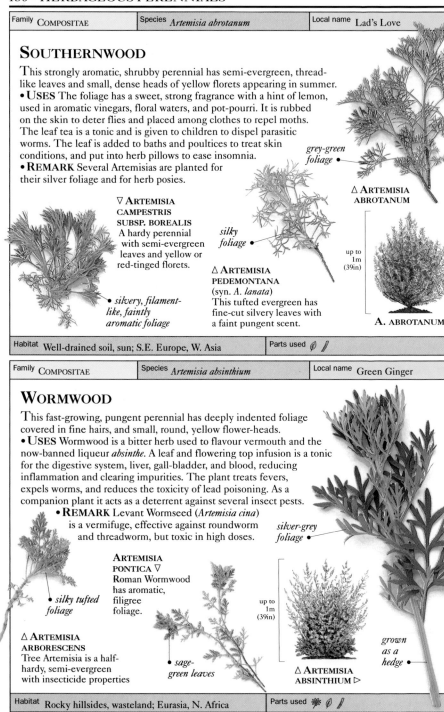

Family COMPOSITAE	Species *Artemisia abrotanum*	Local name Lad's Love

SOUTHERNWOOD

This strongly aromatic, shrubby perennial has semi-evergreen, thread-like leaves and small, dense heads of yellow florets appearing in summer.
• **USES** The foliage has a sweet, strong fragrance with a hint of lemon, used in aromatic vinegars, floral waters, and pot-pourri. It is rubbed on the skin to deter flies and placed among clothes to repel moths. The leaf tea is a tonic and is given to children to dispel parasitic worms. The leaf is added to baths and poultices to treat skin conditions, and put into herb pillows to ease insomnia.
• **REMARK** Several Artemisias are planted for their silver foliage and for herb posies.

grey-green foliage •

△ **ARTEMISIA ABROTANUM**

▽ **ARTEMISIA CAMPESTRIS SUBSP. BOREALIS**
A hardy perennial with semi-evergreen leaves and yellow or red-tinged florets.

silky foliage •

△ **ARTEMISIA PEDEMONTANA** (syn. *A. lanata*)
This tufted evergreen has fine-cut silvery leaves with a faint pungent scent.

• *silvery, filament-like, faintly aromatic foliage*

up to 1m (39in)

A. ABROTANUM

Habitat Well-drained soil, sun; S.E. Europe, W. Asia	Parts used 🌿 ✎

Family COMPOSITAE	Species *Artemisia absinthium*	Local name Green Ginger

WORMWOOD

This fast-growing, pungent perennial has deeply indented foliage covered in fine hairs, and small, round, yellow flower-heads.
• **USES** Wormwood is a bitter herb used to flavour vermouth and the now-banned liqueur *absinthe*. A leaf and flowering top infusion is a tonic for the digestive system, liver, gall-bladder, and blood, reducing inflammation and clearing impurities. The plant treats fevers, expels worms, and reduces the toxicity of lead poisoning. As a companion plant it acts as a deterrent against several insect pests.
• **REMARK** Levant Wormseed (*Artemisia cina*) is a vermifuge, effective against roundworm and threadworm, but toxic in high doses.

silver-grey foliage •

ARTEMISIA PONTICA ▽
Roman Wormwood has aromatic, filigree foliage.

• *silky tufted foliage*

△ **ARTEMISIA ARBORESCENS**
Tree Artemisia is a half-hardy, semi-evergreen with insecticide properties

• *sage-green leaves*

up to 1m (39in)

△ **ARTEMISIA ABSINTHIUM** ▷

grown as a hedge •

Habitat Rocky hillsides, wasteland; Eurasia, N. Africa	Parts used 🌸 🌿 ✎

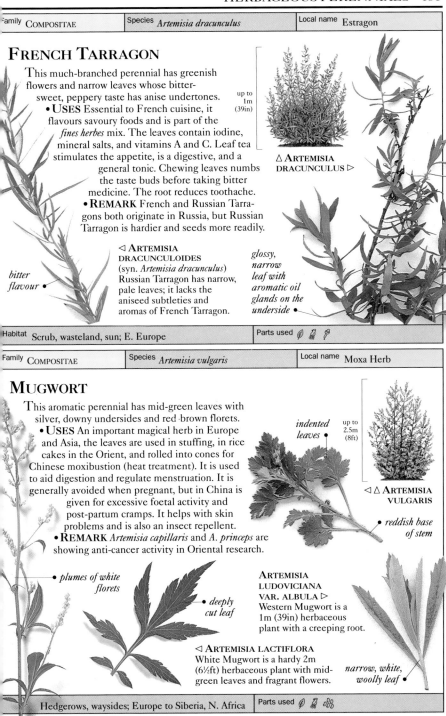

Family COMPOSITAE	Species *Artemisia dracunculus*	Local name Estragon

FRENCH TARRAGON

This much-branched perennial has greenish
flowers and narrow leaves whose bittersweet, peppery taste has anise undertones.
• **USES** Essential to French cuisine, it
flavours savoury foods and is part of the
fines herbes mix. The leaves contain iodine,
mineral salts, and vitamins A and C. Leaf tea
stimulates the appetite, is a digestive, and a
general tonic. Chewing leaves numbs
the taste buds before taking bitter
medicine. The root reduces toothache.
• **REMARK** French and Russian Tarra-
gons both originate in Russia, but Russian
Tarragon is hardier and seeds more readily.

up to
1m
(39in)

△ **ARTEMISIA
DRACUNCULUS** ▷

◁ **ARTEMISIA
DRACUNCULOIDES**
(syn. *Artemisia dracunculus*)
Russian Tarragon has narrow,
pale leaves; it lacks the
aniseed subtleties and
aromas of French Tarragon.

*bitter
flavour* •

*glossy,
narrow
leaf with
aromatic oil
glands on the
underside* •

Habitat Scrub, wasteland, sun; E. Europe	Parts used

Family COMPOSITAE	Species *Artemisia vulgaris*	Local name Moxa Herb

MUGWORT

This aromatic perennial has mid-green leaves with
silver, downy undersides and red ·brown florets.
• **USES** An important magical herb in Europe
and Asia, the leaves are used in stuffing, in rice
cakes in the Orient, and rolled into cones for
Chinese moxibustion (heat treatment). It is used
to aid digestion and regulate menstruation. It is
generally avoided when pregnant, but in China is
given for excessive foetal activity and
post-partum cramps. It helps with skin
problems and is also an insect repellent.
• **REMARK** *Artemisia capillaris* and *A. princeps* are
showing anti-cancer activity in Oriental research.

*indented
leaves* •

up to
2.5m
(8ft)

◁ △ **ARTEMISIA
VULGARIS**

• *reddish base
of stem*

• *plumes of white
florets*

• *deeply
cut leaf*

**ARTEMISIA
LUDOVICIANA
VAR. ALBULA** ▷
Western Mugwort is a
1m (39in) herbaceous
plant with a creeping root.

◁ **ARTEMISIA LACTIFLORA**
White Mugwort is a hardy 2m
(6½ft) herbaceous plant with mid-
green leaves and fragrant flowers.

*narrow, white,
woolly leaf* •

Hedgerows, waysides; Europe to Siberia, N. Africa	Parts used

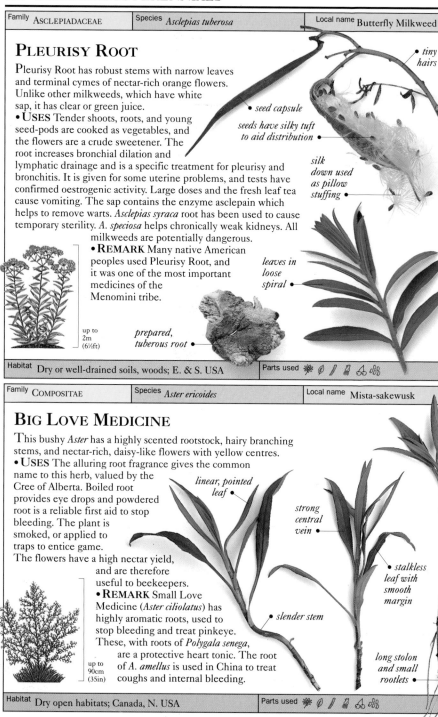

Family ASCLEPIADACEAE	Species *Asclepias tuberosa*	Local name Butterfly Milkweed

PLEURISY ROOT

Pleurisy Root has robust stems with narrow leaves and terminal cymes of nectar-rich orange flowers. Unlike other milkweeds, which have white sap, it has clear or green juice.
• USES Tender shoots, roots, and young seed-pods are cooked as vegetables, and the flowers are a crude sweetener. The root increases bronchial dilation and lymphatic drainage and is a specific treatment for pleurisy and bronchitis. It is given for some uterine problems, and tests have confirmed oestrogenic activity. Large doses and the fresh leaf tea cause vomiting. The sap contains the enzyme asclepain which helps to remove warts. *Asclepias syraca* root has been used to cause temporary sterility. *A. speciosa* helps chronically weak kidneys. All milkweeds are potentially dangerous.
• REMARK Many native American peoples used Pleurisy Root, and it was one of the most important medicines of the Menomini tribe.

tiny hairs

seed capsule

seeds have silky tuft to aid distribution

silk down used as pillow stuffing

leaves in loose spiral

up to 2m (6½ft)

prepared, tuberous root

Habitat Dry or well-drained soils, woods; E. & S. USA	Parts used

Family COMPOSITAE	Species *Aster ericoides*	Local name Mista-sakewusk

BIG LOVE MEDICINE

This bushy *Aster* has a highly scented rootstock, hairy branching stems, and nectar-rich, daisy-like flowers with yellow centres.
• USES The alluring root fragrance gives the common name to this herb, valued by the Cree of Alberta. Boiled root provides eye drops and powdered root is a reliable first aid to stop bleeding. The plant is smoked, or applied to traps to entice game. The flowers have a high nectar yield, and are therefore useful to beekeepers.
• REMARK Small Love Medicine (*Aster ciliolatus*) has highly aromatic roots, used to stop bleeding and treat pinkeye. These, with roots of *Polygala senega*, are a protective heart tonic. The root of *A. amellus* is used in China to treat coughs and internal bleeding.

linear, pointed leaf

strong central vein

stalkless leaf with smooth margin

slender stem

up to 90cm (35in)

long stolon and small rootlets

Habitat Dry open habitats; Canada, N. USA	Parts used

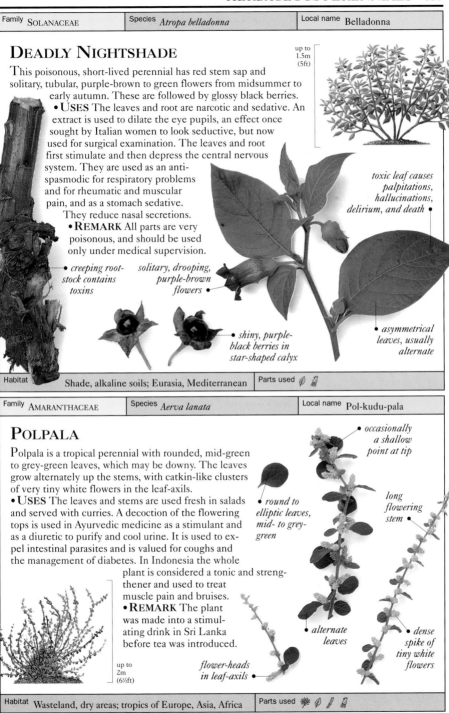

Family SOLANACEAE	Species *Atropa belladonna*	Local name Belladonna

DEADLY NIGHTSHADE

up to 1.5m (5ft)

This poisonous, short-lived perennial has red stem sap and solitary, tubular, purple-brown to green flowers from midsummer to early autumn. These are followed by glossy black berries.

• **USES** The leaves and root are narcotic and sedative. An extract is used to dilate the eye pupils, an effect once sought by Italian women to look seductive, but now used for surgical examination. The leaves and root first stimulate and then depress the central nervous system. They are used as an anti-spasmodic for respiratory problems and for rheumatic and muscular pain, and as a stomach sedative. They reduce nasal secretions.

• **REMARK** All parts are very poisonous, and should be used only under medical supervision.

toxic leaf causes palpitations, hallucinations, delirium, and death •

• creeping root-stock contains toxins

solitary, drooping, purple-brown flowers •

• shiny, purple-black berries in star-shaped calyx

• asymmetrical leaves, usually alternate

Habitat Shade, alkaline soils; Eurasia, Mediterranean	Parts used

Family AMARANTHACEAE	Species *Aerva lanata*	Local name Pol-kudu-pala

POLPALA

Polpala is a tropical perennial with rounded, mid-green to grey-green leaves, which may be downy. The leaves grow alternately up the stems, with catkin-like clusters of very tiny white flowers in the leaf-axils.

• **USES** The leaves and stems are used fresh in salads and served with curries. A decoction of the flowering tops is used in Ayurvedic medicine as a stimulant and as a diuretic to purify and cool urine. It is used to expel intestinal parasites and is valued for coughs and the management of diabetes. In Indonesia the whole plant is considered a tonic and strengthener and used to treat muscle pain and bruises.

• **REMARK** The plant was made into a stimulating drink in Sri Lanka before tea was introduced.

• occasionally a shallow point at tip

long flowering stem •

• round to elliptic leaves, mid- to grey-green

up to 2m (6½ft)

• alternate leaves

• dense spike of tiny white flowers

flower-heads in leaf-axils •

Habitat Wasteland, dry areas; tropics of Europe, Asia, Africa	Parts used

Family SCROPHULARIACEAE	Species *Bacopa monnieri*	Local name Water Hyssop

BACOPA

This perennial forms dense mats of foliage on water-side mud and bears axial clusters of small, bell-shaped, white or pale blue flowers in summer.

up to 50cm (20in)

• **USES** The succulent leaves and stems of Bacopa have a slightly biting taste, enjoyed as a salad herb, and taken to improve the memory. Hindus use an infusion as a nerve tonic, particularly for epilepsy. In Indonesia Bacopa is taken for the tropical disease, filariasis. In China the plant is credited with warming the kidneys and stimulating yang energy. It is prescribed for impotence, premature ejaculation, kidney-related backache, uterine fertility problems, irregular menstruation, and rheumatism.

• leaves are given as brain nourishment in Ayurvedic medicine

• succulent, smooth stems and leaves eaten as salad

• **REMARK** New research has shown that Bacopa has great potential as a nourishing brain tonic.

branching roots and rootlets •

• rounded, obovate leaves with occasional tip indentation

• leaf nodes along prostrate stems frequently take root

Habitat Marshes, pond edges; warm temperate areas, tropics	Parts used ✿ 🌿

Family COMPOSITAE	Species *Bellis perennis*	Local name English Daisy

LAWN DAISY

This cheerful perennial, a symbol of innocence, has flat rosettes of scalloped, basal leaves, and small, composite flower-heads with white ray florets and yellow disc florets.

up to 15cm (6in)

• **USES** Tender young leaves and white petals can be tossed in salads. In spring, the stem sap is applied to spots. A flower infusion added to baths helps revive winter-dulled and sallow skins. It has been used as a skin wash for eczema, a douche for thrush, and an expectorant for coughs. Research has shown that it may slow the growth of breast tumours. In Europe flower tea is given to listless children.

fresh petals without bitter yellow centre •

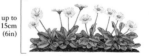

• **REMARK** Lawn Daisy can provoke allergies.

• florets attract bees and butterflies

• flower petals can be added to salads or used as decorative garnish

• golden-centred, compound flowers may be single or double, and produced from spring to autumn

• flowers are used in homeopathy as "bellide oil"

• scalloped leaf margin

• flower-bud popular in posies

boiled or pickled roots were once added to salads •

• leaves have long been used on wounds and bruises

Habitat Grass or meadows; S., W., & C. Europe, W. Asia	Parts used ✿ 🌿

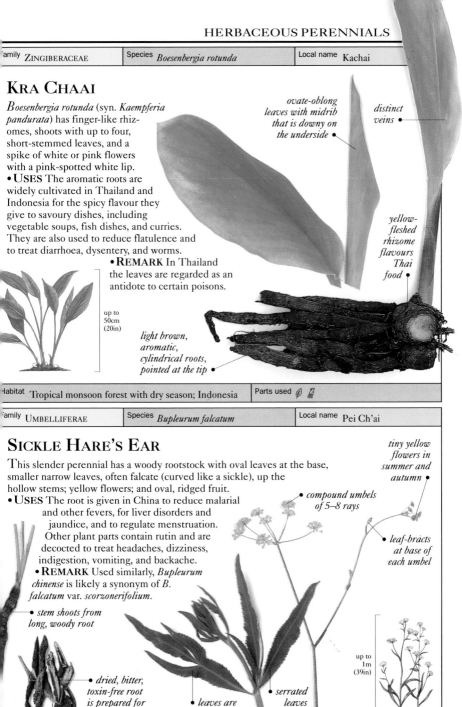

| Family | ZINGIBERACEAE | Species | *Boesenbergia rotunda* | Local name | Kachai |

KRA CHAAI

Boesenbergia rotunda (syn. *Kaempferia pandurata*) has finger-like rhiz-omes, shoots with up to four, short-stemmed leaves, and a spike of white or pink flowers with a pink-spotted white lip.
• USES The aromatic roots are widely cultivated in Thailand and Indonesia for the spicy flavour they give to savoury dishes, including vegetable soups, fish dishes, and curries. They are also used to reduce flatulence and to treat diarrhoea, dysentery, and worms.
    • REMARK In Thailand the leaves are regarded as an antidote to certain poisons.

ovate-oblong leaves with midrib that is downy on the underside •

distinct veins •

yellow-fleshed rhizome flavours Thai food •

up to 50cm (20in)

light brown, aromatic, cylindrical roots, pointed at the tip •

| Habitat | Tropical monsoon forest with dry season; Indonesia | Parts used | 🌿 🫚 |

| Family | UMBELLIFERAE | Species | *Bupleurum falcatum* | Local name | Pei Ch'ai |

SICKLE HARE'S EAR

This slender perennial has a woody rootstock with oval leaves at the base, smaller narrow leaves, often falcate (curved like a sickle), up the hollow stems; yellow flowers; and oval, ridged fruit.
• USES The root is given in China to reduce malarial and other fevers, for liver disorders and jaundice, and to regulate menstruation. Other plant parts contain rutin and are decocted to treat headaches, dizziness, indigestion, vomiting, and backache.
    • REMARK Used similarly, *Bupleurum chinense* is likely a synonym of *B. falcatum* var. *scorzonerifolium*.

tiny yellow flowers in summer and autumn •

• *compound umbels of 5–8 rays*

• *leaf-bracts at base of each umbel*

• *stem shoots from long, woody root*

up to 1m (39in)

• *dried, bitter, toxin-free root is prepared for Chinese medicine*

• *leaves are often falcate*

• *serrated leaves*

| Habitat | Wasteland, hedgebanks; S., C., & E. Europe, Asia | Parts used | 🌼 🌿 🍃 🫚 |

Family LABIATAE	Species *Calamintha grandiflora*	Local name Mountain Balm

LARGE-FLOWERED CALAMINT

This aromatic perennial has a thin, creeping rhizome, deep green, slightly hairy leaves with six teeth on each side, and a flowering spike bearing inflorescences of up to five tubular pink flowers in summer.
• USES Calamint contains camphor-like essential oils. The infused leaves yield a peppermint flavour. They are also made into a decoction or syrup to ease coughs and, when fresh, can be made into a poultice for bruises. The tea is drunk for flatulent colic and as an invigorating tonic recommended by Culpeper for "all afflictions of the brain".
• REMARK The leaves of *Calamintha sylvatica* and *C. nepeta* are used as an expectorant and diaphoretic to promote perspiration.

up to 60cm (24in)

• *leaf with unusual brown fringe*

• *pointed-toothed, dark green leaf*

◁ △ CALAMINTHA GRANDIFLORA

◁ ▽ CALAMINTHA SYLVATICA (syn. *C. ascendens*) Common Calamint has mint-scented leaves, and late-summer flowers.

◁ CALAMINTHA GRANDIFLORA 'VARIEGATA' Has dark green markings.

• *green-splashed gold leaves with 6 teeth on each side*

oval, blunt-ended leaf •

pink-spotted purple flower •

Habitat Mountainous woods; S.E. Europe, Anatolia, N. Iran	Parts used ❋ ✿ ⌇ ↯

Family LILIACEAE	Species *Camassia quamash*	Local name Quamash

CAMASS

This bulbous, shade-tolerant perennial with grass-like leaf blades has showy, blue flowering spikes in late spring.
• USES The bulb was an important native American food source that caused inter-tribal war over possession of its habitat. Camass is high in sugar but low in starch. It is eaten raw, boiled, or slowly baked in special pits to enhance its sweetness. The baked bulbs thicken and flavour gravy; any surplus were sun-dried whole or mashed into cakes with berries for winter use. The water in which the bulbs were boiled provided a sweetish drink.
• REMARK The bulbs of Eastern Camass (*Camassia scilloides* syn. *C. esculenta*) can also be eaten. The cream-flowered Death Camass, (*Zigadenus venenosus*) looks similar but is fatally poisonous.

• *tapered point*

• *lance-shaped leaves emerge from the bulb*

dark green, grass-like blades

• *green, unripe seed capsule*

• *edible rounded bulb with black outer skin and pale flesh*

up to 80cm (32in)

bulbs should be picked when blue flowers appear •

Habitat Mountains, fields, woods; W. North America	Parts used ⌇

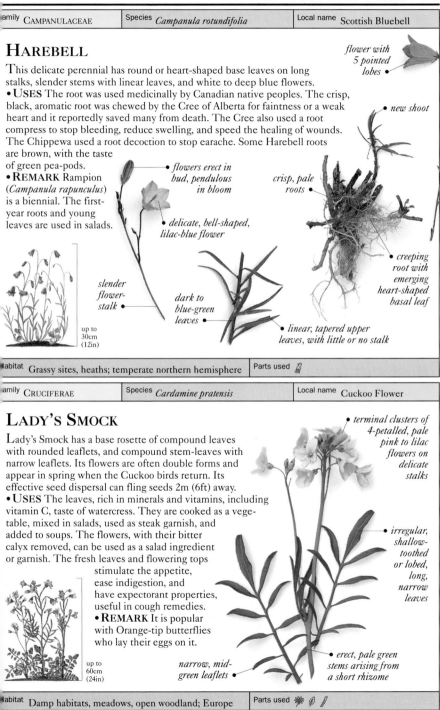

Family CAMPANULACEAE	Species *Campanula rotundifolia*	Local name Scottish Bluebell

HAREBELL

This delicate perennial has round or heart-shaped base leaves on long stalks, slender stems with linear leaves, and white to deep blue flowers.

• USES The root was used medicinally by Canadian native peoples. The crisp, black, aromatic root was chewed by the Cree of Alberta for faintness or a weak heart and it reportedly saved many from death. The Cree also used a root compress to stop bleeding, reduce swelling, and speed the healing of wounds. The Chippewa used a root decoction to stop earache. Some Harebell roots are brown, with the taste of green pea-pods.

• REMARK Rampion (*Campanula rapunculus*) is a biennial. The first-year roots and young leaves are used in salads.

flower with 5 pointed lobes

new shoot

flowers erect in bud, pendulous in bloom

crisp, pale roots

delicate, bell-shaped, lilac-blue flower

creeping root with emerging heart-shaped basal leaf

slender flower-stalk

dark to blue-green leaves

up to 30cm (12in)

linear, tapered upper leaves, with little or no stalk

Habitat Grassy sites, heaths; temperate northern hemisphere	Parts used 🌿

Family CRUCIFERAE	Species *Cardamine pratensis*	Local name Cuckoo Flower

LADY'S SMOCK

Lady's Smock has a base rosette of compound leaves with rounded leaflets, and compound stem-leaves with narrow leaflets. Its flowers are often double forms and appear in spring when the Cuckoo birds return. Its effective seed dispersal can fling seeds 2m (6ft) away.

• USES The leaves, rich in minerals and vitamins, including vitamin C, taste of watercress. They are cooked as a vegetable, mixed in salads, used as steak garnish, and added to soups. The flowers, with their bitter calyx removed, can be used as a salad ingredient or garnish. The fresh leaves and flowering tops stimulate the appetite, ease indigestion, and have expectorant properties, useful in cough remedies.

• REMARK It is popular with Orange-tip butterflies who lay their eggs on it.

terminal clusters of 4-petalled, pale pink to lilac flowers on delicate stalks

irregular, shallow-toothed or lobed, long, narrow leaves

up to 60cm (24in)

narrow, mid-green leaflets

erect, pale green stems arising from a short rhizome

Habitat Damp habitats, meadows, open woodland; Europe	Parts used 🌸 🌿

Family COMPOSITAE	Species *Carlina acaulis*	Dwarf Thistle

STEMLESS CARLINE THISTLE

This stemless thistle has a rosette of spiny leaves and a lilac-brown or white flower-head surrounded by silvery, papery bracts.
• **USES** The flower receptacle is eaten like Artichoke, and the leaves used to curdle milk. The roots, macerated in wine, give a digestive stomach tonic, beneficial for eczema and skin rashes.
A root infusion is diuretic, mildly laxative, an antiseptic gargle and wound wash, a liver tonic, and a worm expellant, and is used by vets to stimulate cattle appetites. A country humidity gauge, the flower bracts close as rain approaches.
• **REMARK** Named *Carlina* after the Emperor Charlemagne who dreamed of it as a plague cure, it became popular in poison and snakebite remedies and protective charms.

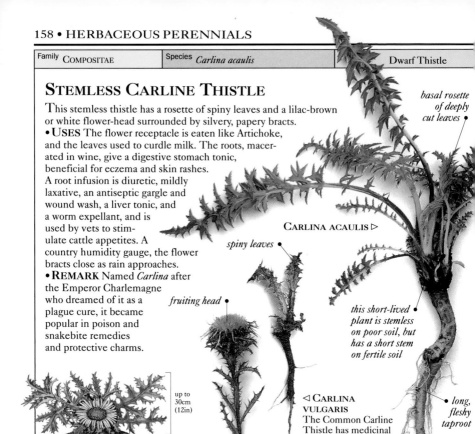

basal rosette of deeply cut leaves

CARLINA ACAULIS ▷

spiny leaves

fruiting head

this short-lived plant is stemless on poor soil, but has a short stem on fertile soil

up to 30cm (12in)

CARLINA ACAULIS

◁ **CARLINA VULGARIS**
The Common Carline Thistle has medicinal properties.

long, fleshy taproot

Habitat Poor pastureland, rocky slopes; S. & E. Europe	Parts used 🌸 🍃 🌱

Family APOCYNACEAE	Species *Catharanthus roseus*	Local name Cayenne Jasmine

MADAGASCAR PERIWINKLE

The toxic Madagascar Periwinkle is a much-branched, fleshy perennial with shiny, dark green foliage and flat, rosy pink flowers.
• **USES** The use of *Catharanthus roseus* (syn. *Vinca rosea*) in folk medicine for diabetes prompted research which found it contained an insulin substitute and 55 active alkaloids. Some affect white blood cells, lymph glands, and the spleen, with significant anti-cancer cell action, and are given for children's leukaemia, Hodgkin's disease, and solid tumours. Unfortunately healthy cells are also affected, causing short-term side-effects.
• **REMARK** The Madagascar Periwinkle plant is poisonous to humans and livestock.

up to 60cm (24in)

fleshy stem

leaves in opposite pairs with pale, distinct central vein

oblong to obovate smooth leaves with smooth margins

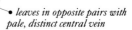

5-petalled, rosy pink, white, or crimson flowers with darker centres

Habitat Sunny, humid tropics; Madagascar	Parts used 🌸 🍃 🌿 🌱

Family UMBELLIFERAE	Species *Centella asiatica*	Local name Gotu-kola

CENTELLA

This slender herb with fan-shaped leaves and small white flowers spreads by rooting along its prostrate stems.

long reddish stems •

• **USES** An Eastern longevity herb and brain food, taken to develop spiritual powers, Centella is enjoying new attention. Research shows it is tonic, anti-inflammatory, wound-healing, diuretic, laxative, and sedative. It treats skin infections including leprosy and skin ulcers, and appears to activate blood-cleansing and immunity while stimulating deep skin replacement. It is a nerve tonic to improve memory and reduce mental fatigue. It treats liver complaints and high blood pressure.

• rounded leaf on long stalk

• bright green cupped leaf with scalloped margin

• **REMARK** Large doses may cause vertigo.

stem-nodes produce small • leaf cluster and roots

up to 50cm (20in)

Habitat Damp grassland; tropics, subtropics	Parts used 🌼 🍃

Family COMPOSITAE	Species *Chamaemelum nobile*	Local name English Chamomile

PERENNIAL CHAMOMILE

Also called Roman Chamomile, this aromatic evergreen has feathery, apple-scented leaves and white flowers with conical, golden centres.

centre of summer flowers contains active ingredients •

• dried flowers as tea relieve indigestion, nausea, nightmares, and insomnia

• **USES** The flowers make a digestive, nervine, and sedative tea which is used for soothing restless children, helps prevent nightmares and insomnia, and suppresses nausea. Used tea bags or flower cream reduce inflammation and fatigue shadows under the eyes and make a poultice to treat eczema and wounds. A flower decoction conditions and lightens fair hair. In reviving baths it softens and whitens sun- or wind-damaged skin. Chamomile's anti-inflammatory, analgesic, and disinfectant qualities treat urinary infections and nappy rash, and soothe toothache, earache, sore nipples, and neuralgia. The flower compounds have shown anti-tumour activity in laboratory tests. In the garden it is a "physician plant", reviving nearby ailing plants.

▽ CHAMAEMELUM NOBILE 'FLORE-PLENO'
Double-flowered Chamomile is a perennial with double cream flowers and apple-scented leaves.

CHAMAEMELUM NOBILE ▷

aromatic leaves used in snuff and pot-pourri •

• **REMARK** Moroccan Chamomile (*Chamaemelum mixta* syn. *Ormenis mixta*) yields essential oil also sold as Chamomile.

revives ailing plants nearby •

• mat-forming, creeping rootstock

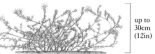

up to 30cm (12in)

C. NOBILE (syn. *Anthemus nobilis*)

CHAMAEMELUM NOBILE 'TRENEAGUE' ▷
This non-flowering cultivar has apple-scented leaves, ideal in lawns and by garden seats.

Habitat Light sandy soils; W. Europe	Parts used 🌼 🍃 🌿

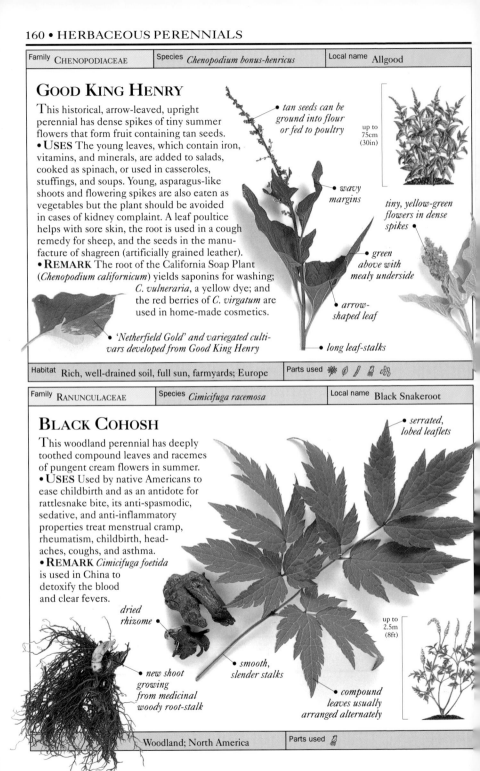

Family CHENOPODIACEAE	Species *Chenopodium bonus-henricus*	Local name Allgood

GOOD KING HENRY

This historical, arrow-leaved, upright perennial has dense spikes of tiny summer flowers that form fruit containing tan seeds.
• **USES** The young leaves, which contain iron, vitamins, and minerals, are added to salads, cooked as spinach, or used in casseroles, stuffings, and soups. Young, asparagus-like shoots and flowering spikes are also eaten as vegetables but the plant should be avoided in cases of kidney complaint. A leaf poultice helps with sore skin, the root is used in a cough remedy for sheep, and the seeds in the manu-facture of shagreen (artificially grained leather).
• **REMARK** The root of the California Soap Plant (*Chenopodium californicum*) yields saponins for washing; *C. vulneraria*, a yellow dye; and the red berries of *C. virgatum* are used in home-made cosmetics.

tan seeds can be ground into flour or fed to poultry

up to 75cm (30in)

wavy margins

tiny, yellow-green flowers in dense spikes

green above with mealy underside

arrow-shaped leaf

'Netherfield Gold' and variegated culti-vars developed from Good King Henry

long leaf-stalks

Habitat Rich, well-drained soil, full sun, farmyards; Europe	Parts used

Family RANUNCULACEAE	Species *Cimicifuga racemosa*	Local name Black Snakeroot

BLACK COHOSH

This woodland perennial has deeply toothed compound leaves and racemes of pungent cream flowers in summer.
• **USES** Used by native Americans to ease childbirth and as an antidote for rattlesnake bite, its anti-spasmodic, sedative, and anti-inflammatory properties treat menstrual cramp, rheumatism, childbirth, head-aches, coughs, and asthma.
• **REMARK** *Cimicifuga foetida* is used in China to detoxify the blood and clear fevers.

serrated, lobed leaflets

dried rhizome

new shoot growing from medicinal woody root-stalk

smooth, slender stalks

up to 2.5m (8ft)

compound leaves usually arranged alternately

Woodland; North America	Parts used

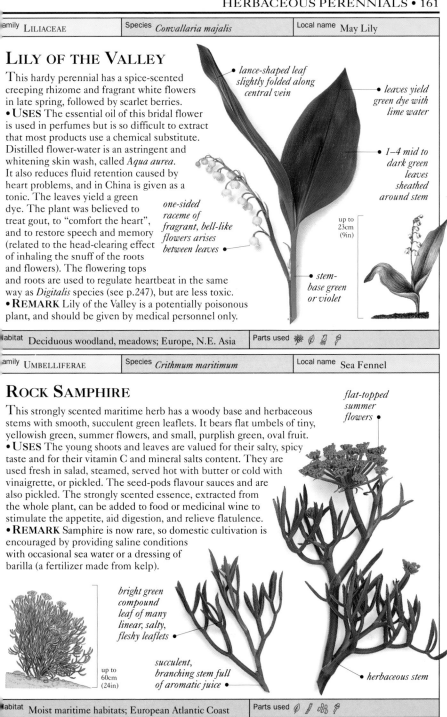

| Family | LILIACEAE | Species | *Convallaria majalis* | Local name | May Lily |

LILY OF THE VALLEY

This hardy perennial has a spice-scented creeping rhizome and fragrant white flowers in late spring, followed by scarlet berries.
• **USES** The essential oil of this bridal flower is used in perfumes but is so difficult to extract that most products use a chemical substitute. Distilled flower-water is an astringent and whitening skin wash, called *Aqua aurea*. It also reduces fluid retention caused by heart problems, and in China is given as a tonic. The leaves yield a green dye. The plant was believed to treat gout, to "comfort the heart", and to restore speech and memory (related to the head-clearing effect of inhaling the snuff of the roots and flowers). The flowering tops and roots are used to regulate heartbeat in the same way as *Digitalis* species (see p.247), but are less toxic.
• **REMARK** Lily of the Valley is a potentially poisonous plant, and should be given by medical personnel only.

lance-shaped leaf slightly folded along central vein

leaves yield green dye with lime water

1–4 mid to dark green leaves sheathed around stem

one-sided raceme of fragrant, bell-like flowers arises between leaves

up to 23cm (9in)

stem-base green or violet

| Habitat | Deciduous woodland, meadows; Europe, N.E. Asia | Parts used ❋ 🍃 🔪 🌿 |

| Family | UMBELLIFERAE | Species | *Crithmum maritimum* | Local name | Sea Fennel |

ROCK SAMPHIRE

This strongly scented maritime herb has a woody base and herbaceous stems with smooth, succulent green leaflets. It bears flat umbels of tiny, yellowish green, summer flowers, and small, purplish green, oval fruit.
• **USES** The young shoots and leaves are valued for their salty, spicy taste and for their vitamin C and mineral salts content. They are used fresh in salad, steamed, served hot with butter or cold with vinaigrette, or pickled. The seed-pods flavour sauces and are also pickled. The strongly scented essence, extracted from the whole plant, can be added to food or medicinal wine to stimulate the appetite, aid digestion, and relieve flatulence.
• **REMARK** Samphire is now rare, so domestic cultivation is encouraged by providing saline conditions with occasional sea water or a dressing of barilla (a fertilizer made from kelp).

flat-topped summer flowers

bright green compound leaf of many linear, salty, fleshy leaflets

succulent, branching stem full of aromatic juice

herbaceous stem

up to 60cm (24in)

| Habitat | Moist maritime habitats; European Atlantic Coast | Parts used 🍃 🍃 🌰 🌿 |

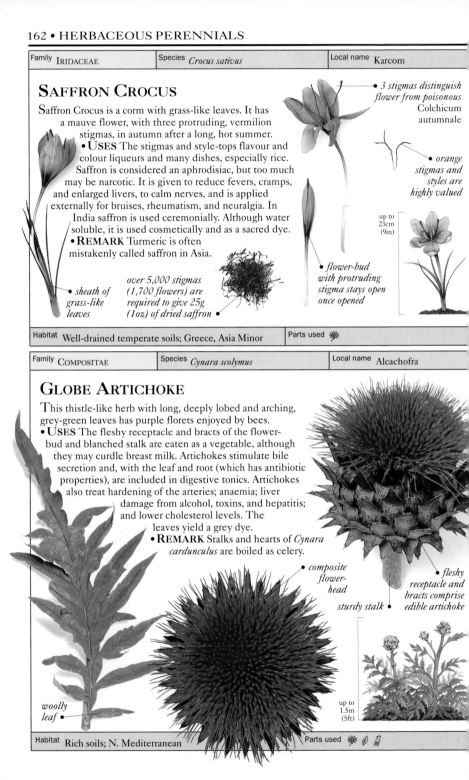

| Family IRIDACEAE | Species *Crocus sativus* | Local name Karcom |

SAFFRON CROCUS

Saffron Crocus is a corm with grass-like leaves. It has
a mauve flower, with three protruding, vermilion
stigmas, in autumn after a long, hot summer.
• **USES** The stigmas and style-tops flavour and
colour liqueurs and many dishes, especially rice.
Saffron is considered an aphrodisiac, but too much
may be narcotic. It is given to reduce fevers, cramps,
and enlarged livers, to calm nerves, and is applied
externally for bruises, rheumatism, and neuralgia. In
India saffron is used ceremonially. Although water
soluble, it is used cosmetically and as a sacred dye.
• **REMARK** Turmeric is often
mistakenly called saffron in Asia.

*• 3 stigmas distinguish
flower from poisonous
Colchicum
autumnale*

*• orange
stigmas and
styles are
highly valued*

up to
23cm
(9in)

*• flower-bud
with protruding
stigma stays open
once opened*

*• sheath of
grass-like
leaves*

*over 5,000 stigmas
(1,700 flowers) are
required to give 25g
(1oz) of dried saffron •*

| Habitat Well-drained temperate soils; Greece, Asia Minor | Parts used ❋ |

| Family COMPOSITAE | Species *Cynara scolymus* | Local name Alcachofra |

GLOBE ARTICHOKE

This thistle-like herb with long, deeply lobed and arching,
grey-green leaves has purple florets enjoyed by bees.
• **USES** The fleshy receptacle and bracts of the flower-
bud and blanched stalk are eaten as a vegetable, although
they may curdle breast milk. Artichokes stimulate bile
secretion and, with the leaf and root (which has antibiotic
properties), are included in digestive tonics. Artichokes
also treat hardening of the arteries; anaemia; liver
damage from alcohol, toxins, and hepatitis;
and lower cholesterol levels. The
leaves yield a grey dye.
• **REMARK** Stalks and hearts of *Cynara
cardunculus* are boiled as celery.

*• composite
flower-
head*

sturdy stalk •

*• fleshy
receptacle and
bracts comprise
edible artichoke*

up to
1.5m
(5ft)

*woolly
leaf •*

| Habitat Rich soils; N. Mediterranean | Parts used ❋ 🌿 |

Family ZINGIBERACEAE	Species *Curcuma longa*	Local name Yu-chin / Besar

TURMERIC

Turmeric has an aromatic rhizome, large leaves, and yellow flowers with pink bracts.

• **USES** The dried root gives flavour and colour to curry powders, many Indian dishes, and piccalilli, and is sometimes sold as saffron. The young shoots and inflorescences are Thai vegetables. In Chinese medicine the root stimulates circulation, resolves bruises and clots, and is a Thai treatment for cobra venom. Research shows Turmeric strengthens the gall-bladder; inhibits dangerous blood-clotting; reduces some liver toxins and helps it metabolize fats (possibly assisting weight loss); and has an anti-inflammatory, non-steroidal action. Turmeric gives a golden fabric dye, and features in Indian ceremonies.

• **REMARK** Zeodary has reduced cervical cancer in trials, and increased the effectiveness of radiotherapy and chemotherapy.

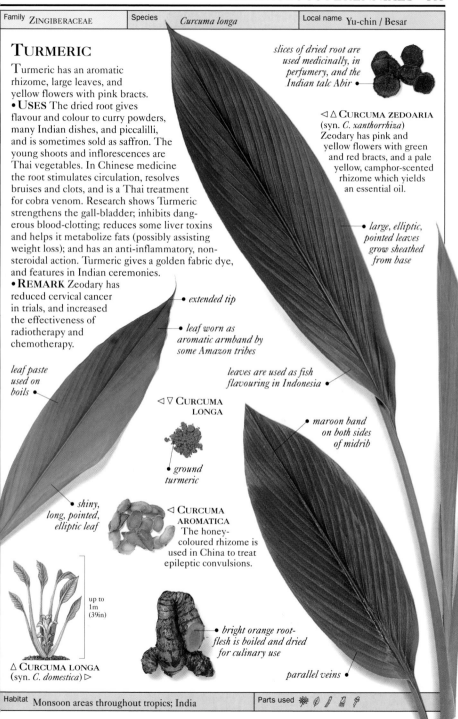

slices of dried root are used medicinally, in perfumery, and the Indian talc Abir •

◁ △ CURCUMA ZEDOARIA (syn. *C. xanthorrhiza*) Zeodary has pink and yellow flowers with green and red bracts, and a pale yellow, camphor-scented rhizome which yields an essential oil.

• large, elliptic, pointed leaves grow sheathed from base

• extended tip

• leaf worn as aromatic armband by some Amazon tribes

leaf paste used on boils •

leaves are used as fish flavouring in Indonesia •

◁ ▽ CURCUMA LONGA

• maroon band on both sides of midrib

• ground turmeric

• shiny, long, pointed, elliptic leaf

◁ CURCUMA AROMATICA The honey-coloured rhizome is used in China to treat epileptic convulsions.

up to 1m (39in)

△ CURCUMA LONGA (syn. *C. domestica*) ▷

• bright orange root-flesh is boiled and dried for culinary use

parallel veins •

Habitat Monsoon areas throughout tropics; India	Parts used 🌼 🍃 🥄 📜 🌾

Family GRAMINEAE	Species *Cymbopogon citratus*	Local name Melissa Grass / Sereh

LEMON GRASS

This aromatic grass has clumped, bulbous stems becoming leaf-blades and a branched panicle of flowers.

• USES The culinary stem and leaf have a distinct lemon flavour. The leaf tea is used for stomachache, diarrhoea, headaches, fevers, and flu, and is antiseptic. The essential oil is used in cosmetics and food, and in aromatherapy to improve circulation and muscle tone. The antiseptic oil treats athlete's foot and acne, and, when sprayed, reduces air-borne infections.

• REMARK *Cymbopogon flexuosus* yields a slightly different Lemon Grass oil *Vervaines des Indes*. *C. martini* leaves yield Palmarosa oil with a gingery-floral scent, said to aid skin cell renewal.

leaf with centre fold

sliced fresh stalks show concentric, sheathed leaves

lower 10–15cm (4–6in) of leek-like stalks have most succulent flavour

△ CYMBOPOGON CITRATUS ▷

◁ CYMBOPOGON NARDUS
Citronella is a coarse grass with lemon-scented stalks used in tropical dishes. Its antiseptic, deodorizing essential oil has various household and cosmetic uses, and deters cats.

long, blue-green grass blades with strong lemon scent

clumped stems become long, pointed blades

roots and root hairs help bind dry soils

up to 1.5m (5ft)

CYMBOPOGON CITRATUS

pale roots

Habitat Open, tropical habitats in dry soil; S. India, Sri Lanka	Parts used

Family CYPERACEAE	Species *Cyperus papyrus*	Local name Egyptian Paper Reed

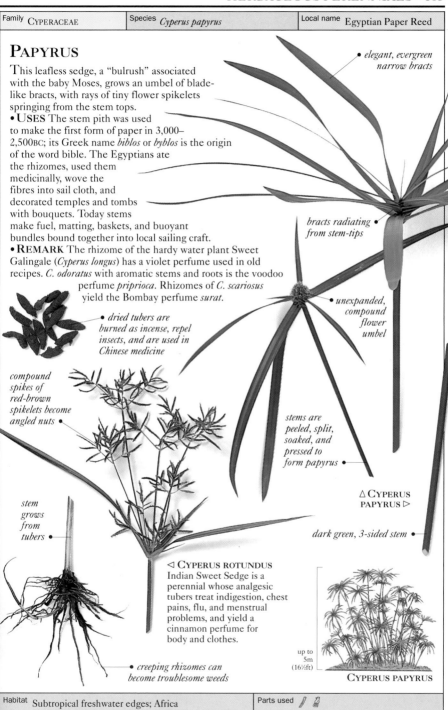

PAPYRUS

This leafless sedge, a "bulrush" associated with the baby Moses, grows an umbel of blade-like bracts, with rays of tiny flower spikelets springing from the stem tops.

• **USES** The stem pith was used to make the first form of paper in 3,000–2,500BC; its Greek name *biblos* or *byblos* is the origin of the word bible. The Egyptians ate the rhizomes, used them medicinally, wove the fibres into sail cloth, and decorated temples and tombs with bouquets. Today stems make fuel, matting, baskets, and buoyant bundles bound together into local sailing craft.

• **REMARK** The rhizome of the hardy water plant Sweet Galingale (*Cyperus longus*) has a violet perfume used in old recipes. *C. odoratus* with aromatic stems and roots is the voodoo perfume *priprioca*. Rhizomes of *C. scariosus* yield the Bombay perfume *surat*.

elegant, evergreen narrow bracts

bracts radiating from stem-tips

unexpanded, compound flower umbel

dried tubers are burned as incense, repel insects, and are used in Chinese medicine

compound spikes of red-brown spikelets become angled nuts

stems are peeled, split, soaked, and pressed to form papyrus

△ CYPERUS PAPYRUS ▷

stem grows from tubers

dark green, 3-sided stem

◁ **CYPERUS ROTUNDUS** Indian Sweet Sedge is a perennial whose analgesic tubers treat indigestion, chest pains, flu, and menstrual problems, and yield a cinnamon perfume for body and clothes.

creeping rhizomes can become troublesome weeds

up to 5m (16½ft)

CYPERUS PAPYRUS

Habitat Subtropical freshwater edges; Africa	Parts used

Family CARYOPHYLLACEAE	Species *Dianthus caryophyllus*	Local name Gillyflower

CLOVE PINK

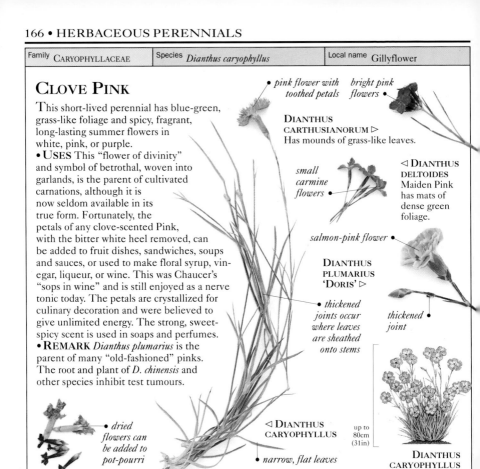

This short-lived perennial has blue-green, grass-like foliage and spicy, fragrant, long-lasting summer flowers in white, pink, or purple.
• USES This "flower of divinity" and symbol of betrothal, woven into garlands, is the parent of cultivated carnations, although it is now seldom available in its true form. Fortunately, the petals of any clove-scented Pink, with the bitter white heel removed, can be added to fruit dishes, sandwiches, soups and sauces, or used to make floral syrup, vinegar, liqueur, or wine. This was Chaucer's "sops in wine" and is still enjoyed as a nerve tonic today. The petals are crystallized for culinary decoration and were believed to give unlimited energy. The strong, sweet-spicy scent is used in soaps and perfumes.
• REMARK *Dianthus plumarius* is the parent of many "old-fashioned" pinks. The root and plant of *D. chinensis* and other species inhibit test tumours.

pink flower with toothed petals

bright pink flowers

DIANTHUS CARTHUSIANORUM ▷
Has mounds of grass-like leaves.

small carmine flowers

◁ **DIANTHUS DELTOIDES**
Maiden Pink has mats of dense green foliage.

salmon-pink flower

DIANTHUS PLUMARIUS 'DORIS' ▷

thickened joints occur where leaves are sheathed onto stems

thickened joint

dried flowers can be added to pot-pourri

◁ **DIANTHUS CARYOPHYLLUS**

narrow, flat leaves

up to 80cm (31in)

DIANTHUS CARYOPHYLLUS

Habitat Well-drained rocky areas, sun; Mediterranean	Parts used ❋ ℘

Family RUTACEAE	Species *Dictamnus albus*	Local name Burning Bush

WHITE DITTANY

Aromatic Dittany has pale roots, large, upright racemes of five-petalled white, pink, or lilac flowers, and star-shaped capsules with black seeds.
• USES The leaves give a digestive, nerve-tonic tea. Flower and root essences flavour liqueurs and perfumes. In homeopathy a leaf and flower tincture treats gynaecological disorders. The diuretic, toxic root causes uterine muscles to contract.
• REMARK All parts are covered with lemon-scented glands which exude sufficient vapour to ignite in hot weather.

compound leaf with heart-shaped terminal leaflet

balsamic-scented glands

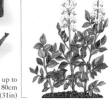

woody stem bases

serrated margin

up to 80cm (31in)

Habitat High altitudes; S.W. Europe, S. & C. Asia	Parts used ❋ ℘ 🍂 ℘

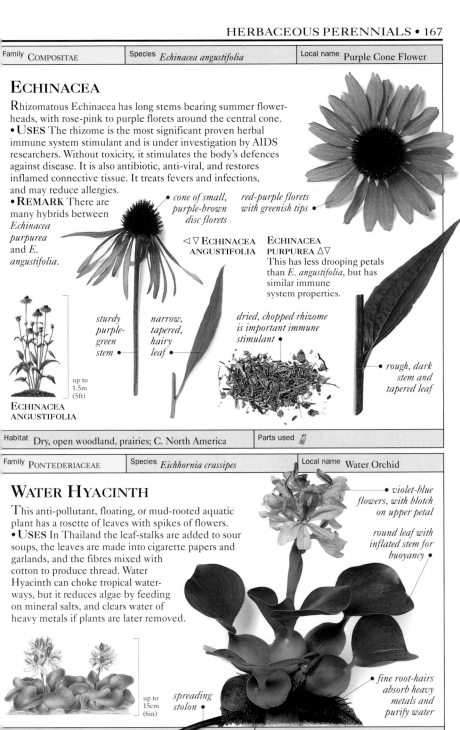

| Family COMPOSITAE | Species *Echinacea angustifolia* | Local name Purple Cone Flower |

ECHINACEA

Rhizomatous Echinacea has long stems bearing summer flower-heads, with rose-pink to purple florets around the central cone.
• **USES** The rhizome is the most significant proven herbal immune system stimulant and is under investigation by AIDS researchers. Without toxicity, it stimulates the body's defences against disease. It is also antibiotic, anti-viral, and restores inflamed connective tissue. It treats fevers and infections, and may reduce allergies.
• **REMARK** There are many hybrids between *Echinacea purpurea* and *E. angustifolia*.

cone of small, purple-brown disc florets •

red-purple florets with greenish tips •

◁ ▽ **ECHINACEA ANGUSTIFOLIA**

ECHINACEA PURPUREA △▽
This has less drooping petals than *E. angustifolia*, but has similar immune system properties.

sturdy purple-green stem •

narrow, tapered, hairy leaf •

dried, chopped rhizome is important immune stimulant •

• rough, dark stem and tapered leaf

up to 1.5m (5ft)

ECHINACEA ANGUSTIFOLIA

| Habitat Dry, open woodland, prairies; C. North America | Parts used 🥔 |

| Family PONTEDERIACEAE | Species *Eichhornia crassipes* | Local name Water Orchid |

WATER HYACINTH

This anti-pollutant, floating, or mud-rooted aquatic plant has a rosette of leaves with spikes of flowers.
• **USES** In Thailand the leaf-stalks are added to sour soups, the leaves are made into cigarette papers and garlands, and the fibres mixed with cotton to produce thread. Water Hyacinth can choke tropical water-ways, but it reduces algae by feeding on mineral salts, and clears water of heavy metals if plants are later removed.

• violet-blue flowers, with blotch on upper petal

round leaf with inflated stem for buoyancy •

• fine root-hairs absorb heavy metals and purify water

up to 15cm (6in)

spreading stolon •

| Habitat Tropical fresh waterways; S. America | Parts used 🥔 🌿 |

Family COMPOSITAE	Species *Eupatorium purpureum*	Local name Gravel Root

SWEET JOE PYE

This stately herb has whorls of three to six leaves which have a faint scent of vanilla or apple peel, and pink flowers in late summer.
• **USES** Named after the native American who cured New Englanders of typhus, the rhizome is still used to induce fever-breaking sweats. It tones the reproductive system, eases menstrual cramps, and helps gout, rheumatism, and kidney and urinary problems. The seeds yield a pink textile dye, used by native Americans.
• **REMARK** Compounds of *Eupatorium perfoliatum*, *E. cannabinum*, and possibly *E. purpureum* have exhibited anti-tumour activity. The green parts of *E. odoratum* are used in China to destroy parasitic worms and to stop bleeding.

up to 3m (10ft)

EUPATORIUM PURPUREUM

panicles of white to mauve florets

divided leaves in opposite pairs

◁ EUPATORIUM CANNABINIUM ▷
The aerial parts of Hemp Agrimony are tonic, diuretic, and stimulate the immune system.

rough, ridged stem from spreading rootstock

dense clusters of rose-pink flowers

leaves coarsely toothed and softly hairy

serrated margin

whorls of 3–6 pointed leaves

◁ EUPATORIUM PURPUREUM ▽

tough rhizome

pairs of leaves

shavings of cream root flesh

EUPATORIUM PERFOLIATUM ▽▷
Boneset bears purplish white florets and narrow, wrinkled leaves with yellow resin dots.

treats "bone-aching" flu and catarrh

dried root and rhizome are diuretic, tonic, stimulant, and anti-rheumatic

bruised leaf has faint apple-peel scent

maroon stems

EUPATORIUM PURPUREUM ▷

dried aerial parts

Habitat Moderately fertile woodland; E. Canada, USA	Parts used

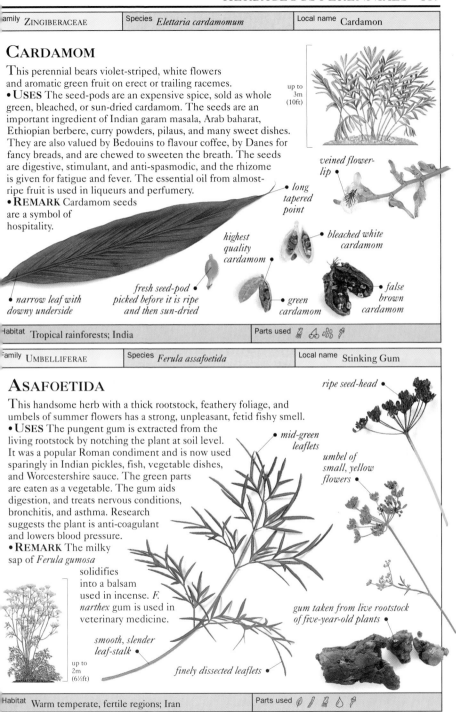

| Family ZINGIBERACEAE | Species *Elettaria cardamomum* | Local name Cardamon |

CARDAMOM

This perennial bears violet-striped, white flowers
and aromatic green fruit on erect or trailing racemes.
• **USES** The seed-pods are an expensive spice, sold as whole
green, bleached, or sun-dried cardamom. The seeds are an
important ingredient of Indian garam masala, Arab baharat,
Ethiopian berbere, curry powders, pilaus, and many sweet dishes.
They are also valued by Bedouins to flavour coffee, by Danes for
fancy breads, and are chewed to sweeten the breath. The seeds
are digestive, stimulant, and anti-spasmodic, and the rhizome
is given for fatigue and fever. The essential oil from almost-
ripe fruit is used in liqueurs and perfumery.
• **REMARK** Cardamom seeds
are a symbol of
hospitality.

up to
3m
(10ft)

veined flower-
lip •

long
tapered
point

highest
quality
cardamom •

• bleached white
cardamom

fresh seed-pod •
picked before it is ripe
and then sun-dried

• narrow leaf with
downy underside

• green
cardamom

• false
brown
cardamom

| Habitat Tropical rainforests; India | Parts used |

| Family UMBELLIFERAE | Species *Ferula assafoetida* | Local name Stinking Gum |

ASAFOETIDA

ripe seed-head •

This handsome herb with a thick rootstock, feathery foliage, and
umbels of summer flowers has a strong, unpleasant, fetid fishy smell.
• **USES** The pungent gum is extracted from the
living rootstock by notching the plant at soil level.
It was a popular Roman condiment and is now used
sparingly in Indian pickles, fish, vegetable dishes,
and Worcestershire sauce. The green parts
are eaten as a vegetable. The gum aids
digestion, and treats nervous conditions,
bronchitis, and asthma. Research
suggests the plant is anti-coagulant
and lowers blood pressure.
• **REMARK** The milky
sap of *Ferula gumosa*
solidifies
into a balsam
used in incense. *F.
narthex* gum is used in
veterinary medicine.

• mid-green
leaflets

umbel of
small, yellow
flowers •

gum taken from live rootstock
of five-year-old plants •

smooth, slender
leaf-stalk •

finely dissected leaflets •

up to
2m
(6½ft)

| Habitat Warm temperate, fertile regions; Iran | Parts used |

Family ROSACEAE	Species *Filipendula ulmaria*	Local name Queen of the Meadow

MEADOWSWEET

This herb has upright stems of wintergreen-scented, divided leaves, topped by frothy corymbs of almond-scented cream flowers.
• **USES** The flowers give an almond flavour to mead, herb wines, jam, and stewed fruit. Dried flowers scent linen and yield an astringent skin tonic. Flower-buds contain salicylic acid from which aspirin was synthesized, but the herb as a whole is gentler on the stomach. Herbalists use flower tea for stomach ulcers and headaches, as an antiseptic diuretic, and for feverish colds, diarrhoea, and heartburn; its mild painkilling, anti-inflammatory action treats rheumatism. The flowering tops yield a greenish yellow dye, the leaf and stem a blue dye, and the root a black dye.
• **REMARK** Meadowsweet was sacred to the Druids and the favoured strewing herb of Elizabeth I.

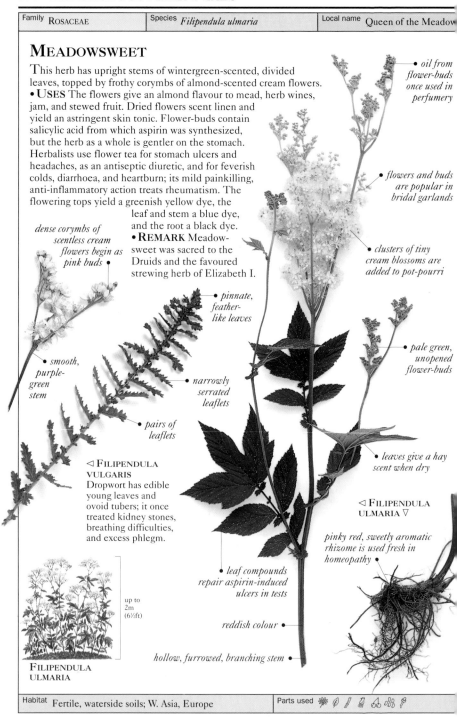

oil from flower-buds once used in perfumery

flowers and buds are popular in bridal garlands

clusters of tiny cream blossoms are added to pot-pourri

dense corymbs of scentless cream flowers begin as pink buds

pinnate, feather-like leaves

pale green, unopened flower-buds

smooth, purple-green stem

narrowly serrated leaflets

pairs of leaflets

leaves give a hay scent when dry

◁ FILIPENDULA VULGARIS
Dropwort has edible young leaves and ovoid tubers; it once treated kidney stones, breathing difficulties, and excess phlegm.

◁ FILIPENDULA ULMARIA ▽

pinky red, sweetly aromatic rhizome is used fresh in homeopathy

leaf compounds repair aspirin-induced ulcers in tests

up to 2m (6½ft)

reddish colour

FILIPENDULA ULMARIA

hollow, furrowed, branching stem

Habitat Fertile, waterside soils; W. Asia, Europe	Parts used

| amily UMBELLIFERAE | Species *Foeniculum vulgare* | Local name Finocchio / Fenouil |

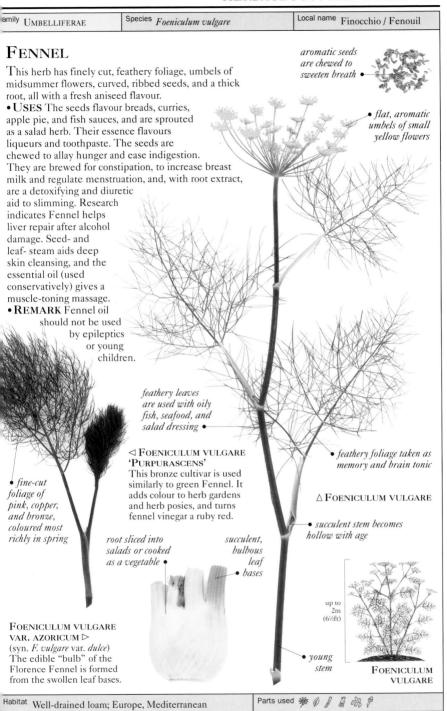

FENNEL

This herb has finely cut, feathery foliage, umbels of midsummer flowers, curved, ribbed seeds, and a thick root, all with a fresh aniseed flavour.

• **USES** The seeds flavour breads, curries, apple pie, and fish sauces, and are sprouted as a salad herb. Their essence flavours liqueurs and toothpaste. The seeds are chewed to allay hunger and ease indigestion. They are brewed for constipation, to increase breast milk and regulate menstruation, and, with root extract, are a detoxifying and diuretic aid to slimming. Research indicates Fennel helps liver repair after alcohol damage. Seed- and leaf- steam aids deep skin cleansing, and the essential oil (used conservatively) gives a muscle-toning massage.

• **REMARK** Fennel oil should not be used by epileptics or young children.

aromatic seeds are chewed to sweeten breath •

• flat, aromatic umbels of small yellow flowers

feathery leaves are used with oily fish, seafood, and salad dressing •

◁ **FOENICULUM VULGARE 'PURPURASCENS'**
This bronze cultivar is used similarly to green Fennel. It adds colour to herb gardens and herb posies, and turns fennel vinegar a ruby red.

• feathery foliage taken as memory and brain tonic

△ **FOENICULUM VULGARE**

• fine-cut foliage of pink, copper, and bronze, coloured most richly in spring

• succulent stem becomes hollow with age

root sliced into salads or cooked as a vegetable •

succulent, bulbous leaf • bases

up to 2m (6½ft)

FOENICULUM VULGARE VAR. AZORICUM ▷
(syn. *F. vulgare* var. *dulce*)
The edible "bulb" of the Florence Fennel is formed from the swollen leaf bases.

• young stem

FOENICULUM VULGARE

| Habitat Well-drained loam; Europe, Mediterranean | Parts used ❋ 🌢 ✏ 🎋 🌰 ⚘ |

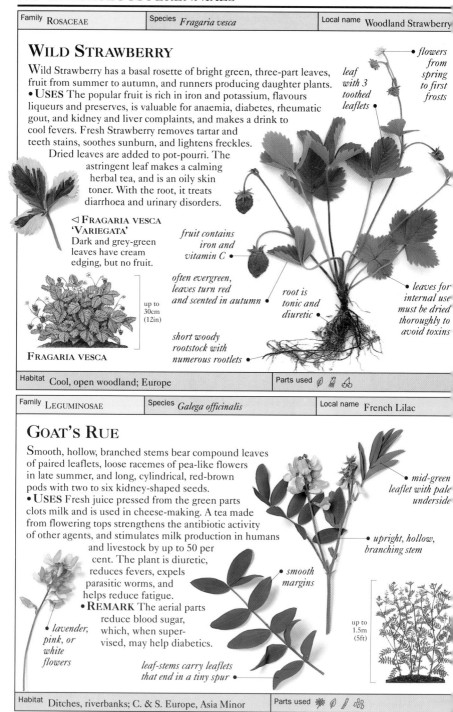

| Family ROSACEAE | Species *Fragaria vesca* | Local name Woodland Strawberry |

WILD STRAWBERRY

Wild Strawberry has a basal rosette of bright green, three-part leaves, fruit from summer to autumn, and runners producing daughter plants.
• **USES** The popular fruit is rich in iron and potassium, flavours liqueurs and preserves, is valuable for anaemia, diabetes, rheumatic gout, and kidney and liver complaints, and makes a drink to cool fevers. Fresh Strawberry removes tartar and teeth stains, soothes sunburn, and lightens freckles.
Dried leaves are added to pot-pourri. The astringent leaf makes a calming herbal tea, and is an oily skin toner. With the root, it treats diarrhoea and urinary disorders.

◁ **FRAGARIA VESCA 'VARIEGATA'**
Dark and grey-green leaves have cream edging, but no fruit.

leaf with 3 toothed leaflets •

flowers from spring to first frosts

fruit contains iron and vitamin C •

often evergreen, leaves turn red and scented in autumn •

root is tonic and diuretic •

leaves for internal use must be dried thoroughly to avoid toxins

short woody rootstock with numerous rootlets •

up to 30cm (12in)

FRAGARIA VESCA

| Habitat Cool, open woodland; Europe | Parts used 🌿 🍓 ⚘ |

| Family LEGUMINOSAE | Species *Galega officinalis* | Local name French Lilac |

GOAT'S RUE

Smooth, hollow, branched stems bear compound leaves of paired leaflets, loose racemes of pea-like flowers in late summer, and long, cylindrical, red-brown pods with two to six kidney-shaped seeds.
• **USES** Fresh juice pressed from the green parts clots milk and is used in cheese-making. A tea made from flowering tops strengthens the antibiotic activity of other agents, and stimulates milk production in humans and livestock by up to 50 per cent. The plant is diuretic, reduces fevers, expels parasitic worms, and helps reduce fatigue.
• **REMARK** The aerial parts reduce blood sugar, which, when supervised, may help diabetics.

mid-green leaflet with pale underside

upright, hollow, branching stem

smooth margins

lavender, pink, or white flowers

leaf-stems carry leaflets that end in a tiny spur •

up to 1.5m (5ft)

| Habitat Ditches, riverbanks; C. & S. Europe, Asia Minor | Parts used ✿ 🌿 ⚘ 🌱 |

| Family RUBIACEAE | Species *Galium odoratum* | Local name Waldmeister |

SWEET WOODRUFF

This woodland herb has a red-brown, creeping rootstock, attractive "ruffs" of six to nine elliptic leaves at intervals on the stem, and small clusters of brilliant white flowers in late spring.
• **USES** The sweet, new-mown-hay scent of coumarin in the leaves develops only as the leaves dry out, so they must be picked several hours before use. They are added to liqueurs, white wines, and German May Bowl punch. They also flavour sorbets, fruit salads, and aromatic snuff. The refreshing leaf tea is a diuretic liver tonic, gives anti-spasmodic relief for stomach pains, and is a gentle sedative for children and elderly people. Bruised fresh leaves are an anti-coagulant for wounds. Dried leaves deter insects, act as a fixative in pot-pourri, and scent linen.
  • **REMARK** All *Galium* rhizomes yield the red dye characteristic of the Rubiaceae family. The powdered herb of *Galium verum* soothes red, inflamed skin.

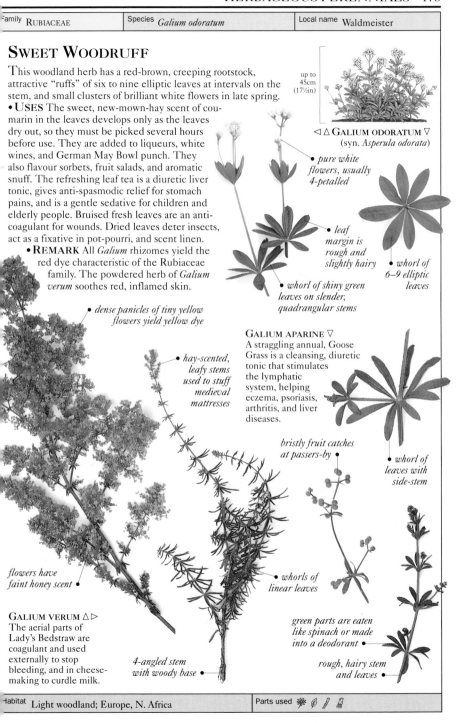

up to 45cm (17½in)

◁ △ **GALIUM ODORATUM** ▽
(syn. *Asperula odorata*)

• *pure white flowers, usually 4-petalled*

• *leaf margin is rough and slightly hairy*

• *whorl of 6–9 elliptic leaves*

• *whorl of shiny green leaves on slender, quadrangular stems*

• *dense panicles of tiny yellow flowers yield yellow dye*

GALIUM APARINE ▽
A straggling annual, Goose Grass is a cleansing, diuretic tonic that stimulates the lymphatic system, helping eczema, psoriasis, arthritis, and liver diseases.

• *hay-scented, leafy stems used to stuff medieval mattresses*

• *bristly fruit catches at passers-by*

• *whorl of leaves with side-stem*

• *flowers have faint honey scent*

GALIUM VERUM △ ▷
The aerial parts of Lady's Bedstraw are coagulant and used externally to stop bleeding, and in cheese-making to curdle milk.

• *4-angled stem with woody base*

• *whorls of linear leaves*

• *green parts are eaten like spinach or made into a deodorant*

• *rough, hairy stem and leaves*

| Habitat Light woodland; Europe, N. Africa | Parts used ✳ 🌿 ✒ 🥄 |

Family GERANIACEAE	Species *Geranium macrorrhizum*	Local name Bigroot Geranium

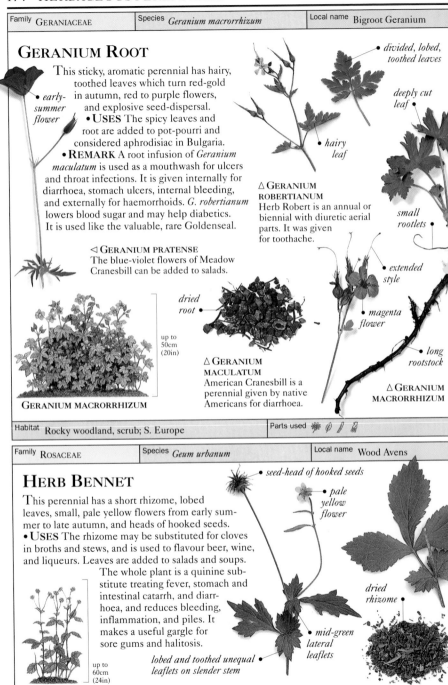

GERANIUM ROOT

This sticky, aromatic perennial has hairy, toothed leaves which turn red-gold in autumn, red to purple flowers, and explosive seed-dispersal.

• early-summer flower

• **USES** The spicy leaves and root are added to pot-pourri and considered aphrodisiac in Bulgaria.

• **REMARK** A root infusion of *Geranium maculatum* is used as a mouthwash for ulcers and throat infections. It is given internally for diarrhoea, stomach ulcers, internal bleeding, and externally for haemorrhoids. *G. robertianum* lowers blood sugar and may help diabetics. It is used like the valuable, rare Goldenseal.

◁ **GERANIUM PRATENSE**
The blue-violet flowers of Meadow Cranesbill can be added to salads.

• divided, lobed, toothed leaves

• deeply cut leaf

• hairy leaf

△ **GERANIUM ROBERTIANUM**
Herb Robert is an annual or biennial with diuretic aerial parts. It was given for toothache.

• small rootlets

• extended style

• magenta flower

dried root •

up to 50cm (20in)

△ **GERANIUM MACULATUM**
American Cranesbill is a perennial given by native Americans for diarrhoea.

• long rootstock

GERANIUM MACRORRHIZUM

△ **GERANIUM MACRORRHIZUM**

Habitat Rocky woodland, scrub; S. Europe	Parts used ✹ ⊘ ∥ ▦

Family ROSACEAE	Species *Geum urbanum*	Local name Wood Avens

HERB BENNET

This perennial has a short rhizome, lobed leaves, small, pale yellow flowers from early summer to late autumn, and heads of hooked seeds.
• **USES** The rhizome may be substituted for cloves in broths and stews, and is used to flavour beer, wine, and liqueurs. Leaves are added to salads and soups. The whole plant is a quinine substitute treating fever, stomach and intestinal catarrh, and diarrhoea, and reduces bleeding, inflammation, and piles. It makes a useful gargle for sore gums and halitosis.

• seed-head of hooked seeds

• pale yellow flower

dried rhizome •

• mid-green lateral leaflets

up to 60cm (24in)

lobed and toothed unequal leaflets on slender stem •

Habitat Woodland; Europe	Parts used ✹ ⊘ ∥ ▦

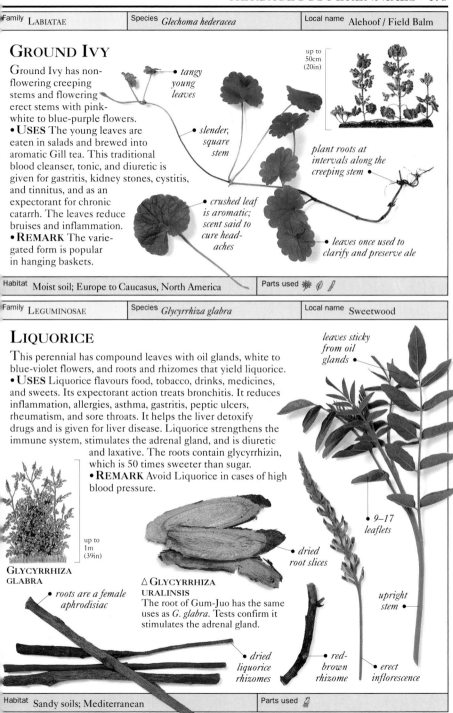

Family LABIATAE	Species *Glechoma hederacea*	Local name Alehoof / Field Balm

GROUND IVY

Ground Ivy has non-flowering creeping stems and flowering erect stems with pink-white to blue-purple flowers.

• **USES** The young leaves are eaten in salads and brewed into aromatic Gill tea. This traditional blood cleanser, tonic, and diuretic is given for gastritis, kidney stones, cystitis, and tinnitus, and as an expectorant for chronic catarrh. The leaves reduce bruises and inflammation.

• **REMARK** The variegated form is popular in hanging baskets.

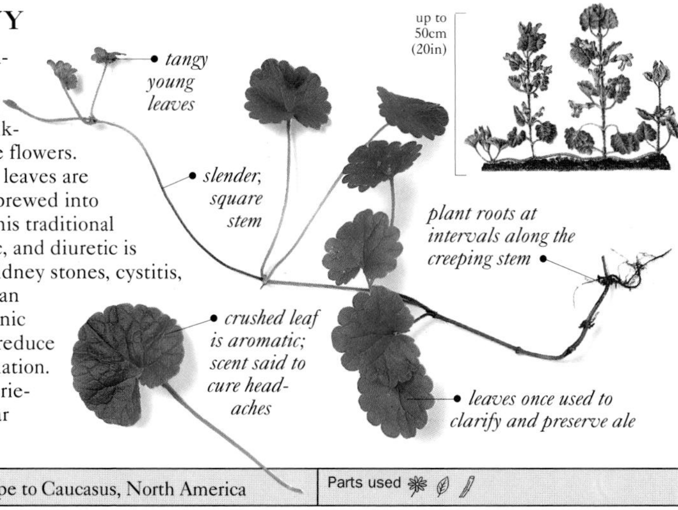
up to
50cm
(20in)
tangy young leaves
slender, square stem
plant roots at intervals along the creeping stem
crushed leaf is aromatic; scent said to cure headaches
leaves once used to clarify and preserve ale

Habitat Moist soil; Europe to Caucasus, North America	Parts used

Family LEGUMINOSAE	Species *Glycyrrhiza glabra*	Local name Sweetwood

LIQUORICE

This perennial has compound leaves with oil glands, white to blue-violet flowers, and roots and rhizomes that yield liquorice.

• **USES** Liquorice flavours food, tobacco, drinks, medicines, and sweets. Its expectorant action treats bronchitis. It reduces inflammation, allergies, asthma, gastritis, peptic ulcers, rheumatism, and sore throats. It helps the liver detoxify drugs and is given for liver disease. Liquorice strengthens the immune system, stimulates the adrenal gland, and is diuretic and laxative. The roots contain glycyrrhizin, which is 50 times sweeter than sugar.

• **REMARK** Avoid Liquorice in cases of high blood pressure.

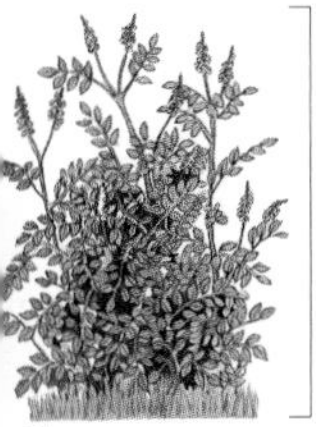
up to
1m
(39in)

GLYCYRRHIZA GLABRA

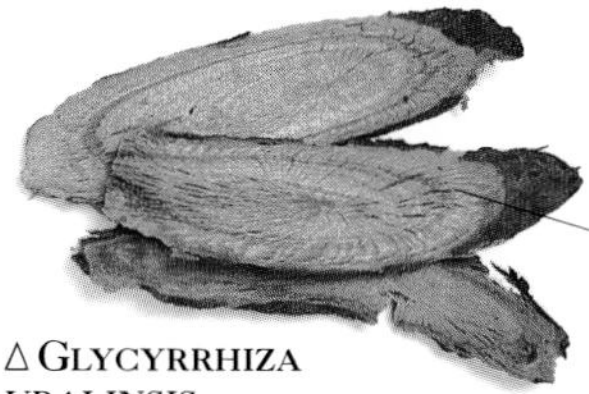
dried root slices

△ GLYCYRRHIZA URALINSIS

The root of Gum-Juo has the same uses as *G. glabra*. Tests confirm it stimulates the adrenal gland.

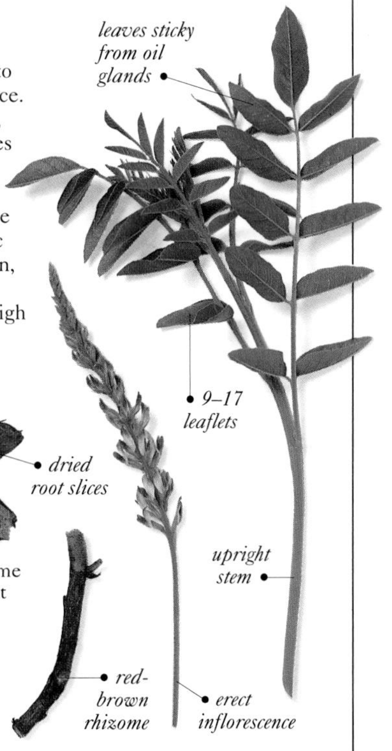
leaves sticky from oil glands
9–17 leaflets
upright stem
erect inflorescence
red-brown rhizome

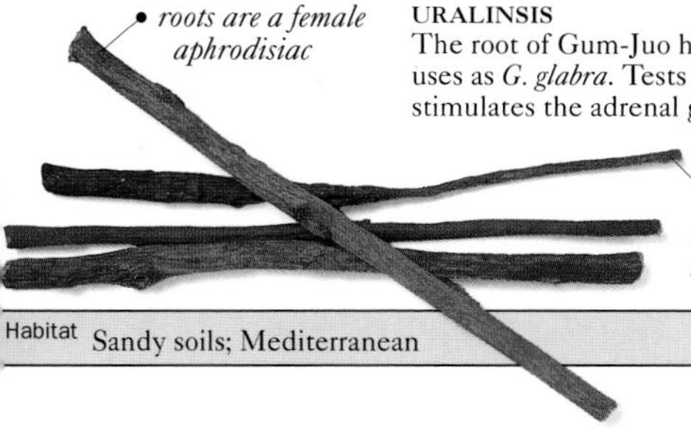
roots are a female aphrodisiac
dried liquorice rhizomes

Habitat Sandy soils; Mediterranean	Parts used

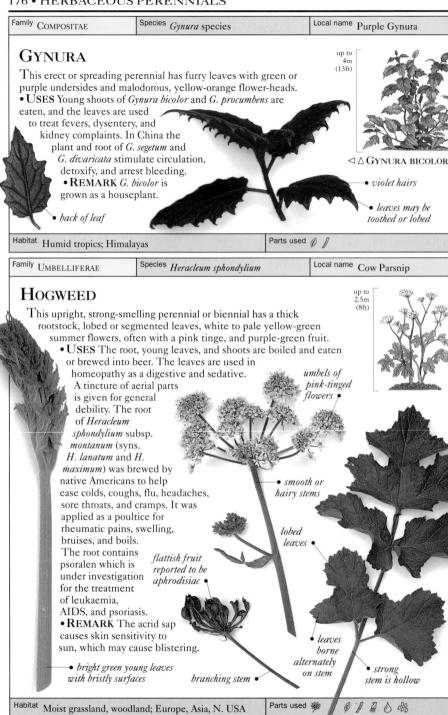

| Family COMPOSITAE | Species *Gynura* species | Local name Purple Gynura |

GYNURA

up to
4m
(13ft)

This erect or spreading perennial has furry leaves with green or purple undersides and malodorous, yellow-orange flower-heads.
• **USES** Young shoots of *Gynura bicolor* and *G. procumbens* are eaten, and the leaves are used to treat fevers, dysentery, and kidney complaints. In China the plant and root of *G. segetum* and *G. divaricata* stimulate circulation, detoxify, and arrest bleeding.
• **REMARK** *G. bicolor* is grown as a houseplant.

◁ △ GYNURA BICOLOR

• *violet hairs*

• *leaves may be toothed or lobed*

• *back of leaf*

| Habitat Humid tropics; Himalayas | Parts used 🌿 🍃 |

| Family UMBELLIFERAE | Species *Heracleum sphondylium* | Local name Cow Parsnip |

HOGWEED

up to
2.5m
(8ft)

This upright, strong-smelling perennial or biennial has a thick rootstock, lobed or segmented leaves, white to pale yellow-green summer flowers, often with a pink tinge, and purple-green fruit.
• **USES** The root, young leaves, and shoots are boiled and eaten or brewed into beer. The leaves are used in homeopathy as a digestive and sedative. A tincture of aerial parts is given for general debility. The root of *Heracleum sphondylium* subsp. *montanum* (syns. *H. lanatum* and *H. maximum*) was brewed by native Americans to help ease colds, coughs, flu, headaches, sore throats, and cramps. It was applied as a poultice for rheumatic pains, swelling, bruises, and boils. The root contains psoralen which is under investigation for the treatment of leukaemia, AIDS, and psoriasis.
• **REMARK** The acrid sap causes skin sensitivity to sun, which may cause blistering.

umbels of pink-tinged flowers

• *smooth or hairy stems*

lobed leaves •

flattish fruit reported to be aphrodisiac •

• *leaves borne alternately on stem*

• *strong stem is hollow*

• *bright green young leaves with bristly surfaces*

branching stem •

| Habitat Moist grassland, woodland; Europe, Asia, N. USA | Parts used 🌼 🌿 🍃 🥄 💧 ✿ |

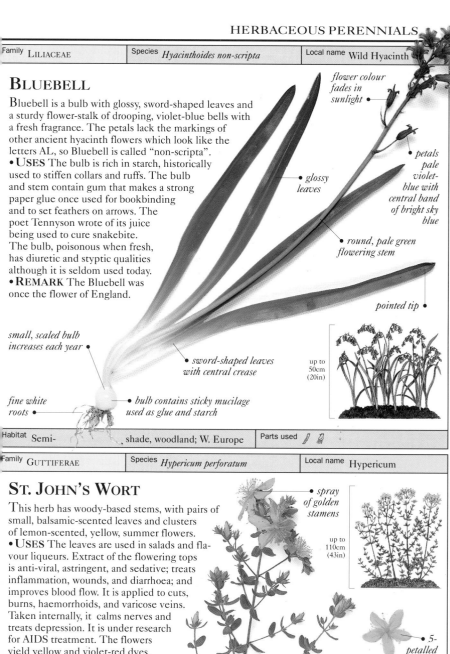

| Family | LILIACEAE | Species | *Hyacinthoides non-scripta* | Local name | Wild Hyacinth |

BLUEBELL

Bluebell is a bulb with glossy, sword-shaped leaves and a sturdy flower-stalk of drooping, violet-blue bells with a fresh fragrance. The petals lack the markings of other ancient hyacinth flowers which look like the letters AL, so Bluebell is called "non-scripta".
• **USES** The bulb is rich in starch, historically used to stiffen collars and ruffs. The bulb and stem contain gum that makes a strong paper glue once used for bookbinding and to set feathers on arrows. The poet Tennyson wrote of its juice being used to cure snakebite. The bulb, poisonous when fresh, has diuretic and styptic qualities although it is seldom used today.
• **REMARK** The Bluebell was once the flower of England.

flower colour fades in sunlight •

• petals pale violet-blue with central band of bright sky blue

• glossy leaves

• round, pale green flowering stem

• pointed tip

small, scaled bulb increases each year •

• sword-shaped leaves with central crease

up to 50cm (20in)

fine white roots •

• bulb contains sticky mucilage used as glue and starch

| Habitat | Semi-shade, woodland; W. Europe | Parts used | 〵 〴 |

| Family | GUTTIFERAE | Species | *Hypericum perforatum* | Local name | Hypericum |

ST. JOHN'S WORT

This herb has woody-based stems, with pairs of small, balsamic-scented leaves and clusters of lemon-scented, yellow, summer flowers.
• **USES** The leaves are used in salads and flavour liqueurs. Extract of the flowering tops is anti-viral, astringent, and sedative; treats inflammation, wounds, and diarrhoea; and improves blood flow. It is applied to cuts, burns, haemorrhoids, and varicose veins. Taken internally, it calms nerves and treats depression. It is under research for AIDS treatment. The flowers yield yellow and violet-red dyes.
• **REMARK** Some consider it unsafe as it can cause dermatitis.

• spray of golden stamens

up to 110cm (43in)

• 5-petalled flower

scented petal •

oil glands along edges •

leaf has translucent oil glands which resemble tiny holes •

| Habitat | Semi-dry soils; Europe to C. China | Parts used | ❋ 〵 〴 ⚬⚬ |

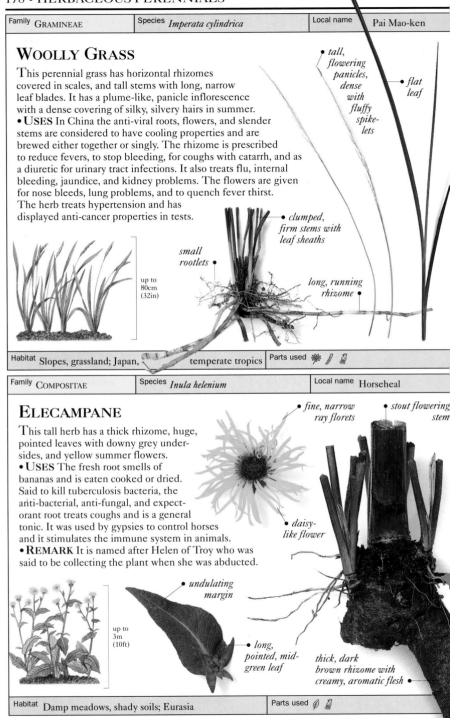

Family GRAMINEAE	Species *Imperata cylindrica*	Local name Pai Mao-ken

WOOLLY GRASS

This perennial grass has horizontal rhizomes
covered in scales, and tall stems with long, narrow
leaf blades. It has a plume-like, panicle inflorescence
with a dense covering of silky, silvery hairs in summer.
• USES In China the anti-viral roots, flowers, and slender
stems are considered to have cooling properties and are
brewed either together or singly. The rhizome is prescribed
to reduce fevers, to stop bleeding, for coughs with catarrh, and as
a diuretic for urinary tract infections. It also treats flu, internal
bleeding, jaundice, and kidney problems. The flowers are given
for nose bleeds, lung problems, and to quench fever thirst.
The herb treats hypertension and has
displayed anti-cancer properties in tests.

• *tall, flowering panicles, dense with fluffy spike-lets*

• *flat leaf*

• *clumped, firm stems with leaf sheaths*

small rootlets •

long, running rhizome •

up to 80cm (32in)

Habitat Slopes, grassland; Japan, temperate tropics	Parts used

Family COMPOSITAE	Species *Inula helenium*	Local name Horseheal

ELECAMPANE

This tall herb has a thick rhizome, huge,
pointed leaves with downy grey undersides, and yellow summer flowers.
• USES The fresh root smells of
bananas and is eaten cooked or dried.
Said to kill tuberculosis bacteria, the
anti-bacterial, anti-fungal, and expectorant root treats coughs and is a general
tonic. It was used by gypsies to control horses
and it stimulates the immune system in animals.
• REMARK It is named after Helen of Troy who was
said to be collecting the plant when she was abducted.

• *fine, narrow ray florets*

• *stout flowering stem*

• *daisy-like flower*

• *undulating margin*

• *long, pointed, mid-green leaf*

thick, dark brown rhizome with creamy, aromatic flesh •

up to 3m (10ft)

Habitat Damp meadows, shady soils; Eurasia	Parts used

Family IRIDACEAE	Species *Iris germanica* var. *florentina*	Local name Fleur-de-lis

ORRIS ROOT

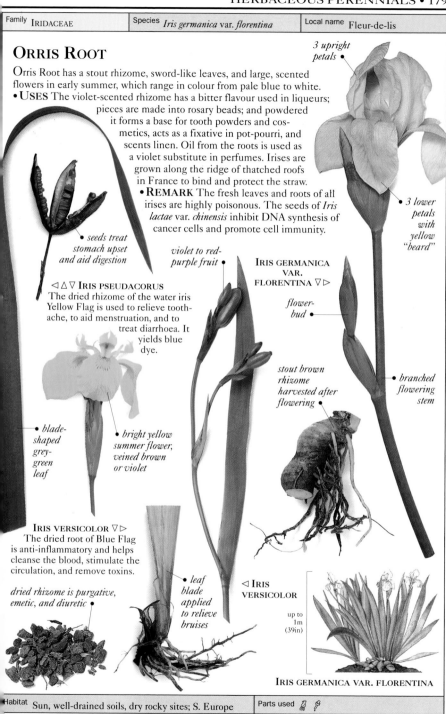

3 upright petals •

Orris Root has a stout rhizome, sword-like leaves, and large, scented flowers in early summer, which range in colour from pale blue to white.
• **USES** The violet-scented rhizome has a bitter flavour used in liqueurs; pieces are made into rosary beads; and powdered it forms a base for tooth powders and cosmetics, acts as a fixative in pot-pourri, and scents linen. Oil from the roots is used as a violet substitute in perfumes. Irises are grown along the ridge of thatched roofs in France to bind and protect the straw.
• **REMARK** The fresh leaves and roots of all irises are highly poisonous. The seeds of *Iris lactae* var. *chinensis* inhibit DNA synthesis of cancer cells and promote cell immunity.

• 3 lower petals with yellow "beard"

• seeds treat stomach upset and aid digestion

violet to red-purple fruit •

◁△▽ **IRIS PSEUDACORUS**
The dried rhizome of the water iris Yellow Flag is used to relieve toothache, to aid menstruation, and to treat diarrhoea. It yields blue dye.

IRIS GERMANICA VAR. FLORENTINA ▽▷

flower-bud •

stout brown rhizome harvested after flowering •

• branched flowering stem

• blade-shaped grey-green leaf

• bright yellow summer flower, veined brown or violet

IRIS VERSICOLOR ▽▷
The dried root of Blue Flag is anti-inflammatory and helps cleanse the blood, stimulate the circulation, and remove toxins.

dried rhizome is purgative, emetic, and diuretic •

• leaf blade applied to relieve bruises

◁ **IRIS VERSICOLOR**

up to 1m (39in)

IRIS GERMANICA VAR. FLORENTINA

Habitat Sun, well-drained soils, dry rocky sites; S. Europe	Parts used 🍂 🌸

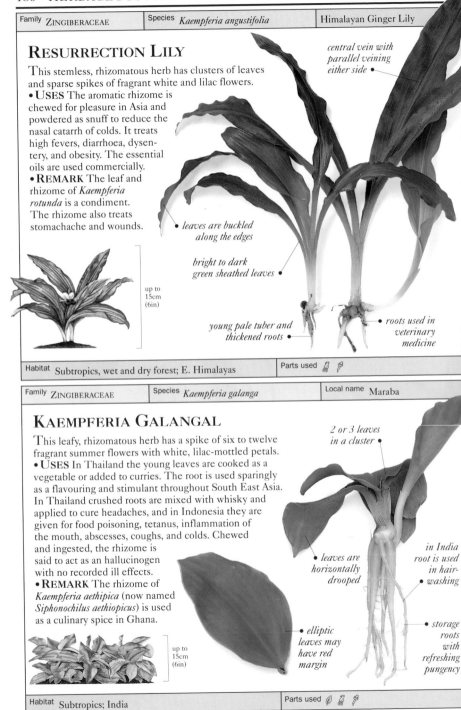

| Family ZINGIBERACEAE | Species *Kaempferia angustifolia* | Himalayan Ginger Lily |

RESURRECTION LILY

This stemless, rhizomatous herb has clusters of leaves and sparse spikes of fragrant white and lilac flowers.
• **USES** The aromatic rhizome is chewed for pleasure in Asia and powdered as snuff to reduce the nasal catarrh of colds. It treats high fevers, diarrhoea, dysentery, and obesity. The essential oils are used commercially.
• **REMARK** The leaf and rhizome of *Kaempferia rotunda* is a condiment. The rhizome also treats stomachache and wounds.

central vein with parallel veining either side •

• leaves are buckled along the edges

bright to dark green sheathed leaves •

up to 15cm (6in)

young pale tuber and thickened roots •

• roots used in veterinary medicine

| Habitat Subtropics, wet and dry forest; E. Himalayas | Parts used |

| Family ZINGIBERACEAE | Species *Kaempferia galanga* | Local name Maraba |

KAEMPFERIA GALANGAL

This leafy, rhizomatous herb has a spike of six to twelve fragrant summer flowers with white, lilac-mottled petals.
• **USES** In Thailand the young leaves are cooked as a vegetable or added to curries. The root is used sparingly as a flavouring and stimulant throughout South East Asia. In Thailand crushed roots are mixed with whisky and applied to cure headaches, and in Indonesia they are given for food poisoning, tetanus, inflammation of the mouth, abscesses, coughs, and colds. Chewed and ingested, the rhizome is said to act as an hallucinogen with no recorded ill effects.
• **REMARK** The rhizome of *Kaempferia aethipica* (now named *Siphonochilus aethiopicus*) is used as a culinary spice in Ghana.

2 or 3 leaves in a cluster •

• leaves are horizontally drooped

in India root is used in hair-washing •

• elliptic leaves may have red margin

• storage roots with refreshing pungency

up to 15cm (6in)

| Habitat Subtropics; India | Parts used |

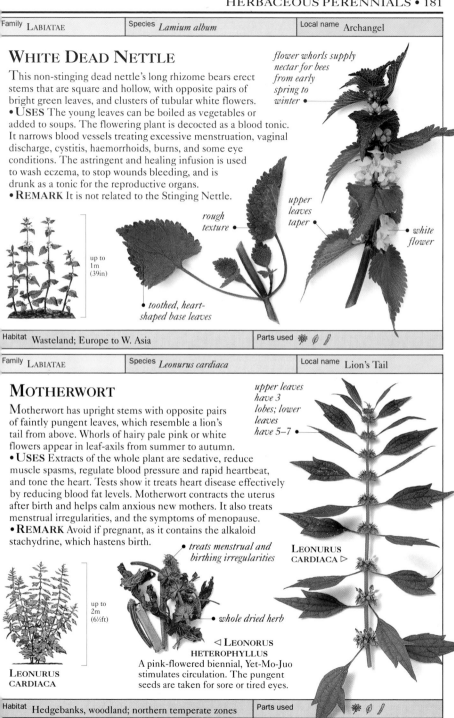

Family LABIATAE	Species *Lamium album*	Local name Archangel

WHITE DEAD NETTLE

This non-stinging dead nettle's long rhizome bears erect stems that are square and hollow, with opposite pairs of bright green leaves, and clusters of tubular white flowers.
• USES The young leaves can be boiled as vegetables or added to soups. The flowering plant is decocted as a blood tonic. It narrows blood vessels treating excessive menstruation, vaginal discharge, cystitis, haemorrhoids, burns, and some eye conditions. The astringent and healing infusion is used to wash eczema, to stop wounds bleeding, and is drunk as a tonic for the reproductive organs.
• REMARK It is not related to the Stinging Nettle.

flower whorls supply nectar for bees from early spring to winter •

upper leaves taper •

• white flower

rough texture •

up to 1m (39in)

• toothed, heart-shaped base leaves

Habitat Wasteland; Europe to W. Asia	Parts used ✳ ✎ ⫽

Family LABIATAE	Species *Leonurus cardiaca*	Local name Lion's Tail

MOTHERWORT

Motherwort has upright stems with opposite pairs of faintly pungent leaves, which resemble a lion's tail from above. Whorls of hairy pale pink or white flowers appear in leaf-axils from summer to autumn.
• USES Extracts of the whole plant are sedative, reduce muscle spasms, regulate blood pressure and rapid heartbeat, and tone the heart. Tests show it treats heart disease effectively by reducing blood fat levels. Motherwort contracts the uterus after birth and helps calm anxious new mothers. It also treats menstrual irregularities, and the symptoms of menopause.
• REMARK Avoid if pregnant, as it contains the alkaloid stachydrine, which hastens birth.

upper leaves have 3 lobes; lower leaves have 5–7 •

LEONURUS CARDIACA ▷

• treats menstrual and birthing irregularities

• whole dried herb

up to 2m (6½ft)

LEONURUS CARDIACA

◁ LEONURUS HETEROPHYLLUS
A pink-flowered biennial, Yet-Mo-Juo stimulates circulation. The pungent seeds are taken for sore or tired eyes.

Habitat Hedgebanks, woodland; northern temperate zones	Parts used ✳ ✎ ⫽

Family COMPOSITAE	Species *Leucanthemum vulgare*	Local name Moon Daisy

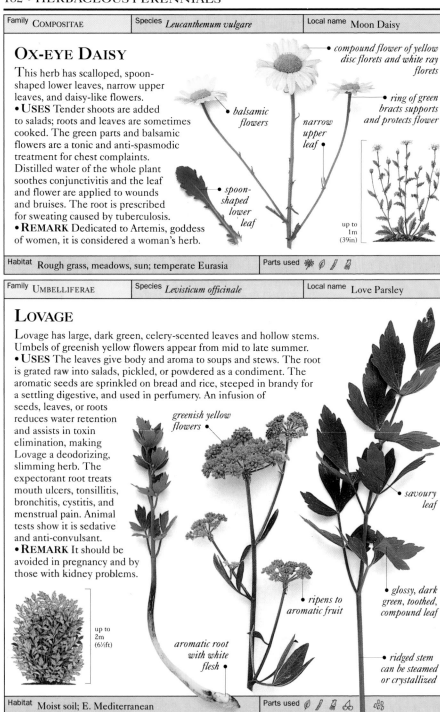

OX-EYE DAISY

This herb has scalloped, spoon-shaped lower leaves, narrow upper leaves, and daisy-like flowers.
• **USES** Tender shoots are added to salads; roots and leaves are sometimes cooked. The green parts and balsamic flowers are a tonic and anti-spasmodic treatment for chest complaints. Distilled water of the whole plant soothes conjunctivitis and the leaf and flower are applied to wounds and bruises. The root is prescribed for sweating caused by tuberculosis.
• **REMARK** Dedicated to Artemis, goddess of women, it is considered a woman's herb.

compound flower of yellow disc florets and white ray florets •

• ring of green bracts supports and protects flower

• *balsamic flowers*

narrow upper leaf •

• *spoon-shaped lower leaf*

up to 1m (39in)

Habitat Rough grass, meadows, sun; temperate Eurasia	Parts used ✱ ✿ ⫽ ⊞

Family UMBELLIFERAE	Species *Levisticum officinale*	Local name Love Parsley

LOVAGE

Lovage has large, dark green, celery-scented leaves and hollow stems. Umbels of greenish yellow flowers appear from mid to late summer.
• **USES** The leaves give body and aroma to soups and stews. The root is grated raw into salads, pickled, or powdered as a condiment. The aromatic seeds are sprinkled on bread and rice, steeped in brandy for a settling digestive, and used in perfumery. An infusion of seeds, leaves, or roots reduces water retention and assists in toxin elimination, making Lovage a deodorizing, slimming herb. The expectorant root treats mouth ulcers, tonsillitis, bronchitis, cystitis, and menstrual pain. Animal tests show it is sedative and anti-convulsant.
• **REMARK** It should be avoided in pregnancy and by those with kidney problems.

greenish yellow flowers •

• *savoury leaf*

• *glossy, dark green, toothed, compound leaf*

• *ripens to aromatic fruit*

up to 2m (6½ft)

aromatic root with white flesh •

• *ridged stem can be steamed or crystallized*

Habitat Moist soil; E. Mediterranean	Parts used ✿ ⫽ ⊞ ⚶ ⚙

Family COMPOSITAE	Species *Liatris spicata*	Local name Button Snakewort

GAY FEATHER

This striking rhizomatous herb has long stems with many thin, radiating leaves, and feathery, compound flowers.
• **USES** The leaves and turpentine-scented root are powdered to repel insects and flavour tobacco. The diuretic, sweat-inducing, and anti-bacterial root is decocted for use as a sore throat gargle and previously treated gonorrhoea.
• **REMARK** *Liatris chapmannii* contains liatrin, which has anti-cancer properties. Vanilla Plant (*L. odoratissima*) leaves contain coumarin which repels moths; they are soothing, and reduce fevers. The root is a strong diuretic.

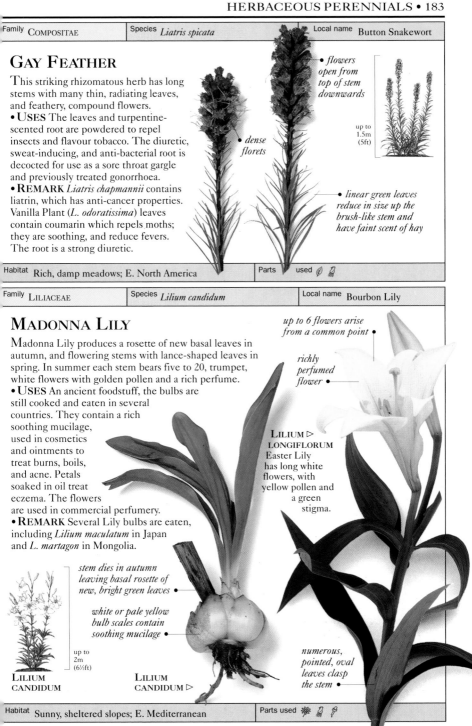

• *flowers open from top of stem downwards*

up to 1.5m (5ft)

• *dense florets*

• *linear green leaves reduce in size up the brush-like stem and have faint scent of hay*

Habitat Rich, damp meadows; E. North America	Parts used 🌿 ✋

Family LILIACEAE	Species *Lilium candidum*	Local name Bourbon Lily

MADONNA LILY

Madonna Lily produces a rosette of new basal leaves in autumn, and flowering stems with lance-shaped leaves in spring. In summer each stem bears five to 20, trumpet, white flowers with golden pollen and a rich perfume.
• **USES** An ancient foodstuff, the bulbs are still cooked and eaten in several countries. They contain a rich soothing mucilage, used in cosmetics and ointments to treat burns, boils, and acne. Petals soaked in oil treat eczema. The flowers are used in commercial perfumery.
• **REMARK** Several Lily bulbs are eaten, including *Lilium maculatum* in Japan and *L. martagon* in Mongolia.

up to 6 flowers arise from a common point •

richly perfumed flower •

LILIUM ▷
LONGIFLORUM
Easter Lily
has long white flowers, with yellow pollen and a green stigma.

stem dies in autumn leaving basal rosette of new, bright green leaves •

white or pale yellow bulb scales contain soothing mucilage •

up to 2m (6½ft)

LILIUM
CANDIDUM

LILIUM
CANDIDUM ▷

numerous, pointed, oval leaves clasp the stem •

Habitat Sunny, sheltered slopes; E. Mediterranean	Parts used 🌸 🌿 🌷

Family CAMPANULACEAE	Species *Lobelia siphilitica*	Local name Blue Cardinal Flower

GIANT LOBELIA

This erect, leafy perennial with lance-shaped leaves
has tubular blue flowers from summer to autumn.
• USES Decocted root was used by Iroquois Indians to
treat syphilis. It is given for fluid retention and is used
in homeopathy for diarrhoea. Powdered root was put in
the bed of arguing Iroquois couples to rekindle love.
• REMARK The leaves and shoots of Cardinal Flower
(*Lobelia cardinalis*) and Indian Tobacco (*L. inflata*) contain
alkaloids that are expectorant and cause vomiting. Cardinal
Flower is milder and a specific treatment for bronchial
spasms. Indian Tobacco is more poisonous with unpleasant
side-effects, but as it stimulates respiration, it is smoked to treat asthma,
bronchitis, and to improve mental clarity. It is added to anti-smoking
mixtures as a nicotine substitute.
Both should be taken in small
doses and given by qualified
medical personnel only.

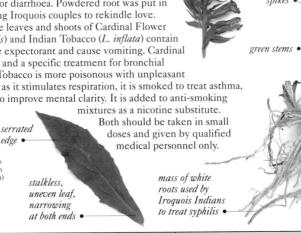

*dense spike
of blue flowers*

*erect leaf-stems bear
flowering
spikes*

green stems

*serrated
edge*

up to
60cm
(24in)

*stalkless,
uneven leaf,
narrowing
at both ends*

*mass of white
roots used by
Iroquois Indians
to treat syphilis*

Habitat Moist woodland, stream banks; E. North America	Parts used

Family LEGUMINOSAE	Species *Lotus corniculatus*	Local name Eggs and Bacon

BIRD'S FOOT TREFOIL

This small perennial herb has a woody taproot, upright
or trailing stems, and a mass of bright yellow spring to
summer flowers which darken to red flecked with orange.
• USES Bird's Foot Trefoil is relatively new to the practice
of herbal medicine and research has found the flowers
have sedative properties. They have been known to
reduce muscle spasms, have been made into a cardiac
tonic, and supply a yellow dye. Indications are that the
whole plant has similar effects to those of Passion Flower
(*Passiflora incarnata*). Externally the plant can be made into a compress to reduce skin inflammation. The flowers are
now included in several herbal preparations for
their therapeutic qualities. The
herb enriches soil as a nitrogen-
fixing, green manure plant.
• REMARK The red streaks
on the bright yellow flowers
give the plant the common
name Eggs and Bacon.

*bright golden
heads of 4–8
flowers*

*good nectar
source*

*pollinated by
bumblebees*

*brown
cylindrical
seed-pods twist
and split to
release oval
brown seeds*

*tiny,
rounded,
smooth
green leaflets*

*long,
upright
flower-
stalk*

up to
40cm
(16in)

angular stem

*hollow or
solid stem*

*compound
leaves*

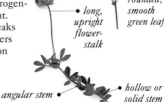

Habitat Pastureland, roadsides, sun; Europe, Asia, Africa	Parts used

Family LEGUMINOSAE	Species *Lupinus polyphyllus*	Local name Many-leaved Lupin

LUPIN

Lupins have long leaf-stems topped by a circle of narrow leaflets, and a handsome flowering raceme.
• USES The powdered seeds of this species and *Lupinus albus* are applied to scabby blemishes, and added to facial steams and exfoliating face masks to reduce oiliness and invigorate tired skin. The seeds of *L. albus*, *L. luteus*, *L. varius*, *L. mutabilis*, and *L. terminis* are roasted to remove toxins and used as flour or coffee substitutes. Lupins fix nitrogen and phosphate and are useful green manure crops. They absorb excess pesticides and other soil poisons.

• REMARK Lupins were planted round Chernobyl, Ukraine, to absorb radiation poison after the nuclear disaster.

• blue, purple, dark pink, or white flowers

• green leaflet may contain toxins

△ LUPINUS PUBESCENS
This annual with a circular, compound leaf is a useful green manure crop.

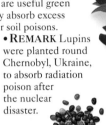

up to 1.5m (5ft)

△ LUPINUS POLYPHYLLUS ▷

• seed-flour used as exfoliant and pore refiner

• sturdy flowering raceme

plant deters rabbits •

Habitat Moist, well-drained grassy sites; W. North America	Parts used

Family LABIATAE	Species *Lycopus europaeus*	Local name Egyptian's Herb

GIPSYWORT

Gipsywort has curled, purple leaves which unfold to green. Hairy, square stems bear whorls of small, white, late-summer flowers with purple dots.
• USES The plant juice gives a black fabric dye, once used by Gipsy fortune tellers to tan their skin and impersonate Egyptians. The aerial parts are astringent and sedative, and a cardiac tonic for anxiety, tuberculosis, and palpitations.
• REMARK The more potent mint-scented *Lycopus virginicus* is sedative, astringent, and narcotic. Both species may have a contraceptive effect.

• pointed, spear-shaped, toothed leaves

• mature green leaf

leaves deeply lobed at base •

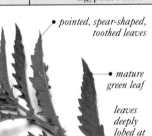

clusters of flowers in leaf-axils •

up to 120cm (47in)

leaves occur in opposite pairs •

Habitat Damp meadows, stream banks; Europe to N.W. Asia	Parts used

Family LYTHRACEAE	Species *Lythrum salicaria*	Local name Spiked Loosestrife

PURPLE LOOSESTRIFE

Purple Loosestrife has a creeping rootstock, angled stems with lance-shaped leaves, and spikes of purple-red flowers.
• **USES** The leaves are eaten as an emergency vegetable and fermented into a mild alcohol. The astringent leaves tighten skin, counter wrinkles, and add sheen to blond hair. The herb adds brightness to eyes and reduces puffiness. It shrinks blood capillaries, reducing over-reddened skin and curbing nose-bleeds. The flowering plant is an intestinal disinfectant, treating diarrhoea and food poisoning. It acts as a typhus antibiotic, a sore throat gargle, and is given for fevers, liver problems, to cleanse sores, and stop bleeding wounds.
• **REMARK** *Lythrum verticillatum* has similar uses, and is planted in pastures to prevent abortion in cows and mares.

spike of long-lasting, late-summer flowers

clustered whorls of purple-red flowers in bract-axils

angled stem covered in soft, fine hairs

opposite leaves with smooth margin

up to 120cm (47in)

narrow, pointed leaves

Habitat Water-retentive land; temperate Europe, Asia, Africa	Parts used ✳ ⊘ ∥

Family MALVACEAE	Species *Malva moschata*	Local name Cut-leaf Mallow

MUSK MALLOW

Musk Mallow has faintly musky, elegantly cut leaves on branching stems and rounded, shallow-lobed base leaves with large, white or pink flowers throughout summer.
• **USES** The flowers are used in salads, and the leaves and young shoots containing vitamins A, B, and C are boiled as a vegetable. The leaves and roots are added to soothing skin ointments and cough syrups.
• **REMARK** Common Mallow is used like Musk Mallow and is more potent. The leaves, flowers, and roots soothe membranes, reduce inflammation, and are given for bronchitis and gastro-intestinal irritations.

long flowering season

5 petals

◁ **MALVA MOSCHATA** ▷

musky scent when bruised

veined mauve flowers

◁ **MALVA SYLVESTRIS**
Common Mallow is a perennial with a pulpy taproot, and emollient, expectorant, vitamin-rich leaves.

up to 60cm (24in)

toothed leaf with soft hairs

a leaf poultice soothes insect bites

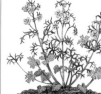

MALVA MOSCHATA

Habitat Wasteland, sun; Europe, N.W. Africa	Parts used ✳ ⊘ ∥ ⚘

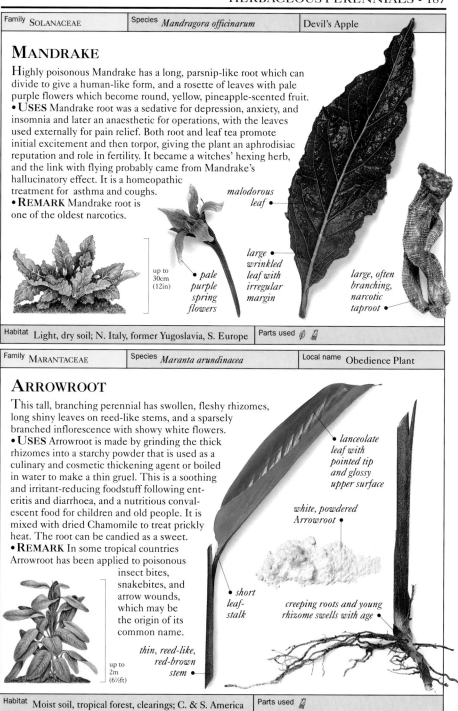

| Family SOLANACEAE | Species *Mandragora officinarum* | Devil's Apple |

MANDRAKE

Highly poisonous Mandrake has a long, parsnip-like root which can divide to give a human-like form, and a rosette of leaves with pale purple flowers which become round, yellow, pineapple-scented fruit.
• **USES** Mandrake root was a sedative for depression, anxiety, and insomnia and later an anaesthetic for operations, with the leaves used externally for pain relief. Both root and leaf tea promote initial excitement and then torpor, giving the plant an aphrodisiac reputation and role in fertility. It became a witches' hexing herb, and the link with flying probably came from Mandrake's hallucinatory effect. It is a homeopathic treatment for asthma and coughs.
• **REMARK** Mandrake root is one of the oldest narcotics.

malodorous leaf •

up to 30cm (12in)

• *pale purple spring flowers*

large • wrinkled leaf with irregular margin

large, often branching, narcotic taproot •

| Habitat Light, dry soil; N. Italy, former Yugoslavia, S. Europe | Parts used 🌿 |

| Family MARANTACEAE | Species *Maranta arundinacea* | Local name Obedience Plant |

ARROWROOT

This tall, branching perennial has swollen, fleshy rhizomes, long shiny leaves on reed-like stems, and a sparsely branched inflorescence with showy white flowers.
• **USES** Arrowroot is made by grinding the thick rhizomes into a starchy powder that is used as a culinary and cosmetic thickening agent or boiled in water to make a thin gruel. This is a soothing and irritant-reducing foodstuff following enteritis and diarrhoea, and a nutritious convalescent food for children and old people. It is mixed with dried Chamomile to treat prickly heat. The root can be candied as a sweet.
• **REMARK** In some tropical countries Arrowroot has been applied to poisonous insect bites, snakebites, and arrow wounds, which may be the origin of its common name.

• *lanceolate leaf with pointed tip and glossy upper surface*

white, powdered Arrowroot •

• *short leaf-stalk*

creeping roots and young rhizome swells with age •

thin, reed-like, red-brown stem •

up to 2m (6½ft)

| Habitat Moist soil, tropical forest, clearings; C. & S. America | Parts used 🌿 |

Family LABIATAE	Species *Marrubium vulgare*	Local name White Horehound

HOREHOUND

Horehound is a woolly herb with a faint scent of Wormwood, hairy leaves, and flowering stems with whorls of small white blossoms.

• **USES** The leaves are used in tonics, liqueurs, and ales, and are made into expectorant and antiseptic cough sweets. An infusion relaxes muscles and helps expel mucus, treating bronchitis, croup, and asthma. It destroys intestinal worms and acts as a digestive and liver tonic and a laxative. The tea was used internally and externally for eczema and shingles. Its sedative action allows small amounts to control rapid irregular heartbeats. A hot infusion helps to break fevers and treats malaria when quinine is ineffective. It helps heal skin lesions. The Navaho Indians gave mothers a root decoction before and after childbirth.

• **REMARK** Horehound's woolly leaves were once used to clean milk pails, and the dried flower remains floated on oil as candle wicks.

• *pairs of ovate, wrinkled, green leaves covered in fine white hairs*

• *a pincushion whorl of small, 2-lipped, white flowers in leaf-axils*

• *Horehound honey soothes coughs*

• *rounded leaf with serrated margins*

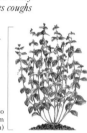

up to 45cm (17¾in)

Habitat Grassy, well-drained soil; Europe, N. Africa, Asia	Parts used ✻ ⌀ ∥ ⧄ ⚲

Family LEGUMINOSAE	Species *Medicago sativa*	Local name Lucerne

ALFALFA

This deeply rooting, nitrogen-fixing herb with trifoliate leaves has racemes of violet-blue, cloverlike flowers, followed by spiralling seed-pods.

• **USES** The tonic leaves and sprouted seeds with the flavour of fresh garden peas are eaten in salads or blended into a health drink valued by athletes. Alfalfa provides a nutritious appetite stimulant for convalescents. Arabs feed it to racehorses to increase their speed, and it is a quality fodder, said to increase cow's milk. Growing wild, the plant indicates relatively mineral-rich soil and on poor soil it is an excellent green manure. The leaves are a commercial source of chlorophyll, and the seeds yield yellow dye.

• **REMARK** Snail Clover (*Medicago sculetta*) has similar virtues and is grown for its remarkably snail-like, curled seed-pods.

flowers provide nectar and pollen for butterflies and bees •

• *3-part leaf*

• *raceme of violet flowers*

• *serrated leaf-tips*

• *whole plant used as green, nutrient-rich manure*

upright flower-stalks •

ripening seeds •

edible, sprouted seeds are rich in vitamins and minerals •

seeds sprout in 3–5 days •

• *seeds yield oil*

up to 80cm (32in)

• *green spiral seed-pods*

Habitat Grassland on chalk soils; S.W. Asia, Europe, USA	Parts used ✻ ⌀ ∥ ⚙

Family LABIATAE	Species *Melissa officinalis*	Local name Melissa

LEMON BALM

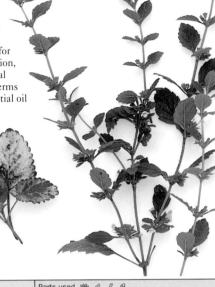

MELISSA
OFFICINALIS ▽

*soft, crinkled
pairs of ovate
leaves*

This bushy herb has square stems, lemon-scented foliage, and late-summer flowers that mature from white or yellow to pale blue.
• **USES** Fresh leaves add a delicate flavour to many dishes, oils, vinegars, and liqueurs, provide a relaxing bath, soothe insect bites, and make a sedative and tonic tea. This tea has a reputation for giving longevity and soothes headaches, indigestion, and nausea. Extracts of Lemon Balm are anti-viral and assist clean wound healing by starving the germs of oxygen. The refreshing, anti-depressant essential oil helps some eczema and allergy sufferers.
• **REMARK** It attracts bees, and if rubbed on empty hives will encourage new tenants.

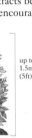

up to
1.5m
(5ft)

scalloped edge •

MELISSA OFFICINALIS

**MELISSA
OFFICINALIS
'VARIEGATA'** △
Requires moist
semi-shade.

Habitat Sunny, well-drained soil, scrub; S. Europe	Parts used ✳ ⌀ ∥ ⸙

Family MENYANTHACEAE	Species *Menyanthes trifoliata*	Local name Marsh Trefoil

BOGBEAN

• *pink-tinged
white flowers*

This marsh and aquatic plant has creeping black rhizomes, leaf-stalks tipped by three thick leaflets, and a raceme of short-lived bearded and fringed, early-summer, whitish flowers with five petals.
• **USES** Bogbean has been used as emergency food, and the leaves dried as a tea substitute. In Sweden the leaves are used commercially as a hop substitute. The Inuit of Arctic Canada grind the rhizomes into flour. The whole plant provides a tonic infusion which cleanses the blood. It is sometimes given to stimulate the appetite, and has a reputation for lowering fevers, easing rheumatic pains, and stabilizing irregular menstruation. Bruised leaves are applied to swellings.
• **REMARK** Excess doses of the whole plant may cause vomiting and diarrhoea.

*indented
margins*

• *purple-
green
colouring*

up to
25cm
(10in)

*leaf-stalk bearing 3 leaflets
sheaths onto rhizome* •

Habitat Water and water margins; northern temperate zones	Parts used ✳ ⌀ ∥ ⸙

Family LABIATAE	Species *Mentha* species	Local name Erba Santa Maria

MINTS

Most mints, including the best known Spearmint and Peppermint, are creeping plants that hybridize easily, producing infinite variations. They have erect, square, branching stems, aromatic foliage, and flowers in leaf-axils.
• USES Spearmint, Peppermint, and Applemint flavour sauces, vinegar, vegetables, desserts, and julep, and are crystallized. Their teas are popular in the alcohol-free Arab world. Spearmint and Peppermint oils have a mild anaesthetic action, and a cool, refreshing taste. They flavour confectionery, drinks, cigarettes, toothpastes, and medicines. Mints are stimulant, aid digestion, and reduce flatulence. Peppermint has additional antiseptic, anti-parasitic, anti-viral, and sweat-inducing properties. It is included in ointments, cold remedies, and is given for headaches and other aches and pains. In an inhalation the essential oil treats shock and nausea, and improves concentration.

• *excellent clean spearmint flavour*

up to 120cm (47in)

wrinkly leaf

▽ △ MENTHA SPICATA

△ MENTHA SPICATA 'MOROCCAN' Moroccan Spearmint relieves spasms.

▽ MENTHA REQUIENII Corsican Mint forms a cushion of tiny, peppermint-scented leaves with miniature flowers.

serrated margin •

◁ MENTHA SUAVEOLENS 'VARIEGATA' Variegated Applemint has cream-edged leaves. Continues growing into early winter.

lilac flower •

• *bright green leaf*

squa • *ste*

appl scente le

MENTHA SUAVEOLENS ▷ Applemint has regularly toothed, bright green leaves, good in fruit salads.

cream edging •

MENTHA X SMITHIANA 'RUBRA' ▽ Red Raripila Mint has leaves with a sweet spearmint flavour, used in salads, desserts, and drinks.

hairy leaf •

gold splash •

• *pointed, dark green leaves*

▽ MENTHA SPICATA 'CRISPA' Curly Mint has attractively crinkle deep green leaves, wi a subtle savoury spearmint flavou

• *smooth leaves*

• *toothed leaves*

△ MENTHA X GRACILIS 'VARIEGATA' Ginger Mint has gold-splashed leaves, with a mild fruity, ginger flavour.

• *healthy purple stem*

curled margin •

Habitat Rich soils, sun, moisture;	Eurasia, Africa	Parts used

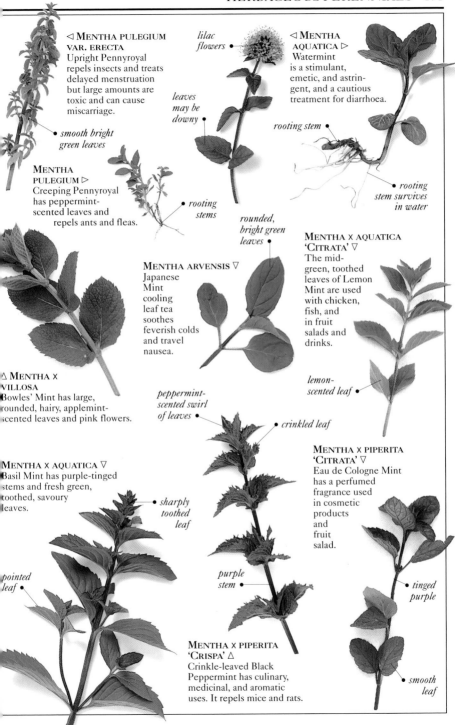

◁ **MENTHA PULEGIUM VAR. ERECTA**
Upright Pennyroyal repels insects and treats delayed menstruation but large amounts are toxic and can cause miscarriage.

smooth bright green leaves

MENTHA PULEGIUM ▷
Creeping Pennyroyal has peppermint-scented leaves and repels ants and fleas.

rooting stems

lilac flowers

leaves may be downy

◁ **MENTHA AQUATICA** ▷
Watermint is a stimulant, emetic, and astringent, and a cautious treatment for diarrhoea.

rooting stem

rooting stem survives in water

rounded, bright green leaves

MENTHA ARVENSIS ▽
Japanese Mint cooling leaf tea soothes feverish colds and travel nausea.

MENTHA X AQUATICA 'CITRATA' ▽
The mid-green, toothed leaves of Lemon Mint are used with chicken, fish, and in fruit salads and drinks.

lemon-scented leaf

△ **MENTHA X VILLOSA**
Bowles' Mint has large, rounded, hairy, applemint-scented leaves and pink flowers.

peppermint-scented swirl of leaves

crinkled leaf

MENTHA X AQUATICA ▽
Basil Mint has purple-tinged stems and fresh green, toothed, savoury leaves.

sharply toothed leaf

MENTHA X PIPERITA 'CITRATA' ▽
Eau de Cologne Mint has a perfumed fragrance used in cosmetic products and fruit salad.

pointed leaf

purple stem

tinged purple

MENTHA X PIPERITA 'CRISPA' △
Crinkle-leaved Black Peppermint has culinary, medicinal, and aromatic uses. It repels mice and rats.

smooth leaf

Family NYCTAGINACEAE	Species *Mirabilis jalapa*	Local name Four O'Clock Plant

MARVEL OF PERU

crimson flower used as food dye

This herb has fragrant crimson, purple, yellow, or white, elongated tubular flowers which open in the late afternoon, hence the local common name.
• USES The Nepalese eat the leaves, and the Japanese use the powdered seeds in cosmetics. The purgative and diuretic root is considered aphrodisiac, reduces inflammation, and promotes circulation. It is used to treat tonsillitis, urinary infections, fluid retention, scabies, and eczema. A leaf poultice is applied to abscesses, and white flower juice is given for spitting up blood.
• REMARK This herb should not be used during pregnancy.

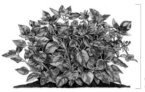

up to 60cm (24in)

leaf with pale veining and wavy margin

Habitat Dry, frost-free climate; S. America	Parts used ❀ 🌿 ⚕ ⚘

Family LABIATAE	Species *Monarda didyma*	Local name Bee Balm

BERGAMOT

This striking, clump-forming herb has aromatic leaves and shaggy heads of scarlet flowers above red bracts in late summer.
• USES The common name was given for its scented likeness to the Bergamot Orange (*Citrus bergamia*). Young leaves flavour wine, drinks, salads, and stuffing, and native Americans brewed them as Oswego tea. They used the leaves of lemon-scented *Monarda citriodora*, lemon-oregano-scented *M. pectina* and *M. fistulosa*, and mint-scented *M. menthifolia* and *M. punctata* as seasoning. Bergamot leaves were infused in oil for use in hair. They contain antiseptic thymol and are applied to pimples, steam-inhaled for colds, and brewed for nausea, flatulence, and insomnia.
• REMARK Horsemint (*M. punctata*) leaves are taken for digestive problems.

up to 120cm (48in)

MONARDA DIDYMA

extended stamens

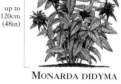

flowering head

▽ MONARDA DIDYMA 'BLUE STOCKING'
Has a long flower tube that gives nectar only to large bees.

purple form

serrated leaf

mauve flowers

◁ MONARDA DIDYMA
Young leaves have eau-de-cologne scent.

MONARDA DIDYMA 'CROFTWAY PINK' ▽
Bears clear pink flowers with mildly scented leaves.

red bracts

shrimp-like flowers

purple stem hosts galls

leaves in pairs

△ MONARDA FISTULOSA
Wild Bergamot leaves treat headaches and fevers.

oval, pointed, serrated leaf

Habitat Woodland; E. North America	Parts used ❀ 🌿 ⚕ ⚘

| Family LILIACEAE | Species *Muscari comosum* | Local name Purse Tassel |

TASSEL HYACINTH

Three to seven narrow, channelled, fleshy leaves arise from the Tassel Hyacinth bulb. In spring a thin flowering stem grows with olive-brown fertile flowers, topped by a plume of violet-blue, sterile flowers.
• USES In Greece the edible bulbs are gathered in spring and boiled to remove their bitterness. They have similar qualities to onions and are pickled in vinegar. Medicinally they are stimulant and diuretic.
• REMARK The edible bulb is sold in the USA as *cipollino*.

infertile flowers

fertile flowers

conspicuous terminal tuft of bright violet flowers

narrow leaf

pinkish brown skin

up to 35cm (14in)

| Habitat Hedgerows, fields; Europe, N. Africa, S.W. Asia | Parts used |

| Family UMBELLIFERAE | Species *Myrrhis odorata* | Local name Garden Myrrh |

SWEET CICELY

The aromatic, fern-like leaves are among the earliest to unfold in spring, followed by umbels of small, white, nectarous flowers which ripen to large, narrow fruit.
• USES The sweet, anise-flavoured, green seeds are eaten raw, sprinkled on fruit salads, and used to flavour liqueurs; they make an aromatic furniture polish. The fresh leaves are chopped into omelettes, soups, and stews and are cooked with acid fruits to reduce their tartness. The root is grated into salads, pickled, or cooked. A root infusion in brandy is a general tonic, a mild antiseptic, and is digestive. Leaf infusions are prescribed for anaemia in the elderly.
• REMARK North American Sweet Cicely (*Osmorhiza longistylis*) is used as bait to catch wild horses.

fern-like leaf

whole, unripe, nutty, green fruit are eaten raw

anise-scented leaf

ripe fruit used for flavouring but is not eaten

glossy, hard, ripe fruit

up to 2m (6½ft)

leaves are dried to decorate paper and candles

hollow, furrowed stem

| Habitat Light woodland, grassy places, moist shade; Europe | Parts used |

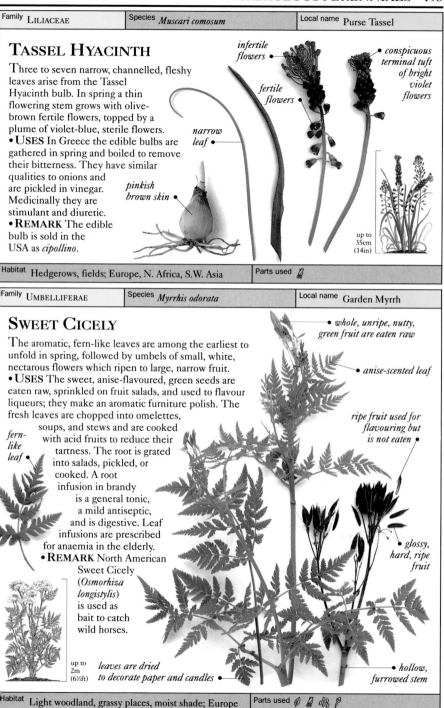

Family CRUCIFERAE	Species *Nasturtium officinale*	Local name Water Pepper

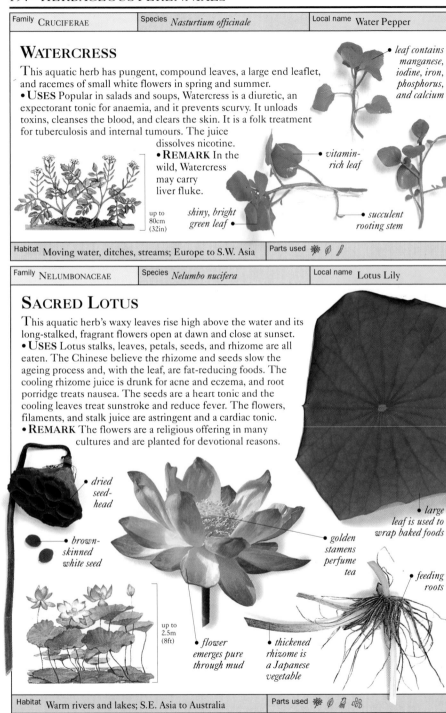

WATERCRESS

This aquatic herb has pungent, compound leaves, a large end leaflet, and racemes of small white flowers in spring and summer.
• **USES** Popular in salads and soups, Watercress is a diuretic, an expectorant tonic for anaemia, and it prevents scurvy. It unloads toxins, cleanses the blood, and clears the skin. It is a folk treatment for tuberculosis and internal tumours. The juice dissolves nicotine.
• **REMARK** In the wild, Watercress may carry liver fluke.

leaf contains manganese, iodine, iron, phosphorus, and calcium

vitamin-rich leaf

up to 80cm (32in)

shiny, bright green leaf

succulent rooting stem

Habitat Moving water, ditches, streams; Europe to S.W. Asia	Parts used

Family NELUMBONACEAE	Species *Nelumbo nucifera*	Local name Lotus Lily

SACRED LOTUS

This aquatic herb's waxy leaves rise high above the water and its long-stalked, fragrant flowers open at dawn and close at sunset.
• **USES** Lotus stalks, leaves, petals, seeds, and rhizome are all eaten. The Chinese believe the rhizome and seeds slow the ageing process and, with the leaf, are fat-reducing foods. The cooling rhizome juice is drunk for acne and eczema, and root porridge treats nausea. The seeds are a heart tonic and the cooling leaves treat sunstroke and reduce fever. The flowers, filaments, and stalk juice are astringent and a cardiac tonic.
• **REMARK** The flowers are a religious offering in many cultures and are planted for devotional reasons.

dried seed-head

brown-skinned white seed

large leaf is used to wrap baked foods

golden stamens perfume tea

feeding roots

up to 2.5m (8ft)

flower emerges pure through mud

thickened rhizome is a Japanese vegetable

Habitat Warm rivers and lakes; S.E. Asia to Australia	Parts used

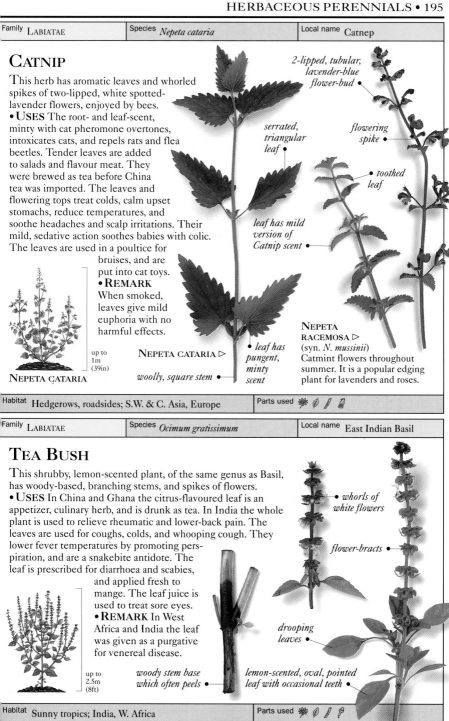

| Family LABIATAE | Species *Nepeta cataria* | Local name Catnep |

CATNIP

This herb has aromatic leaves and whorled spikes of two-lipped, white spotted-lavender flowers, enjoyed by bees.
• USES The root- and leaf-scent, minty with cat pheromone overtones, intoxicates cats, and repels rats and flea beetles. Tender leaves are added to salads and flavour meat. They were brewed as tea before China tea was imported. The leaves and flowering tops treat colds, calm upset stomachs, reduce temperatures, and soothe headaches and scalp irritations. Their mild, sedative action soothes babies with colic. The leaves are used in a poultice for bruises, and are put into cat toys.
• REMARK When smoked, leaves give mild euphoria with no harmful effects.

2-lipped, tubular, lavender-blue flower-bud •

serrated, triangular leaf •

flowering spike •

• *toothed leaf*

leaf has mild version of Catnip scent •

NEPETA RACEMOSA ▷
(syn. *N. mussinii*)
Catmint flowers throughout summer. It is a popular edging plant for lavenders and roses.

up to 1m (39in)

NEPETA CATARIA

NEPETA CATARIA ▷

woolly, square stem •

• *leaf has pungent, minty scent*

| Habitat Hedgerows, roadsides; S.W. & C. Asia, Europe | Parts used |

| Family LABIATAE | Species *Ocimum gratissimum* | Local name East Indian Basil |

TEA BUSH

This shrubby, lemon-scented plant, of the same genus as Basil, has woody-based, branching stems, and spikes of flowers.
• USES In China and Ghana the citrus-flavoured leaf is an appetizer, culinary herb, and is drunk as tea. In India the whole plant is used to relieve rheumatic and lower-back pain. The leaves are used for coughs, colds, and whooping cough. They lower fever temperatures by promoting perspiration, and are a snakebite antidote. The leaf is prescribed for diarrhoea and scabies, and applied fresh to mange. The leaf juice is used to treat sore eyes.
• REMARK In West Africa and India the leaf was given as a purgative for venereal disease.

• *whorls of white flowers*

flower-bracts •

drooping leaves •

up to 2.5m (8ft)

woody stem base which often peels •

lemon-scented, oval, pointed leaf with occasional teeth •

| Habitat Sunny tropics; India, W. Africa | Parts used |

Family ORCHIDACEAE	Species *Orchis mascula*	Local name Salep / Cuckoos

EARLY PURPLE ORCHID

The Early Purple Orchid has narrow leaves, often spotted purple-black, and a spike of purple flowers. *Orchis*, from the Greek word for testicle, refers to the double tubers.
• **USES** The starchy, mucilaginous tubers are one of the most concentrated plant foods known; one feeds the plant, then withers, the other stores surplus food. They were a vital food supply for sea voyages. In India they are made into sweetmeats or eaten raw with honey. The plant made the famous energizing and aphrodisiac drink salep, widely sold before the advent of coffee. It is a good nutritive and soothing tonic.
• **REMARK** The plant has long been associated with sex: the fleshy tuber is eaten as an aphrodisiac, the withered tuber taken to curb passions.

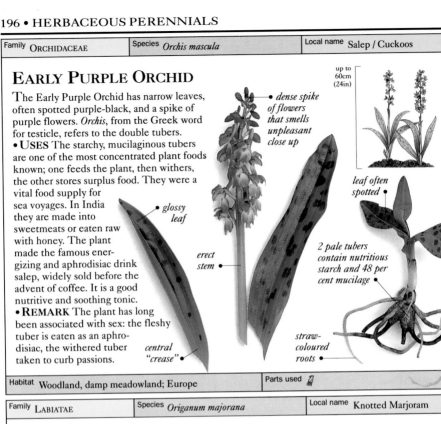

up to 60cm (24in)

dense spike of flowers that smells unpleasant close up

leaf often spotted

glossy leaf

erect stem

2 pale tubers contain nutritious starch and 48 per cent mucilage

central "crease"

straw-coloured roots

Habitat Woodland, damp meadowland; Europe	Parts used

Family LABIATAE	Species *Origanum majorana*	Local name Knotted Marjoram

SWEET MARJORAM

This half-hardy perennial, biennial, or annual has rooting stems, aromatic, hairy leaves, and white to mauve flowers producing knot-like seed clusters.
• **USES** Sweet Marjoram leaves have a sweeter, spicier taste than Oregano and Pot Marjoram. It is a popular culinary herb used in salads, sauces, meats, cheese, and liqueurs, and as part of *herbes de Provence*. As an aromatic tea Sweet Marjoram aids digestion, relieves flatulence, colds, and headaches, soothes nerves, and encourages menstruation. The leaves are enjoyed in scented sachets, sweet waters, and were once rubbed on oak floors as a fragrant polish.
• **REMARK** Marjoram essential oil, distilled from the leaves and flowering tops, is anti-oxidative, reducing skin-ageing. It is also anti-viral, eases spasms, and stimulates local circulation. The oil is added to perfumes and cosmetics.

densely grouped, small, bright green leaves with culinary and fragrant uses

◁ ORIGANUM HERACLEOTICUM Winter Marjoram has sweet, spicy, aromatic leaves and pink flowers.

leaf contains vitamin A

up to 60cm (24in)

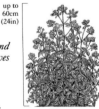

ground leaves

hairy grey-green leaf

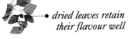

dried leaves retain their flavour well

rooting stems

◁ ORIGANUM MAJORANA ▷

ORIGANUM MAJORANA

Habitat Well-drained soil, hillsides; Mediterranean, Turkey	Parts used

| Family LABIATAE | Species *Origanum onites* | Local name French Marjoram |

POT MARJORAM

This mound-forming, small, shrubby perennial has reddish stems, late summer flowers, and aromatic, savoury green leaves of a colour that comes between the grey-green of Sweet Marjoram and the darker Oregano. The new spring leaves tend towards golden green.
• USES The leaves are generally milder than Oregano, especially in hot countries. They are included in *bouquet garni*, rubbed onto roasting meat, blended with chilli and garlic, and used with tomatoes, cheese, egg, and fish. Stems laid across barbecue embers add a faint flavour to food.
• REMARK The flowers will encourage butterflies and bees into the garden, and seed-heads provide winter fare for birds.

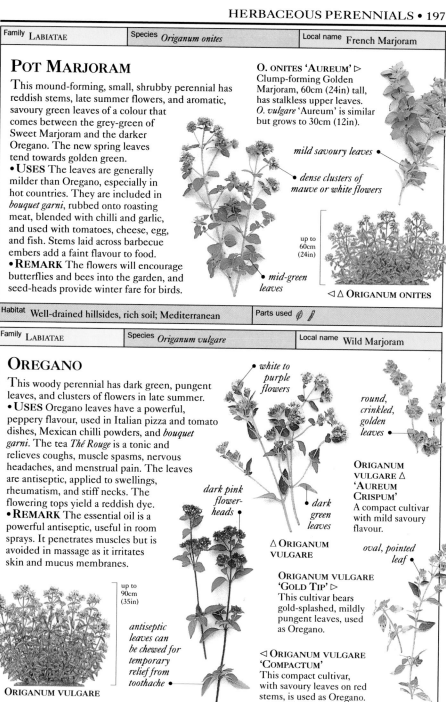

O. ONITES 'AUREUM' ▷
Clump-forming Golden
Marjoram, 60cm (24in) tall,
has stalkless upper leaves.
O. vulgare 'Aureum' is similar
but grows to 30cm (12in).

mild savoury leaves •

• dense clusters of
mauve or white flowers

up to
60cm
(24in)

• mid-green
leaves

◁ △ ORIGANUM ONITES

| Habitat Well-drained hillsides, rich soil; Mediterranean | Parts used 🌿 🍃 |

| Family LABIATAE | Species *Origanum vulgare* | Local name Wild Marjoram |

OREGANO

This woody perennial has dark green, pungent leaves, and clusters of flowers in late summer.
• USES Oregano leaves have a powerful, peppery flavour, used in Italian pizza and tomato dishes, Mexican chilli powders, and *bouquet garni*. The tea *Thé Rouge* is a tonic and relieves coughs, muscle spasms, nervous headaches, and menstrual pain. The leaves are antiseptic, applied to swellings, rheumatism, and stiff necks. The flowering tops yield a reddish dye.
• REMARK The essential oil is a powerful antiseptic, useful in room sprays. It penetrates muscles but is avoided in massage as it irritates skin and mucus membranes.

white to
purple
flowers

round,
crinkled,
golden
leaves •

ORIGANUM
VULGARE △
'AUREUM
CRISPUM'
A compact cultivar
with mild savoury
flavour.

dark pink
flower-
heads •

• dark
green
leaves

△ ORIGANUM
VULGARE

oval, pointed
leaf •

ORIGANUM VULGARE
'GOLD TIP' ▷
This cultivar bears
gold-splashed, mildly
pungent leaves, used
as Oregano.

◁ ORIGANUM VULGARE
'COMPACTUM'
This compact cultivar,
with savoury leaves on red
stems, is used as Oregano.

up to
90cm
(35in)

antiseptic
leaves can
be chewed for
temporary
relief from
toothache •

ORIGANUM VULGARE

| Habitat Open woodland, hillsides, rough grassland; Europe | Parts used 🌸 🌿 🍃 🌱 |

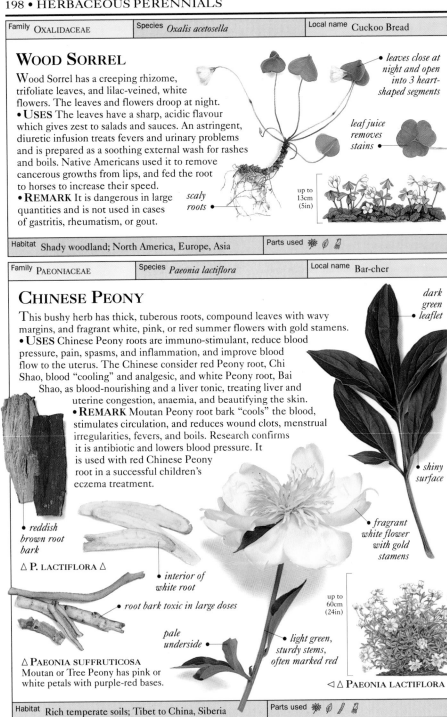

| Family OXALIDACEAE | Species *Oxalis acetosella* | Local name Cuckoo Bread |

WOOD SORREL

Wood Sorrel has a creeping rhizome, trifoliate leaves, and lilac-veined, white flowers. The leaves and flowers droop at night.
• **USES** The leaves have a sharp, acidic flavour which gives zest to salads and sauces. An astringent, diuretic infusion treats fevers and urinary problems and is prepared as a soothing external wash for rashes and boils. Native Americans used it to remove cancerous growths from lips, and fed the root to horses to increase their speed.
• **REMARK** It is dangerous in large quantities and is not used in cases of gastritis, rheumatism, or gout.

• *leaves close at night and open into 3 heart-shaped segments*

leaf juice removes stains •

scaly roots •

up to 13cm (5in)

| Habitat Shady woodland; North America, Europe, Asia | Parts used |

| Family PAEONIACEAE | Species *Paeonia lactiflora* | Local name Bar-cher |

CHINESE PEONY

This bushy herb has thick, tuberous roots, compound leaves with wavy margins, and fragrant white, pink, or red summer flowers with gold stamens.
• **USES** Chinese Peony roots are immuno-stimulant, reduce blood pressure, pain, spasms, and inflammation, and improve blood flow to the uterus. The Chinese consider red Peony root, Chi Shao, blood "cooling" and analgesic, and white Peony root, Bai Shao, as blood-nourishing and a liver tonic, treating liver and uterine congestion, anaemia, and beautifying the skin.
• **REMARK** Moutan Peony root bark "cools" the blood, stimulates circulation, and reduces wound clots, menstrual irregularities, fevers, and boils. Research confirms it is antibiotic and lowers blood pressure. It is used with red Chinese Peony root in a successful children's eczema treatment.

dark green leaflet •

• *shiny surface*

• *reddish brown root bark*

△ P. LACTIFLORA △

• *interior of white root*

• *root bark toxic in large doses*

pale underside •

• *fragrant white flower with gold stamens*

up to 60cm (24in)

• *light green, sturdy stems, often marked red*

△ PAEONIA SUFFRUTICOSA
Moutan or Tree Peony has pink or white petals with purple-red bases.

◁ △ PAEONIA LACTIFLORA

| Habitat Rich temperate soils; Tibet to China, Siberia | Parts used |

| Family PAEONIACEAE | Species *Paeonia officinalis* | Local name King of Flowers |

PEONY

This herb has mid-green, indented foliage, and sumptuous, fragrant, summer blossoms in purple-red, pink, or white. Peony derives its name from Pæon, the celebrated physician of the Greek gods.

• **USES** In Japan, where the plant is considered the "food of dragons", the flowers are eaten as a vegetable. In 14th-century England the seeds were used as a culinary spice, infused in mead for a drink to prevent nightmares, and strung in a necklace as a protective charm. The root was made into beads on which children cut their teeth. The roots are a tonic and anti-spasmodic, and became a popular treatment for head and nerve disorders, including epilepsy. The dried petals are added to pot-pourri.

• **REMARK** Peony can be poisonous and should be given by qualified personnel.

flower-bud •

• double flower

up to 60cm (24in)

deeply indented, pointed leaflets •

| Habitat Bushy areas, meadows; Europe | Parts used |

| Family ARALIACEAE | Species *Panax ginseng* | Local name Nin-sin |

ORIENTAL GINSENG

Deciduous Oriental Ginseng has an aromatic, fleshy taproot and a long stem topped by leaves. Older plants have more stalks, and after three years produce an umbel and two or three red berries.

• **USES** Roots older than two years are a famous "yang" stimulant. Rather than treating specific problems, Ginseng strengthens the body by increasing the efficiency of the endocrine, metabolic, circulatory, and digestive systems. It reduces physical, mental, and emotional stress by increasing oxygen-carrying red blood cells, immune-strengthening white blood cells, and toxin elimination. Tests show Ginseng inhibits cancer cells and increases alertness, reflex actions, and stamina.

• **REMARK** Ginseng should not be taken continuously.

rootlets are less potent •

◁ **PANAX GINSENG** ▷

• *oval leaflet with double-toothed margin*

cigar-shaped root •

• *neck has one wrinkle for each year's growth*

△ **PANAX QUINQUEFOLIUM** North American Ginseng has similar uses to the Oriental kind, but it is less stimulating and more relaxing.

up to 80cm (32in)

PANAX GINSENG

| Habitat Mountains, humus-rich soil; N.E. China, Korea | Parts used |

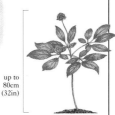
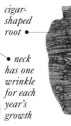

Family LILIACEAE	Species *Paris quadrifolia*	Local name One Berry

HERB PARIS

This rhizomatous herb has a single stalk crowned by a whorl of four leaves through which grow a yellow-green flower and a purple berry.
• USES The root is a toxic narcotic once used to treat gout, cramp, rheumatism, and spasms. Seed and leaf juice were applied to tumours. The fresh plant is an antidote to arsenic, and is now used in homeopathy.
• REMARK The root of *Paris chinensis* treats asthma, tubercular meningitis, and is undergoing lung cancer therapy trials.

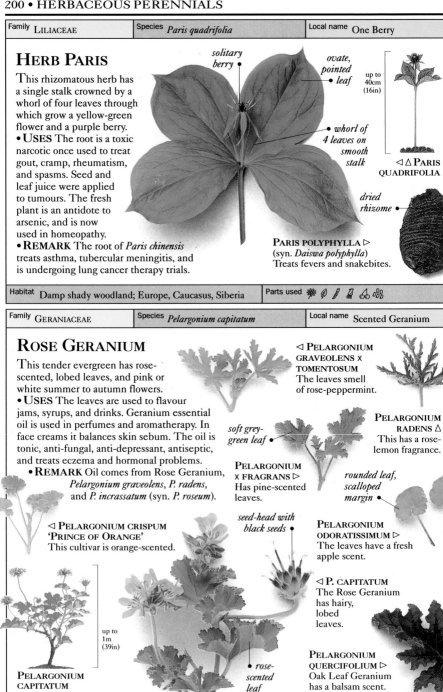

solitary berry

ovate, pointed leaf

up to 40cm (16in)

◁ △ PARIS QUADRIFOLIA

whorl of 4 leaves on smooth stalk

dried rhizome •

PARIS POLYPHYLLA ▷
(syn. *Daiswa polyphylla*)
Treats fevers and snakebites.

Habitat Damp shady woodland; Europe, Caucasus, Siberia	Parts used ✳ 🌰 ⟋ 🗡 ⚘

Family GERANIACEAE	Species *Pelargonium capitatum*	Local name Scented Geranium

ROSE GERANIUM

This tender evergreen has rose-scented, lobed leaves, and pink or white summer to autumn flowers.
• USES The leaves are used to flavour jams, syrups, and drinks. Geranium essential oil is used in perfumes and aromatherapy. In face creams it balances skin sebum. The oil is tonic, anti-fungal, anti-depressant, antiseptic, and treats eczema and hormonal problems.
• REMARK Oil comes from Rose Geranium, *Pelargonium graveolens, P. radens,* and *P. incrassatum* (syn. *P. roseum*).

◁ PELARGONIUM GRAVEOLENS X TOMENTOSUM
The leaves smell of rose-peppermint.

PELARGONIUM RADENS △
This has a rose-lemon fragrance.

soft grey-green leaf •

PELARGONIUM X FRAGRANS ▷
Has pine-scented leaves.

rounded leaf, scalloped margin •

PELARGONIUM ODORATISSIMUM ▷
The leaves have a fresh apple scent.

◁ PELARGONIUM CRISPUM 'PRINCE OF ORANGE'
This cultivar is orange-scented.

seed-head with black seeds •

◁ P. CAPITATUM
The Rose Geranium has hairy, lobed leaves.

up to 1m (39in)

PELARGONIUM CAPITATUM

rose-scented leaf

PELARGONIUM QUERCIFOLIUM ▷
Oak Leaf Geranium has a balsam scent.

Habitat Sand dunes, coastal hillsides, sun; S. Africa	Parts used ✳ 🌰 ⟋ 🍃

Family COMPOSITAE	Species *Petasites fragrans*	Local name Sweet Coltsfoot

WINTER HELIOTROPE

This small herb with deep and extensive rhizomes has heart-shaped basal leaves and vanilla-scented flowers.
• **USES** The perfumed flowers are gathered for their midwinter fragrance, and they provide nectar for the earliest bees.
• **REMARK** The long leaf-stalk of *Petasites japonicus*, peeled and pickled, is a Japanese treat called "Fuki". The pleasantly bitter flower-buds are used as a condiment. In the Arctic, the leaves of *P. frigidus* are eaten, and further south the plants of *P. palmatus* and *P. speciosa* are burned to use the ashes as salt.

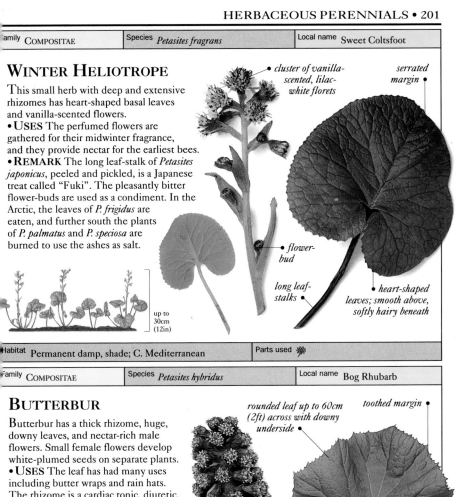

cluster of vanilla-scented, lilac-white florets

serrated margin •

• flower-bud

long leaf-stalks •

• heart-shaped leaves; smooth above, softly hairy beneath

up to 30cm (12in)

Habitat Permanent damp, shade; C. Mediterranean	Parts used ✳

Family COMPOSITAE	Species *Petasites hybridus*	Local name Bog Rhubarb

BUTTERBUR

Butterbur has a thick rhizome, huge, downy leaves, and nectar-rich male flowers. Small female flowers develop white-plumed seeds on separate plants.
• **USES** The leaf has had many uses including butter wraps and rain hats. The rhizome is a cardiac tonic, diuretic, and expectorant, and once treated coughs. The astringent leaves and flowers reduce bleeding and swollen veins. It is rarely used today because of its toxic alkaloids, except for eruptive skin conditions, and in homeopathy as a specific for lower-back pain and loin neuralgia.

rounded leaf up to 60cm (2ft) across with downy underside •

toothed margin •

flower-bud •

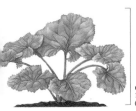

known as "Plague Flower", was considered a sovereign remedy •

dense pink flowering spike bearing male flowers

up to 1m (39in)

Habitat Riverbanks, wet meadows; Europe, N. & W. Asia	Parts used ✳ ⬤ ∥ 📷 ⚶ ⚙

Family GRAMINEAE	Species *Phragmites australis*	Local name Carrizo

REED GRASS

Reed Grass (syn. *Phragmites communis*) has sturdy stems with a long leaf blade and plumes of silky, purple-brown flowers.
• **USES** Native Americans use the tiny reddish seeds to make gruel; boil young shoots as vegetables; grind the roots into flour; toast powdered, moistened stems which puff like marshmallows; and eat the sweet, edible sap. In China the rhizome and roots are given for nausea, urinary problems, arthritis, and fever thirst.
• **REMARK** It has an important future in organic sewage treatment as it absorbs impurities from water.

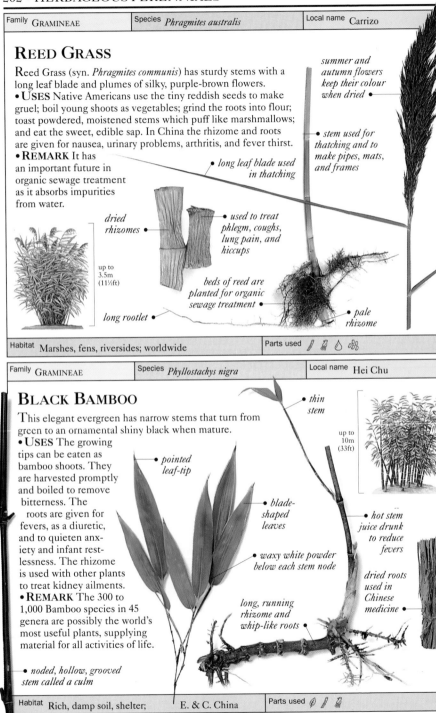

summer and autumn flowers keep their colour when dried

stem used for thatching and to make pipes, mats, and frames

long leaf blade used in thatching

dried rhizomes

used to treat phlegm, coughs, lung pain, and hiccups

up to 3.5m (11½ft)

beds of reed are planted for organic sewage treatment

long rootlet

pale rhizome

Habitat Marshes, fens, riversides; worldwide	Parts used

Family GRAMINEAE	Species *Phyllostachys nigra*	Local name Hei Chu

BLACK BAMBOO

This elegant evergreen has narrow stems that turn from green to an ornamental shiny black when mature.
• **USES** The growing tips can be eaten as bamboo shoots. They are harvested promptly and boiled to remove bitterness. The roots are given for fevers, as a diuretic, and to quieten anxiety and infant restlessness. The rhizome is used with other plants to treat kidney ailments.
• **REMARK** The 300 to 1,000 Bamboo species in 45 genera are possibly the world's most useful plants, supplying material for all activities of life.

thin stem

up to 10m (33ft)

pointed leaf-tip

blade-shaped leaves

hot stem juice drunk to reduce fevers

waxy white powder below each stem node

dried roots used in Chinese medicine

long, running rhizome and whip-like roots

noded, hollow, grooved stem called a culm

Habitat Rich, damp soil, shelter;	E. & C. China	Parts used

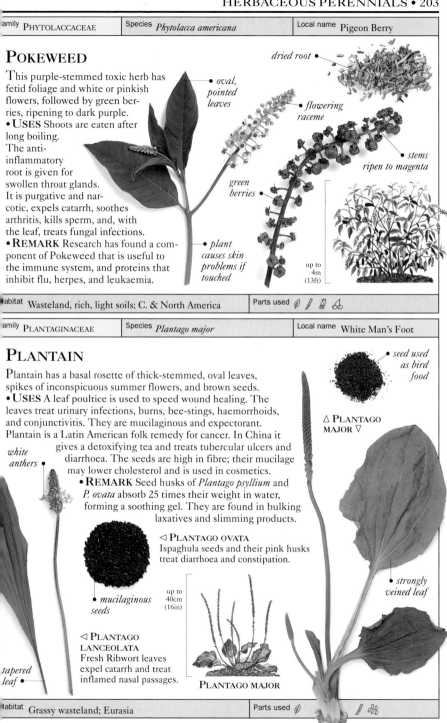

| Family | PHYTOLACCACEAE | Species | *Phytolacca americana* | Local name | Pigeon Berry |

POKEWEED

This purple-stemmed toxic herb has fetid foliage and white or pinkish flowers, followed by green berries, ripening to dark purple.
• USES Shoots are eaten after long boiling.
The anti-inflammatory root is given for swollen throat glands. It is purgative and narcotic, expels catarrh, soothes arthritis, kills sperm, and, with the leaf, treats fungal infections.
• REMARK Research has found a component of Pokeweed that is useful to the immune system, and proteins that inhibit flu, herpes, and leukaemia.

dried root

oval, pointed leaves

flowering raceme

stems ripen to magenta

green berries

plant causes skin problems if touched

up to 4m (13ft)

| Habitat | Wasteland, rich, light soils; C. & North America | Parts used |

| Family | PLANTAGINACEAE | Species | *Plantago major* | Local name | White Man's Foot |

PLANTAIN

Plantain has a basal rosette of thick-stemmed, oval leaves, spikes of inconspicuous summer flowers, and brown seeds.
• USES A leaf poultice is used to speed wound healing. The leaves treat urinary infections, burns, bee-stings, haemorrhoids, and conjunctivitis. They are mucilaginous and expectorant. Plantain is a Latin American folk remedy for cancer. In China it gives a detoxifying tea and treats tubercular ulcers and diarrhoea. The seeds are high in fibre; their mucilage may lower cholesterol and is used in cosmetics.
• REMARK Seed husks of *Plantago psyllium* and *P. ovata* absorb 25 times their weight in water, forming a soothing gel. They are found in bulking laxatives and slimming products.

seed used as bird food

△ PLANTAGO MAJOR ▽

white anthers

◁ PLANTAGO OVATA
Ispaghula seeds and their pink husks treat diarrhoea and constipation.

strongly veined leaf

mucilaginous seeds

up to 40cm (16in)

◁ PLANTAGO LANCEOLATA
Fresh Ribwort leaves expel catarrh and treat inflamed nasal passages.

PLANTAGO MAJOR

tapered leaf

| Habitat | Grassy wasteland; Eurasia | Parts used |

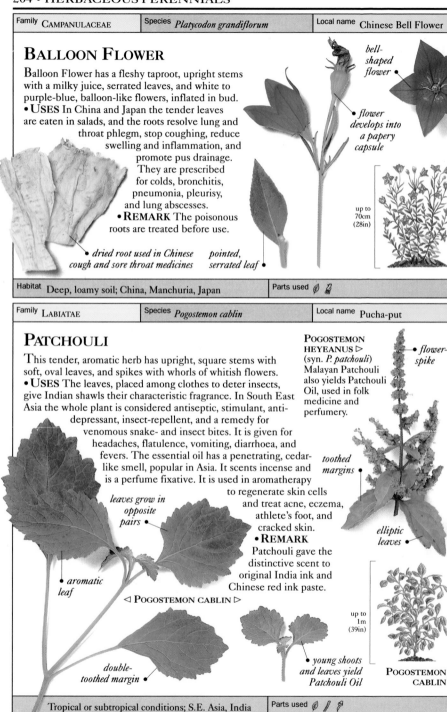

| Family CAMPANULACEAE | Species *Platycodon grandiflorum* | Local name Chinese Bell Flower |

BALLOON FLOWER

Balloon Flower has a fleshy taproot, upright stems with a milky juice, serrated leaves, and white to purple-blue, balloon-like flowers, inflated in bud.
• USES In China and Japan the tender leaves are eaten in salads, and the roots resolve lung and throat phlegm, stop coughing, reduce swelling and inflammation, and promote pus drainage. They are prescribed for colds, bronchitis, pneumonia, pleurisy, and lung abscesses.
• REMARK The poisonous roots are treated before use.

bell-shaped flower

flower develops into a papery capsule

up to 70cm (28in)

dried root used in Chinese cough and sore throat medicines

pointed, serrated leaf

| Habitat Deep, loamy soil; China, Manchuria, Japan | Parts used |

| Family LABIATAE | Species *Pogostemon cablin* | Local name Pucha-put |

PATCHOULI

This tender, aromatic herb has upright, square stems with soft, oval leaves, and spikes with whorls of whitish flowers.
• USES The leaves, placed among clothes to deter insects, give Indian shawls their characteristic fragrance. In South East Asia the whole plant is considered antiseptic, stimulant, anti-depressant, insect-repellent, and a remedy for venomous snake- and insect bites. It is given for headaches, flatulence, vomiting, diarrhoea, and fevers. The essential oil has a penetrating, cedar-like smell, popular in Asia. It scents incense and is a perfume fixative. It is used in aromatherapy to regenerate skin cells and treat acne, eczema, athlete's foot, and cracked skin.
• REMARK Patchouli gave the distinctive scent to original India ink and Chinese red ink paste.

POGOSTEMON HEYEANUS ▷ (syn. *P. patchouli*) Malayan Patchouli also yields Patchouli Oil, used in folk medicine and perfumery.

flower-spike

toothed margins

leaves grow in opposite pairs

elliptic leaves

aromatic leaf

◁ POGOSTEMON CABLIN ▷

double-toothed margin

young shoots and leaves yield Patchouli Oil

up to 1m (39in)

POGOSTEMON CABLIN

| Tropical or subtropical conditions; S.E. Asia, India | Parts used |

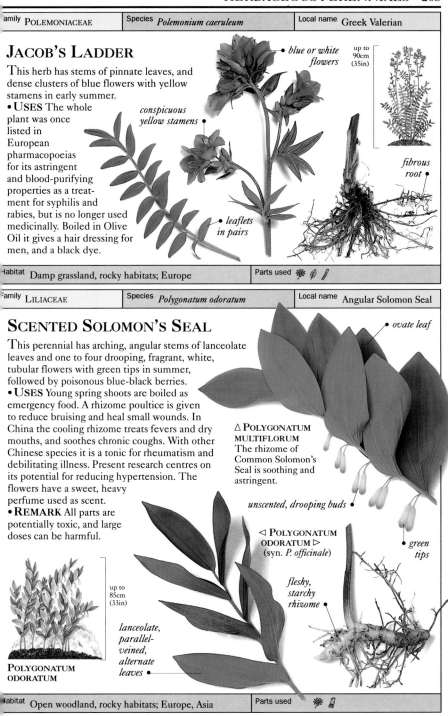

Family POLEMONIACEAE	Species *Polemonium caeruleum*	Local name Greek Valerian

JACOB'S LADDER

This herb has stems of pinnate leaves, and dense clusters of blue flowers with yellow stamens in early summer.
• **USES** The whole plant was once listed in European pharmacopoeias for its astringent and blood-purifying properties as a treatment for syphilis and rabies, but is no longer used medicinally. Boiled in Olive Oil it gives a hair dressing for men, and a black dye.

blue or white flowers

up to 90cm (35in)

conspicuous yellow stamens

fibrous root

leaflets in pairs

Habitat Damp grassland, rocky habitats; Europe	Parts used

Family LILIACEAE	Species *Polygonatum odoratum*	Local name Angular Solomon Seal

SCENTED SOLOMON'S SEAL

This perennial has arching, angular stems of lanceolate leaves and one to four drooping, fragrant, white, tubular flowers with green tips in summer, followed by poisonous blue-black berries.
• **USES** Young spring shoots are boiled as emergency food. A rhizome poultice is given to reduce bruising and heal small wounds. In China the cooling rhizome treats fevers and dry mouths, and soothes chronic coughs. With other Chinese species it is a tonic for rheumatism and debilitating illness. Present research centres on its potential for reducing hypertension. The flowers have a sweet, heavy perfume used as scent.
• **REMARK** All parts are potentially toxic, and large doses can be harmful.

ovate leaf

△ **POLYGONATUM MULTIFLORUM**
The rhizome of Common Solomon's Seal is soothing and astringent.

unscented, drooping buds

◁ **POLYGONATUM ODORATUM** ▷
(syn. *P. officinale*)

green tips

fleshy, starchy rhizome

up to 85cm (33in)

POLYGONATUM ODORATUM

lanceolate, parallel-veined, alternate leaves

Habitat Open woodland, rocky habitats; Europe, Asia	Parts used

Family POLYGONACEAE	Species *Polygonum bistorta*	Local name Snakeweed

BISTORT

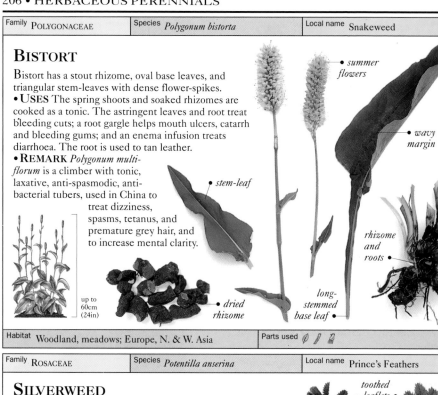

Bistort has a stout rhizome, oval base leaves, and triangular stem-leaves with dense flower-spikes.
• **USES** The spring shoots and soaked rhizomes are cooked as a tonic. The astringent leaves and root treat bleeding cuts; a root gargle helps mouth ulcers, catarrh and bleeding gums; and an enema infusion treats diarrhoea. The root is used to tan leather.
• **REMARK** *Polygonum multiflorum* is a climber with tonic, laxative, anti-spasmodic, antibacterial tubers, used in China to treat dizziness, spasms, tetanus, and premature grey hair, and to increase mental clarity.

summer flowers

wavy margin

stem-leaf

rhizome and roots

up to 60cm (24in)

dried rhizome

long-stemmed base leaf

Habitat Woodland, meadows; Europe, N. & W. Asia	Parts used

Family ROSACEAE	Species *Potentilla anserina*	Local name Prince's Feathers

SILVERWEED

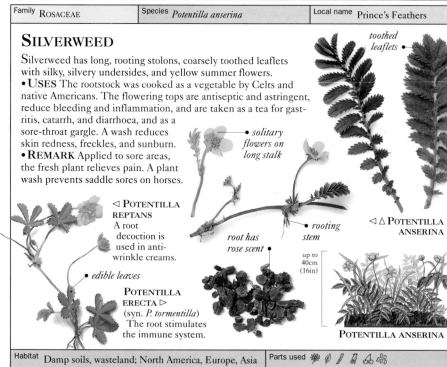

Silverweed has long, rooting stolons, coarsely toothed leaflets with silky, silvery undersides, and yellow summer flowers.
• **USES** The rootstock was cooked as a vegetable by Celts and native Americans. The flowering tops are antiseptic and astringent, reduce bleeding and inflammation, and are taken as a tea for gastritis, catarrh, and diarrhoea, and as a sore-throat gargle. A wash reduces skin redness, freckles, and sunburn.
• **REMARK** Applied to sore areas, the fresh plant relieves pain. A plant wash prevents saddle sores on horses.

toothed leaflets

solitary flowers on long stalk

◁ **POTENTILLA REPTANS**
A root decoction is used in antiwrinkle creams.

rooting stem

root has rose scent

◁△ **POTENTILLA ANSERINA**

edible leaves

POTENTILLA ERECTA ▷
(syn. *P. tormentilla*)
The root stimulates the immune system.

up to 40cm (16in)

POTENTILLA ANSERINA

Habitat Damp soils, wasteland; North America, Europe, Asia	Parts used

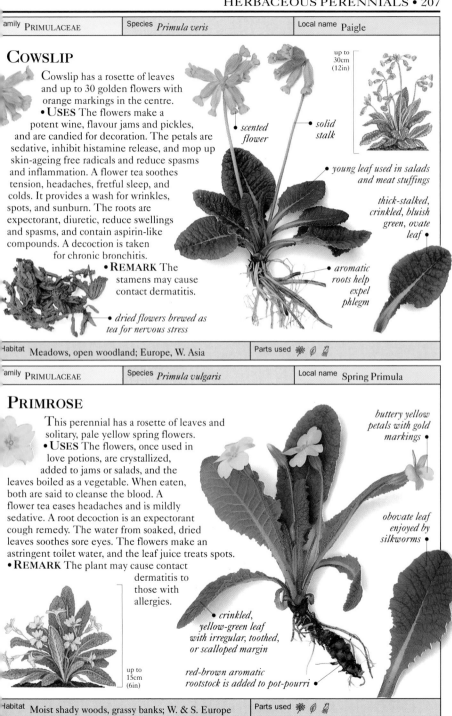

| Family PRIMULACEAE | Species *Primula veris* | Local name Paigle |

COWSLIP

Cowslip has a rosette of leaves and up to 30 golden flowers with orange markings in the centre.
• **USES** The flowers make a potent wine, flavour jams and pickles, and are candied for decoration. The petals are sedative, inhibit histamine release, and mop up skin-ageing free radicals and reduce spasms and inflammation. A flower tea soothes tension, headaches, fretful sleep, and colds. It provides a wash for wrinkles, spots, and sunburn. The roots are expectorant, diuretic, reduce swellings and spasms, and contain aspirin-like compounds. A decoction is taken for chronic bronchitis.
• **REMARK** The stamens may cause contact dermatitis.

up to 30cm (12in)

scented flower

solid stalk

young leaf used in salads and meat stuffings

thick-stalked, crinkled, bluish green, ovate leaf

aromatic roots help expel phlegm

dried flowers brewed as tea for nervous stress

| Habitat Meadows, open woodland; Europe, W. Asia | Parts used 🌼 🍃 🥀 |

| Family PRIMULACEAE | Species *Primula vulgaris* | Local name Spring Primula |

PRIMROSE

This perennial has a rosette of leaves and solitary, pale yellow spring flowers.
• **USES** The flowers, once used in love potions, are crystallized, added to jams or salads, and the leaves boiled as a vegetable. When eaten, both are said to cleanse the blood. A flower tea eases headaches and is mildly sedative. A root decoction is an expectorant cough remedy. The water from soaked, dried leaves soothes sore eyes. The flowers make an astringent toilet water, and the leaf juice treats spots.
• **REMARK** The plant may cause contact dermatitis to those with allergies.

buttery yellow petals with gold markings

obovate leaf enjoyed by silkworms

crinkled, yellow-green leaf with irregular, toothed, or scalloped margin

up to 15cm (6in)

red-brown aromatic rootstock is added to pot-pourri

| Habitat Moist shady woods, grassy banks; W. & S. Europe | Parts used 🌼 🍃 🥀 |

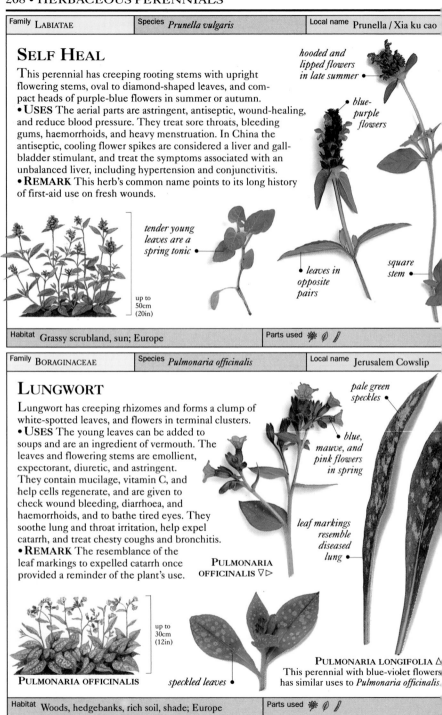

| Family LABIATAE | Species *Prunella vulgaris* | Local name Prunella / Xia ku cao |

SELF HEAL

This perennial has creeping rooting stems with upright flowering stems, oval to diamond-shaped leaves, and compact heads of purple-blue flowers in summer or autumn.
• USES The aerial parts are astringent, antiseptic, wound-healing, and reduce blood pressure. They treat sore throats, bleeding gums, haemorrhoids, and heavy menstruation. In China the antiseptic, cooling flower spikes are considered a liver and gall-bladder stimulant, and treat the symptoms associated with an unbalanced liver, including hypertension and conjunctivitis.
• REMARK This herb's common name points to its long history of first-aid use on fresh wounds.

hooded and lipped flowers in late summer

blue-purple flowers

tender young leaves are a spring tonic

leaves in opposite pairs

square stem

up to 50cm (20in)

| Habitat Grassy scrubland, sun; Europe | Parts used 🌼 ∅ ∥ |

| Family BORAGINACEAE | Species *Pulmonaria officinalis* | Local name Jerusalem Cowslip |

LUNGWORT

Lungwort has creeping rhizomes and forms a clump of white-spotted leaves, and flowers in terminal clusters.
• USES The young leaves can be added to soups and are an ingredient of vermouth. The leaves and flowering stems are emollient, expectorant, diuretic, and astringent. They contain mucilage, vitamin C, and help cells regenerate, and are given to check wound bleeding, diarrhoea, and haemorrhoids, and to bathe tired eyes. They soothe lung and throat irritation, help expel catarrh, and treat chesty coughs and bronchitis.
• REMARK The resemblance of the leaf markings to expelled catarrh once provided a reminder of the plant's use.

pale green speckles

blue, mauve, and pink flowers in spring

leaf markings resemble diseased lung

PULMONARIA OFFICINALIS ▽▷

up to 30cm (12in)

PULMONARIA OFFICINALIS

speckled leaves

PULMONARIA LONGIFOLIA △
This perennial with blue-violet flowers has similar uses to *Pulmonaria officinalis*.

| Habitat Woods, hedgebanks, rich soil, shade; Europe | Parts used 🌼 ∅ ∥ |

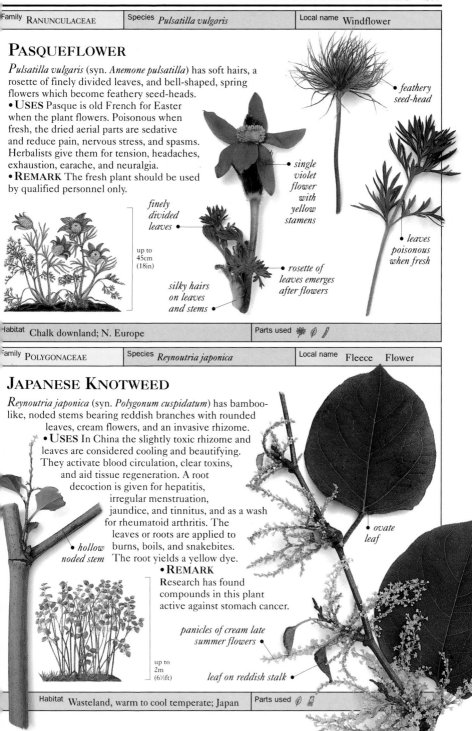

| Family RANUNCULACEAE | Species *Pulsatilla vulgaris* | Local name Windflower |

PASQUEFLOWER

Pulsatilla vulgaris (syn. *Anemone pulsatilla*) has soft hairs, a rosette of finely divided leaves, and bell-shaped, spring flowers which become feathery seed-heads.

• **USES** Pasque is old French for Easter when the plant flowers. Poisonous when fresh, the dried aerial parts are sedative and reduce pain, nervous stress, and spasms. Herbalists give them for tension, headaches, exhaustion, earache, and neuralgia.

• **REMARK** The fresh plant should be used by qualified personnel only.

feathery seed-head

single violet flower with yellow stamens

leaves poisonous when fresh

finely divided leaves

up to 45cm (18in)

silky hairs on leaves and stems

rosette of leaves emerges after flowers

| Habitat Chalk downland; N. Europe | Parts used ✳ ⊘ ∥ |

| Family POLYGONACEAE | Species *Reynoutria japonica* | Local name Fleece Flower |

JAPANESE KNOTWEED

Reynoutria japonica (syn. *Polygonum cuspidatum*) has bamboo-like, noded stems bearing reddish branches with rounded leaves, cream flowers, and an invasive rhizome.

• **USES** In China the slightly toxic rhizome and leaves are considered cooling and beautifying. They activate blood circulation, clear toxins, and aid tissue regeneration. A root decoction is given for hepatitis, irregular menstruation, jaundice, and tinnitus, and as a wash for rheumatoid arthritis. The leaves or roots are applied to burns, boils, and snakebites. The root yields a yellow dye.

• **REMARK** Research has found compounds in this plant active against stomach cancer.

hollow noded stem

ovate leaf

panicles of cream late summer flowers

up to 2m (6½ft)

leaf on reddish stalk

| Habitat Wasteland, warm to cool temperate; Japan | Parts used ⊘ ⬚ |

Family POLYGONACEAE	Species *Rheum officinale*	Local name Chinese Rhubarb

MEDICINAL RHUBARB

crinkled margin with pointed tip •

This thick-rhizomed perennial has large, long-stalked leaves and a tall, branched stem of densely clustered, small, green-white flowers in summer.

• USES The leaf-stalks are edible and mildly laxative, but this variety is not the usual garden rhubarb (*Rheum x cultorum*). The rhizome is a purgative used for constipation, although in small amounts its astringency treats diarrhoea and is an appetite and digestive stimulant added to tonic wines. In Chinese medicine the rhizome disperses blood clots, cleanses the liver, and treats jaundice, fevers, and abdominal pain. It is applied as an antiseptic, anti-inflammatory compress for boils, ulcers, and burns. Chinese research has identified properties that inhibit cancer cells. The rhizome removes rust stains, descales pans, and yields a yellow dye. Rhubarb (*Rheum palmatum*) shares the same medicinal properties.

• REMARK The Rhubarb rhizome has been used in Chinese medicine for almost 3,000 years.

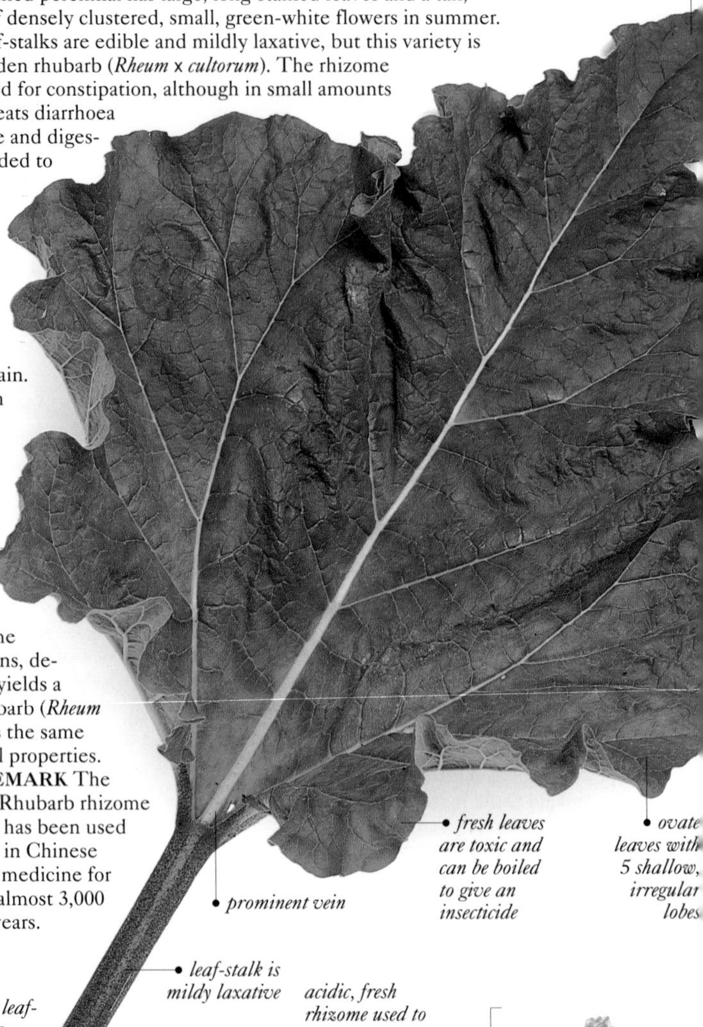

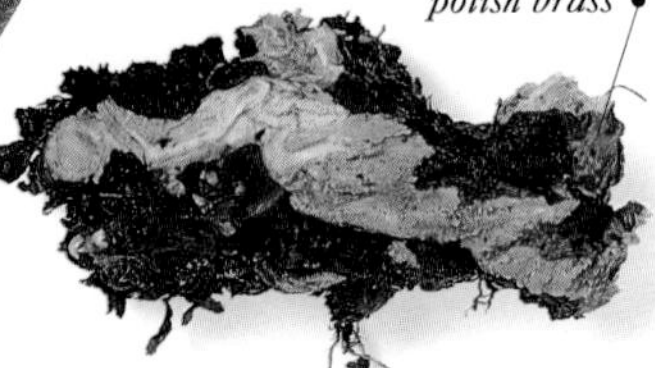

• *dried rhizome*

• *fresh leaves are toxic and can be boiled to give an insecticide*

• *ovate leaves with 5 shallow, irregular lobes*

• *prominent vein*

• *leaf-stalk is mildy laxative*

acidic, fresh rhizome used to polish brass •

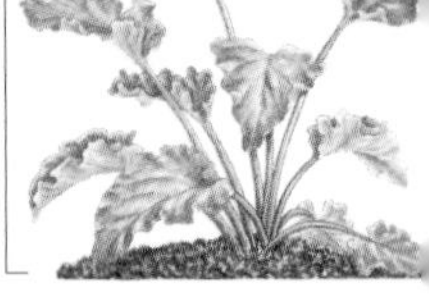

edible leaf-stalk •

green-speckled, pink leaf-stalk •

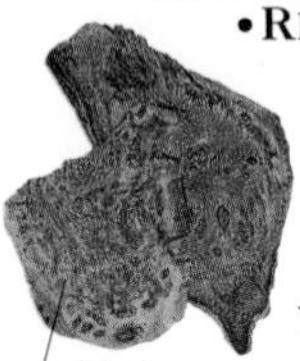

up to 3m (10ft)

Habitat	Rich, moist, deep soil; W. China, Tibet	Parts used

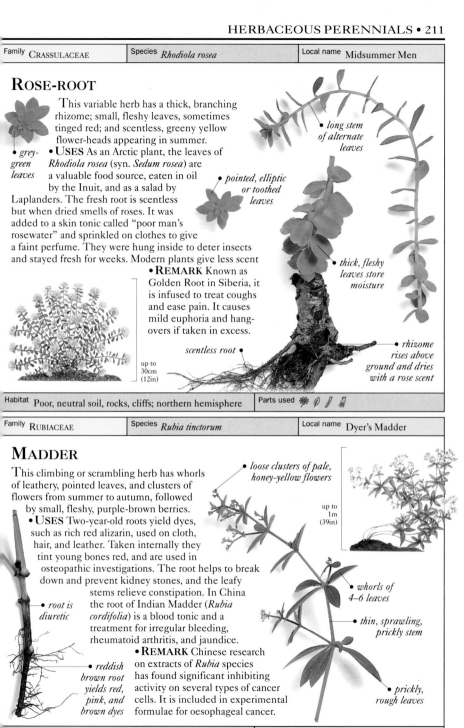

| Family CRASSULACEAE | Species *Rhodiola rosea* | Local name Midsummer Men |

ROSE-ROOT

This variable herb has a thick, branching rhizome; small, fleshy leaves, sometimes tinged red; and scentless, greeny yellow flower-heads appearing in summer.
• **USES** As an Arctic plant, the leaves of *Rhodiola rosea* (syn. *Sedum rosea*) are a valuable food source, eaten in oil by the Inuit, and as a salad by Laplanders. The fresh root is scentless but when dried smells of roses. It was added to a skin tonic called "poor man's rosewater" and sprinkled on clothes to give a faint perfume. They were hung inside to deter insects and stayed fresh for weeks. Modern plants give less scent
• **REMARK** Known as Golden Root in Siberia, it is infused to treat coughs and ease pain. It causes mild euphoria and hangovers if taken in excess.

• grey-green leaves

• long stem of alternate leaves

• pointed, elliptic or toothed leaves

• thick, fleshy leaves store moisture

scentless root •

up to 30cm (12in)

• rhizome rises above ground and dries with a rose scent

| Habitat Poor, neutral soil, rocks, cliffs; northern hemisphere | Parts used |

| Family RUBIACEAE | Species *Rubia tinctorum* | Local name Dyer's Madder |

MADDER

This climbing or scrambling herb has whorls of leathery, pointed leaves, and clusters of flowers from summer to autumn, followed by small, fleshy, purple-brown berries.
• **USES** Two-year-old roots yield dyes, such as rich red alizarin, used on cloth, hair, and leather. Taken internally they tint young bones red, and are used in osteopathic investigations. The root helps to break down and prevent kidney stones, and the leafy stems relieve constipation. In China the root of Indian Madder (*Rubia cordifolia*) is a blood tonic and a treatment for irregular bleeding, rheumatoid arthritis, and jaundice.
• **REMARK** Chinese research on extracts of *Rubia* species has found significant inhibiting activity on several types of cancer cells. It is included in experimental formulae for oesophageal cancer.

• loose clusters of pale, honey-yellow flowers

up to 1m (39in)

• root is diuretic

• reddish brown root yields red, pink, and brown dyes

• whorls of 4–6 leaves

• thin, sprawling, prickly stem

• prickly, rough leaves

| Habitat Wasteland; E. Mediterranean to C. Asia | Parts used |

Family POLYGONACEAE	Species *Rumex acetosa*	Local name Little Vinegar Plant

BROAD-LEAF SORREL

Broad-leaf Sorrel has tall stems with fresh green, arrow-shaped leaves, and red-green flower spikes in summer.
• **USES** The vitamin-rich leaves are bland in spring, but as their sharp, refreshing taste develops they offer zest to salads, soups, sauces, omelettes, meat, fish, and poultry; they can be cooked like spinach with one change of water. The leaves quench thirst, reduce fevers, and are taken as a diuretic tea for some kidney and liver problems. A leaf poultice treats acne, mouth ulcers, boils, and infected wounds, and the root is a mild laxative. Leaf juice will bleach rust, mould, and ink stains from linen, wicker, and silver.
• **REMARK** The root of Yellow Dock (*Rumex crispus*) treats psoriasis and constipation.

◁ ▽ **RUMEX CRISPUS**
The roots of Yellow Dock stimulate liver bile, clear toxins, and are used for chronic skin disorders. The leaves soothe nettle stings.

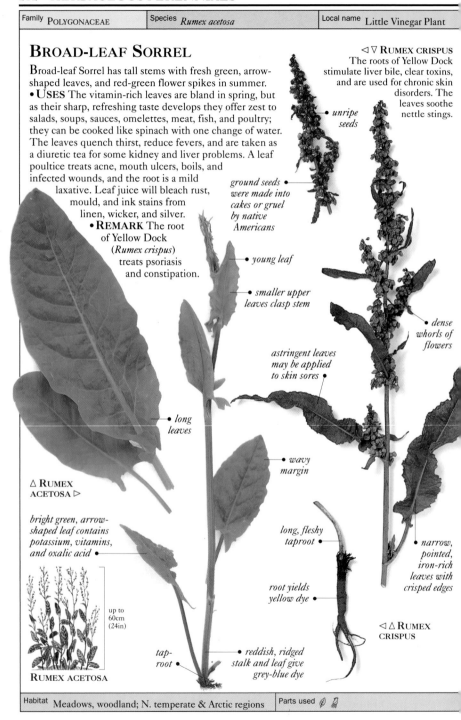

unripe seeds

ground seeds were made into cakes or gruel by native Americans

young leaf

smaller upper leaves clasp stem

astringent leaves may be applied to skin sores

dense whorls of flowers

long leaves

wavy margin

△ **RUMEX ACETOSA** ▷

bright green, arrow-shaped leaf contains potassium, vitamins, and oxalic acid

long, fleshy taproot

narrow, pointed, iron-rich leaves with crisped edges

root yields yellow dye

◁ △ **RUMEX CRISPUS**

up to 60cm (24in)

RUMEX ACETOSA

tap-root

reddish, ridged stalk and leaf give grey-blue dye

Habitat Meadows, woodland; N. temperate & Arctic regions	Parts used 🌿 🗡

Family POLYGONACEAE	Species *Rumex scutatus*	Local name French Sorrel

BUCKLER-LEAF SORREL

This low-growing herb has prostrate and upright stems of shield-shaped leaves with occasional silver patches and pointed lobes. Insignificant summer flower spikes ripen with pinky brown fruit.

light green, edible leaf •

• **USES** Buckler-leaf Sorrel is popular in salads for its mild but succulent lemon piquancy and its attractive leaf size. It is used as Broad-leaf Sorrel and favoured for sorrel soup, sandwiches, and blending into yoghurt drinks.

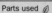 *• small fruit*

up to 45cm (18in)

• **REMARK** It should be avoided by those with arthritis or kidney stones.

Habitat Well-drained soil, pastures; Europe, W. Asia	Parts used 🌿

Family GRAMINEAE	Species *Saccharum officinarum*	Local name Ka-thee

SUGAR CANE

This clump-forming, rhizomatous, perennial grass has stout, cane-like stems; long, pointed, green leaf-blades; and a plumed inflorescence of whitish spikelets in summer.

tough rind surrounds a fibrous core full of sweet juice, which is refined to make sugar •

• **USES** The peeled cane is chewed as a sweet snack and added to Thai fish stews; the cooling stem juice (extracted by rollers) is drunk. The juice contains sucrose and yields brown sugar, refined white sugar, and the by-products mineral-rich molasses, golden syrup, and rum. Cane sugar sweetens, flavours, and preserves food by inhibiting micro-organisms. Cane juice soothes the symptoms of asthma and expels phlegm. In Asia it is applied to wounds and boils, and, with the roots, is a diuretic. The stem residue is made into ethanol, fuel (mainly to power sugar factories and for car engines in Brazil), wax for polish, and paper coating.

cane-like, jointed stem; nodes indicate old leaf joints •

• leaves at the top of ripened stems are often burned off to facilitate stem harvest

green stems can become brown with age •

new shoots or "ratoons" can be more than 7cm (2¾in) in diameter •

• **REMARK** Consumed in excess, cane sugar causes tooth decay and nutritional problems.

• leaf blade

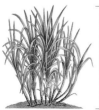

young leaves grow from and sheathe the top of the stems •

long, sword-shaped, sharply pointed leaf •

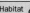 up to 6m (20ft)

Habitat Cultivated land, rich soils; tropical S.E. Asia	Parts used 🌿 🎋

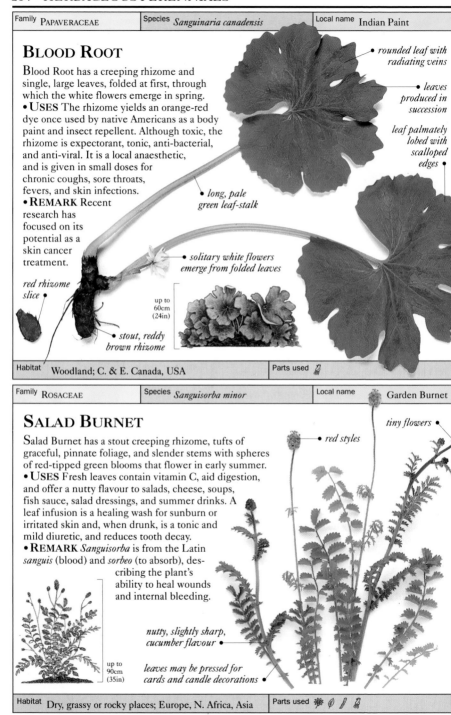

| Family PAPAVERACEAE | Species *Sanguinaria canadensis* | Local name Indian Paint |

BLOOD ROOT

Blood Root has a creeping rhizome and single, large leaves, folded at first, through which the white flowers emerge in spring.
• USES The rhizome yields an orange-red dye once used by native Americans as a body paint and insect repellent. Although toxic, the rhizome is expectorant, tonic, anti-bacterial, and anti-viral. It is a local anaesthetic, and is given in small doses for chronic coughs, sore throats, fevers, and skin infections.
• REMARK Recent research has focused on its potential as a skin cancer treatment.

rounded leaf with radiating veins

leaves produced in succession

leaf palmately lobed with scalloped edges

long, pale green leaf-stalk

solitary white flowers emerge from folded leaves

red rhizome slice

up to 60cm (24in)

stout, reddy brown rhizome

| Habitat Woodland; C. & E. Canada, USA | Parts used |

| Family ROSACEAE | Species *Sanguisorba minor* | Local name Garden Burnet |

SALAD BURNET

Salad Burnet has a stout creeping rhizome, tufts of graceful, pinnate foliage, and slender stems with spheres of red-tipped green blooms that flower in early summer.
• USES Fresh leaves contain vitamin C, aid digestion, and offer a nutty flavour to salads, cheese, soups, fish sauce, salad dressings, and summer drinks. A leaf infusion is a healing wash for sunburn or irritated skin and, when drunk, is a tonic and mild diuretic, and reduces tooth decay.
• REMARK *Sanguisorba* is from the Latin *sanguis* (blood) and *sorbeo* (to absorb), describing the plant's ability to heal wounds and internal bleeding.

tiny flowers

red styles

up to 90cm (35in)

nutty, slightly sharp, cucumber flavour

leaves may be pressed for cards and candle decorations

| Habitat Dry, grassy or rocky places; Europe, N. Africa, Asia | Parts used |

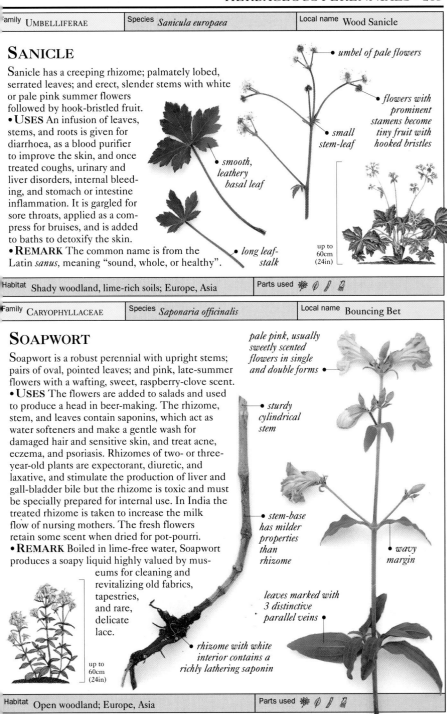

| Family UMBELLIFERAE | Species *Sanicula europaea* | Local name Wood Sanicle |

SANICLE

Sanicle has a creeping rhizome; palmately lobed, serrated leaves; and erect, slender stems with white or pale pink summer flowers followed by hook-bristled fruit.

• **USES** An infusion of leaves, stems, and roots is given for diarrhoea, as a blood purifier to improve the skin, and once treated coughs, urinary and liver disorders, internal bleeding, and stomach or intestine inflammation. It is gargled for sore throats, applied as a compress for bruises, and is added to baths to detoxify the skin.

• **REMARK** The common name is from the Latin *sanus*, meaning "sound, whole, or healthy".

• *umbel of pale flowers*

• *flowers with prominent stamens become tiny fruit with hooked bristles*

• *small stem-leaf*

• *smooth, leathery basal leaf*

• *long leaf-stalk*

up to 60cm (24in)

| Habitat Shady woodland, lime-rich soils; Europe, Asia | Parts used |

| Family CARYOPHYLLACEAE | Species *Saponaria officinalis* | Local name Bouncing Bet |

SOAPWORT

Soapwort is a robust perennial with upright stems; pairs of oval, pointed leaves; and pink, late-summer flowers with a wafting, sweet, raspberry-clove scent.

• **USES** The flowers are added to salads and used to produce a head in beer-making. The rhizome, stem, and leaves contain saponins, which act as water softeners and make a gentle wash for damaged hair and sensitive skin, and treat acne, eczema, and psoriasis. Rhizomes of two- or three-year-old plants are expectorant, diuretic, and laxative, and stimulate the production of liver and gall-bladder bile but the rhizome is toxic and must be specially prepared for internal use. In India the treated rhizome is taken to increase the milk flow of nursing mothers. The fresh flowers retain some scent when dried for pot-pourri.

• **REMARK** Boiled in lime-free water, Soapwort produces a soapy liquid highly valued by museums for cleaning and revitalizing old fabrics, tapestries, and rare, delicate lace.

pale pink, usually sweetly scented flowers in single and double forms •

• *sturdy cylindrical stem*

• *stem-base has milder properties than rhizome*

• *wavy margin*

leaves marked with 3 distinctive parallel veins •

• *rhizome with white interior contains a richly lathering saponin*

up to 60cm (24in)

| Habitat Open woodland; Europe, Asia | Parts used |

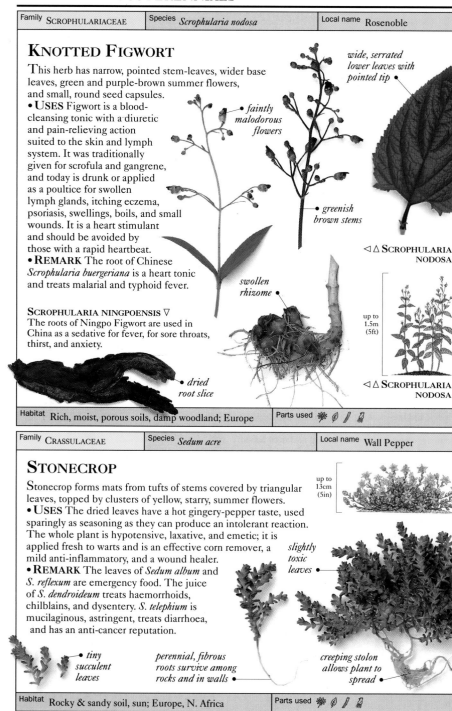

| Family SCROPHULARIACEAE | Species *Scrophularia nodosa* | Local name Rosenoble |

KNOTTED FIGWORT

This herb has narrow, pointed stem-leaves, wider base leaves, green and purple-brown summer flowers, and small, round seed capsules.
• **USES** Figwort is a blood-cleansing tonic with a diuretic and pain-relieving action suited to the skin and lymph system. It was traditionally given for scrofula and gangrene, and today is drunk or applied as a poultice for swollen lymph glands, itching eczema, psoriasis, swellings, boils, and small wounds. It is a heart stimulant and should be avoided by those with a rapid heartbeat.
• **REMARK** The root of Chinese *Scrophularia buergeriana* is a heart tonic and treats malarial and typhoid fever.

SCROPHULARIA NINGPOENSIS ▽
The roots of Ningpo Figwort are used in China as a sedative for fever, for sore throats, thirst, and anxiety.

wide, serrated lower leaves with pointed tip

faintly malodorous flowers

greenish brown stems

◁ △ **SCROPHULARIA NODOSA**

swollen rhizome

up to 1.5m (5ft)

dried root slice

◁ △ **SCROPHULARIA NODOSA**

| Habitat Rich, moist, porous soils, damp woodland; Europe | Parts used ❋ ⌀ ⁄ ⌇ |

| Family CRASSULACEAE | Species *Sedum acre* | Local name Wall Pepper |

STONECROP

Stonecrop forms mats from tufts of stems covered by triangular leaves, topped by clusters of yellow, starry, summer flowers.
• **USES** The dried leaves have a hot gingery-pepper taste, used sparingly as seasoning as they can produce an intolerant reaction. The whole plant is hypotensive, laxative, and emetic; it is applied fresh to warts and is an effective corn remover, a mild anti-inflammatory, and a wound healer.
• **REMARK** The leaves of *Sedum album* and *S. reflexum* are emergency food. The juice of *S. dendroideum* treats haemorrhoids, chilblains, and dysentery. *S. telephium* is mucilaginous, astringent, treats diarrhoea, and has an anti-cancer reputation.

up to 13cm (5in)

slightly toxic leaves

tiny succulent leaves

perennial, fibrous roots survive among rocks and in walls

creeping stolon allows plant to spread

| Habitat Rocky & sandy soil, sun; Europe, N. Africa | Parts used ❋ ⌀ ⁄ ⌇ |

Family LABIATAE	Species *Scutellaria lateriflora*	Local name Quaker Bonnet

VIRGINIA SKULLCAP

This hardy perennial has branching stems of oval to triangular leaves and tubular, blue summer flowers.
• **USES** Virginia Skullcap calms the nerves and is a tonic. The aerial parts are sedative and anti-spasmodic, and were once given for epilepsy and rabies. A tea is now taken for anxiety, depression, nervous exhaustion, premenstrual syndrome, rheumatism, and neuralgia. It has potential in reducing the withdrawal symptoms of Valium and other barbiturates, of alcohol, and in easing the pain of multiple sclerosis.
• **REMARK** Tests on the root of Baikal Skullcap, Huang Qin, confirm it lowers blood pressure. *Scutellaria barbata* inhibits some cancer cells.

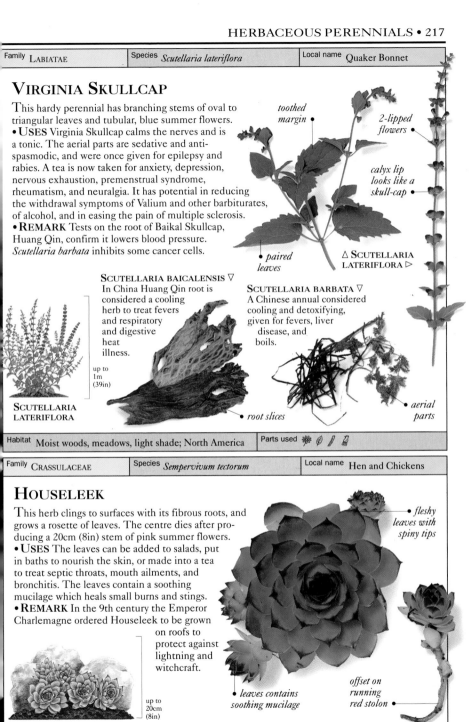

toothed margin

2-lipped flowers

calyx lip looks like a skull-cap

paired leaves

△ SCUTELLARIA LATERIFLORA ▷

SCUTELLARIA BAICALENSIS ▽
In China Huang Qin root is considered a cooling herb to treat fevers and respiratory and digestive heat illness.

SCUTELLARIA BARBATA ▽
A Chinese annual considered cooling and detoxifying, given for fevers, liver disease, and boils.

up to 1m (39in)

SCUTELLARIA LATERIFLORA

root slices

aerial parts

Habitat Moist woods, meadows, light shade; North America	Parts used ❀ ⊘ ∥ 𝕭

Family CRASSULACEAE	Species *Sempervivum tectorum*	Local name Hen and Chickens

HOUSELEEK

This herb clings to surfaces with its fibrous roots, and grows a rosette of leaves. The centre dies after pro-ducing a 20cm (8in) stem of pink summer flowers.
• **USES** The leaves can be added to salads, put in baths to nourish the skin, or made into a tea to treat septic throats, mouth ailments, and bronchitis. The leaves contain a soothing mucilage which heals small burns and stings.
• **REMARK** In the 9th century the Emperor Charlemagne ordered Houseleek to be grown on roofs to protect against lightning and witchcraft.

fleshy leaves with spiny tips

up to 20cm (8in)

leaves contains soothing mucilage

offset on running red stolon

Habitat Dry, thin, well-drained soil; C. Europe	Parts used ⊘

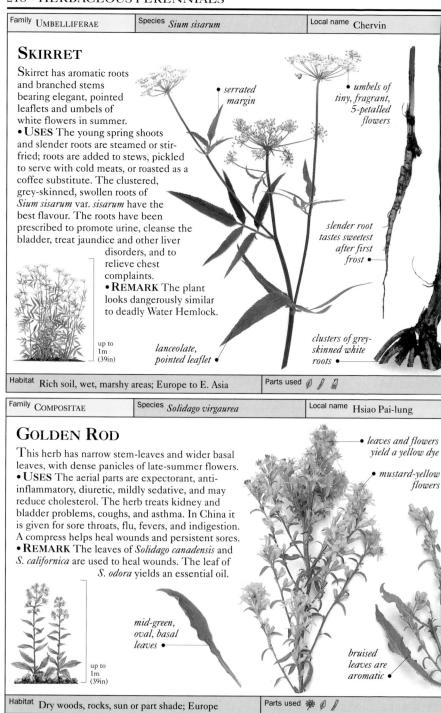

| Family UMBELLIFERAE | Species *Sium sisarum* | Local name Chervin |

SKIRRET

Skirret has aromatic roots and branched stems bearing elegant, pointed leaflets and umbels of white flowers in summer.
• **USES** The young spring shoots and slender roots are steamed or stir-fried; roots are added to stews, pickled to serve with cold meats, or roasted as a coffee substitute. The clustered, grey-skinned, swollen roots of *Sium sisarum* var. *sisarum* have the best flavour. The roots have been prescribed to promote urine, cleanse the bladder, treat jaundice and other liver disorders, and to relieve chest complaints.
• **REMARK** The plant looks dangerously similar to deadly Water Hemlock.

serrated margin

umbels of tiny, fragrant, 5-petalled flowers

slender root tastes sweetest after first frost

clusters of grey-skinned white roots

up to 1m (39in)

lanceolate, pointed leaflet

| Habitat Rich soil, wet, marshy areas; Europe to E. Asia | Parts used |

| Family COMPOSITAE | Species *Solidago virgaurea* | Local name Hsiao Pai-lung |

GOLDEN ROD

This herb has narrow stem-leaves and wider basal leaves, with dense panicles of late-summer flowers.
• **USES** The aerial parts are expectorant, anti-inflammatory, diuretic, mildly sedative, and may reduce cholesterol. The herb treats kidney and bladder problems, coughs, and asthma. In China it is given for sore throats, flu, fevers, and indigestion. A compress helps heal wounds and persistent sores.
• **REMARK** The leaves of *Solidago canadensis* and *S. californica* are used to heal wounds. The leaf of *S. odora* yields an essential oil.

leaves and flowers yield a yellow dye

mustard-yellow flowers

mid-green, oval, basal leaves

bruised leaves are aromatic

up to 1m (39in)

| Habitat Dry woods, rocks, sun or part shade; Europe | Parts used |

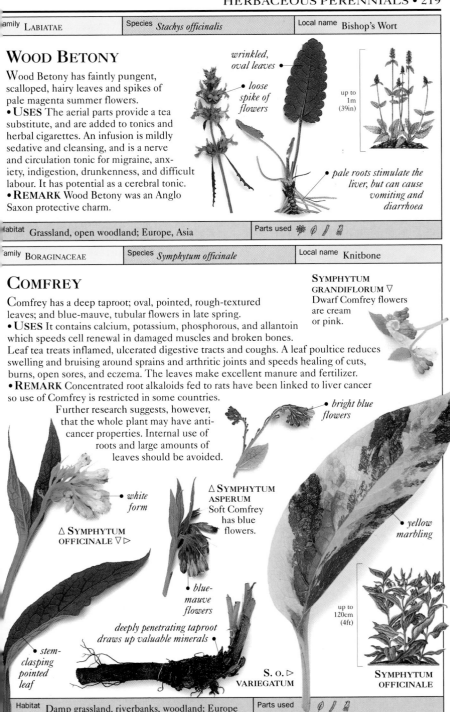

Family LABIATAE	Species *Stachys officinalis*	Local name Bishop's Wort

WOOD BETONY

Wood Betony has faintly pungent,
scalloped, hairy leaves and spikes of
pale magenta summer flowers.
• **USES** The aerial parts provide a tea
substitute, and are added to tonics and
herbal cigarettes. An infusion is mildly
sedative and cleansing, and is a nerve
and circulation tonic for migraine, anxiety, indigestion, drunkenness, and difficult
labour. It has potential as a cerebral tonic.
• **REMARK** Wood Betony was an Anglo
Saxon protective charm.

wrinkled, oval leaves

loose spike of flowers

up to 1m (39in)

pale roots stimulate the liver, but can cause vomiting and diarrhoea

Habitat Grassland, open woodland; Europe, Asia	Parts used

Family BORAGINACEAE	Species *Symphytum officinale*	Local name Knitbone

COMFREY

Comfrey has a deep taproot; oval, pointed, rough-textured
leaves; and blue-mauve, tubular flowers in late spring.
• **USES** It contains calcium, potassium, phosphorous, and allantoin
which speeds cell renewal in damaged muscles and broken bones.
Leaf tea treats inflamed, ulcerated digestive tracts and coughs. A leaf poultice reduces
swelling and bruising around sprains and arthritic joints and speeds healing of cuts,
burns, open sores, and eczema. The leaves make excellent manure and fertilizer.
• **REMARK** Concentrated root alkaloids fed to rats have been linked to liver cancer
so use of Comfrey is restricted in some countries.
Further research suggests, however,
that the whole plant may have anti-
cancer properties. Internal use of
roots and large amounts of
leaves should be avoided.

SYMPHYTUM GRANDIFLORUM ▽
Dwarf Comfrey flowers
are cream
or pink.

bright blue flowers

△ **SYMPHYTUM ASPERUM**
Soft Comfrey
has blue
flowers.

yellow marbling

white form

△ **SYMPHYTUM OFFICINALE** ▽ ▷

blue-mauve flowers

deeply penetrating taproot draws up valuable minerals

stem-clasping pointed leaf

S. O. ▷
VARIEGATUM

up to 120cm (4ft)

SYMPHYTUM OFFICINALE

Habitat Damp grassland, riverbanks, woodland; Europe	Parts used

Family COMPOSITAE	Species *Tanacetum balsamita*	Local name Costmary / Bible Leaf

ALECOST

Alecost has pointed, oval, scalloped, silvery green leaves and small heads of yellow disc florets, sometimes with white outer ray florets.
• **USES** The leaves give a sharp tang to salads, soups, game stuffing, and fruit cakes and have a refreshing, spearmint scent. Before the use of hops they were used to clear, flavour, and preserve ale. The leaves scent linen and pot-pourri; they are balsamic, preservative, and antiseptic. A leaf rinse or crushed leaf soothes burns and stings. The tea relieves colds, catarrh, upset stomachs, and cramps, and was taken to ease childbirth.
• **REMARK** Puritans carried the minty leaf in their Bibles to allay hunger during long sermons.

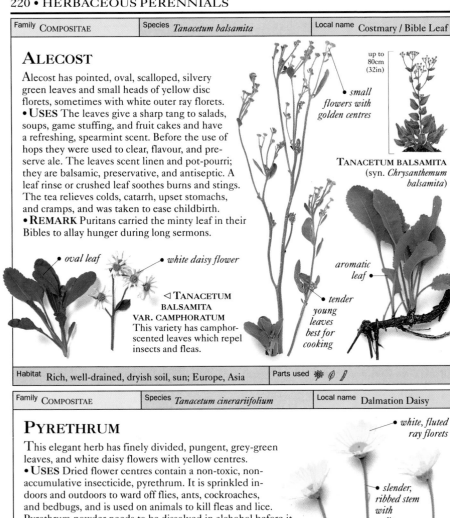

up to 80cm (32in)

small flowers with golden centres

TANACETUM BALSAMITA (syn. *Chrysanthemum balsamita*)

aromatic leaf

oval leaf • *white daisy flower*

◁ **TANACETUM BALSAMITA VAR. CAMPHORATUM** This variety has camphor-scented leaves which repel insects and fleas.

tender young leaves best for cooking

Habitat Rich, well-drained, dryish soil; sun; Europe, Asia	Parts used ❋ ⌀ ∥

Family COMPOSITAE	Species *Tanacetum cinerariifolium*	Local name Dalmation Daisy

PYRETHRUM

This elegant herb has finely divided, pungent, grey-green leaves, and white daisy flowers with yellow centres.
• **USES** Dried flower centres contain a non-toxic, non-accumulative insecticide, pyrethrum. It is sprinkled indoors and outdoors to ward off flies, ants, cockroaches, and bedbugs, and is used on animals to kill fleas and lice. Pyrethrum powder needs to be dissolved in alchohol before it can be diluted with water for garden use. To avoid harming useful insects it should be sprayed at dusk as it decomposes overnight.
• **REMARK** The active ingredients only become toxic if they are extracted and concentrated.

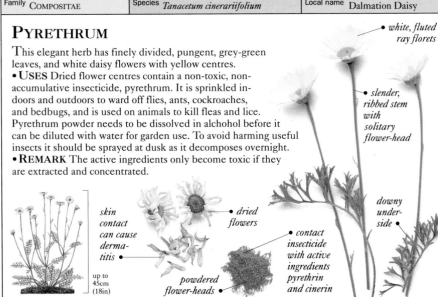

white, fluted ray florets

slender, ribbed stem with solitary flower-head

downy under-side

skin contact can cause derma-titis

up to 45cm (18in)

dried flowers

powdered flower-heads

contact insecticide with active ingredients pyrethrin and cinerin

Habitat Alkaline, well-drained, rocky soil; sun; S.E. Europe	Parts used ❋

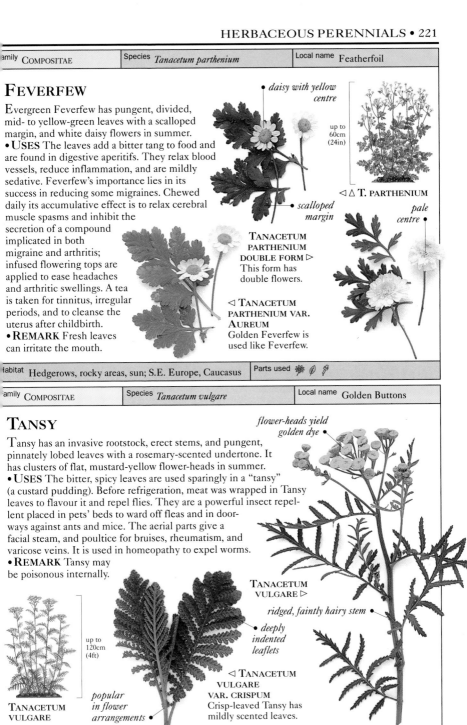

Family COMPOSITAE	Species *Tanacetum parthenium*	Local name Featherfoil

FEVERFEW

Evergreen Feverfew has pungent, divided, mid- to yellow-green leaves with a scalloped margin, and white daisy flowers in summer.
• USES The leaves add a bitter tang to food and are found in digestive aperitifs. They relax blood vessels, reduce inflammation, and are mildly sedative. Feverfew's importance lies in its success in reducing some migraines. Chewed daily its accumulative effect is to relax cerebral muscle spasms and inhibit the secretion of a compound implicated in both migraine and arthritis; infused flowering tops are applied to ease headaches and arthritic swellings. A tea is taken for tinnitus, irregular periods, and to cleanse the uterus after childbirth.
• REMARK Fresh leaves can irritate the mouth.

• *daisy with yellow centre*

up to 60cm (24in)

◁ △ **T. PARTHENIUM**

• *scalloped margin*

pale centre •

TANACETUM PARTHENIUM DOUBLE FORM ▷ This form has double flowers.

◁ **TANACETUM PARTHENIUM VAR. AUREUM** Golden Feverfew is used like Feverfew.

Habitat Hedgerows, rocky areas, sun; S.E. Europe, Caucasus	Parts used ❀ ∅ ℘

Family COMPOSITAE	Species *Tanacetum vulgare*	Local name Golden Buttons

TANSY

Tansy has an invasive rootstock, erect stems, and pungent, pinnately lobed leaves with a rosemary-scented undertone. It has clusters of flat, mustard-yellow flower-heads in summer.
• USES The bitter, spicy leaves are used sparingly in a "tansy" (a custard pudding). Before refrigeration, meat was wrapped in Tansy leaves to flavour it and repel flies. They are a powerful insect repellent placed in pets' beds to ward off fleas and in doorways against ants and mice. The aerial parts give a facial steam, and poultice for bruises, rheumatism, and varicose veins. It is used in homeopathy to expel worms.
• REMARK Tansy may be poisonous internally.

flower-heads yield golden dye •

TANACETUM VULGARE ▷

ridged, faintly hairy stem •

• *deeply indented leaflets*

up to 120cm (4ft)

TANACETUM VULGARE

popular in flower arrangements •

◁ **TANACETUM VULGARE VAR. CRISPUM** Crisp-leaved Tansy has mildly scented leaves.

Habitat Hedgerows, dry soil, sun or light shade; Europe	Parts used ❀ ∅ ⫽ ⚭ ⚘

| Family COMPOSITAE | Species *Taraxacum sect. Ruderalia* species | Local name Fairy Clock |

DANDELION

This hardy herb has rosettes of oblong, deeply toothed leaves. Golden flowers, often striped with brown, appear from from spring to autumn, and are followed by balls of tufted seeds.
• **USES** The flowers are made into wine, the buds are pickled, and the leaves, rich in vitamins A and C and minerals, are eaten in salads. The leaves are a powerful diuretic, treating urinary disorders and fluid retention without depleting body potassium. They detoxify the blood, so are given for acne and eczema. The white sap treats warts, corns, and verrucas. The root reduces inflammation and is a liver stimulant, used for jaundice, gall-stones, and rheumatism. The roots yield a magenta dye.

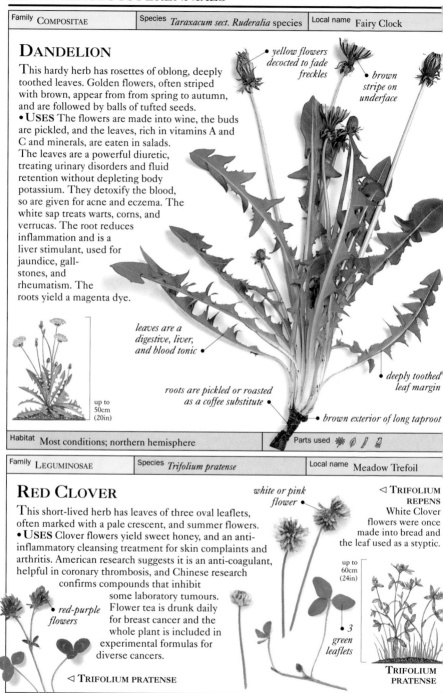

yellow flowers decocted to fade freckles

brown stripe on underface

leaves are a digestive, liver, and blood tonic

roots are pickled or roasted as a coffee substitute

deeply toothed leaf margin

brown exterior of long taproot

up to 50cm (20in)

| Habitat Most conditions; northern hemisphere | Parts used ❋ ⊘ ∥ ⵣ |

| Family LEGUMINOSAE | Species *Trifolium pratense* | Local name Meadow Trefoil |

RED CLOVER

This short-lived herb has leaves of three oval leaflets, often marked with a pale crescent, and summer flowers.
• **USES** Clover flowers yield sweet honey, and an anti-inflammatory cleansing treatment for skin complaints and arthritis. American research suggests it is an anti-coagulant, helpful in coronary thrombosis, and Chinese research confirms compounds that inhibit some laboratory tumours. Flower tea is drunk daily for breast cancer and the whole plant is included in experimental formulas for diverse cancers.

white or pink flower

◁ **TRIFOLIUM REPENS**
White Clover flowers were once made into bread and the leaf used as a styptic.

up to 60cm (24in)

red-purple flowers

3 green leaflets

◁ **TRIFOLIUM PRATENSE**

TRIFOLIUM PRATENSE

| Habitat Moist, grassy places, cultivated land; Europe | Parts used ❋ ⊘ ∥ ⵣ ⬡ |

Family LABIATAE	Species *Teucrium chamaedrys*	Local name Common Germander

WALL GERMANDER

TEUCRIUM
CHAMAEDRYS ▷

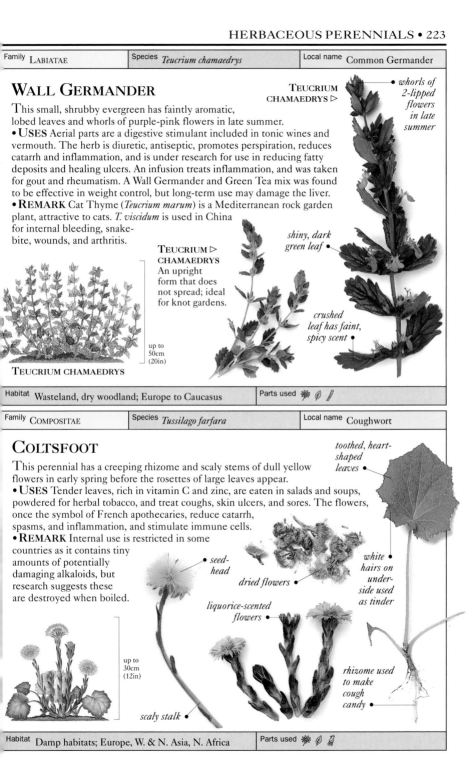

This small, shrubby evergreen has faintly aromatic, lobed leaves and whorls of purple-pink flowers in late summer.
• USES Aerial parts are a digestive stimulant included in tonic wines and vermouth. The herb is diuretic, antiseptic, promotes perspiration, reduces catarrh and inflammation, and is under research for use in reducing fatty deposits and healing ulcers. An infusion treats inflammation, and was taken for gout and rheumatism. A Wall Germander and Green Tea mix was found to be effective in weight control, but long-term use may damage the liver.
• REMARK Cat Thyme (*Teucrium marum*) is a Mediterranean rock garden plant, attractive to cats. *T. viscidum* is used in China for internal bleeding, snake-bite, wounds, and arthritis.

whorls of 2-lipped flowers in late summer

TEUCRIUM ▷
CHAMAEDRYS
An upright form that does not spread; ideal for knot gardens.

shiny, dark green leaf •

crushed leaf has faint, spicy scent •

up to
50cm
(20in)

TEUCRIUM CHAMAEDRYS

Habitat Wasteland, dry woodland; Europe to Caucasus	Parts used ✳ ⌀ ∥

Family COMPOSITAE	Species *Tussilago farfara*	Local name Coughwort

COLTSFOOT

This perennial has a creeping rhizome and scaly stems of dull yellow flowers in early spring before the rosettes of large leaves appear.
• USES Tender leaves, rich in vitamin C and zinc, are eaten in salads and soups, powdered for herbal tobacco, and treat coughs, skin ulcers, and sores. The flowers, once the symbol of French apothecaries, reduce catarrh, spasms, and inflammation, and stimulate immune cells.
• REMARK Internal use is restricted in some countries as it contains tiny amounts of potentially damaging alkaloids, but research suggests these are destroyed when boiled.

toothed, heart-shaped leaves •

• seed-head

dried flowers •

white • hairs on under-side used as tinder

liquorice-scented flowers •

up to
30cm
(12in)

rhizome used to make cough candy •

scaly stalk •

Habitat Damp habitats; Europe, W. & N. Asia, N. Africa	Parts used ✳ ⌀ ∥

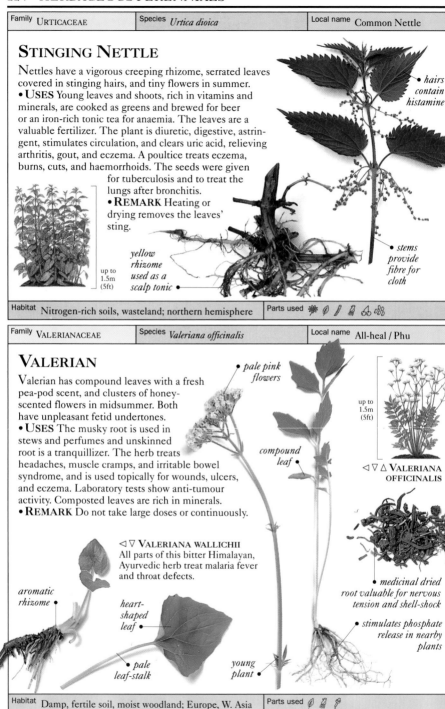

Family URTICACEAE	Species *Urtica dioica*	Local name Common Nettle

STINGING NETTLE

Nettles have a vigorous creeping rhizome, serrated leaves
covered in stinging hairs, and tiny flowers in summer.
• USES Young leaves and shoots, rich in vitamins and
minerals, are cooked as greens and brewed for beer
or an iron-rich tonic tea for anaemia. The leaves are a
valuable fertilizer. The plant is diuretic, digestive, astringent, stimulates circulation, and clears uric acid, relieving
arthritis, gout, and eczema. A poultice treats eczema,
burns, cuts, and haemorrhoids. The seeds were given
for tuberculosis and to treat the
lungs after bronchitis.
• REMARK Heating or
drying removes the leaves'
sting.

hairs contain histamine

stems provide fibre for cloth

up to 1.5m (5ft)

yellow rhizome used as a scalp tonic

Habitat Nitrogen-rich soils, wasteland; northern hemisphere	Parts used

Family VALERIANACEAE	Species *Valeriana officinalis*	Local name All-heal / Phu

VALERIAN

Valerian has compound leaves with a fresh
pea-pod scent, and clusters of honey-
scented flowers in midsummer. Both
have unpleasant fetid undertones.
• USES The musky root is used in
stews and perfumes and unskinned
root is a tranquillizer. The herb treats
headaches, muscle cramps, and irritable bowel
syndrome, and is used topically for wounds, ulcers,
and eczema. Laboratory tests show anti-tumour
activity. Composted leaves are rich in minerals.
• REMARK Do not take large doses or continuously.

pale pink flowers

compound leaf

up to 1.5m (5ft)

◁ ▽ △ VALERIANA
OFFICINALIS

◁ ▽ VALERIANA WALLICHII
All parts of this bitter Himalayan,
Ayurvedic herb treat malaria fever
and throat defects.

aromatic rhizome

heart-shaped leaf

pale leaf-stalk

young plant

medicinal dried root valuable for nervous tension and shell-shock

stimulates phosphate release in nearby plants

Habitat Damp, fertile soil, moist woodland; Europe, W. Asia	Parts used

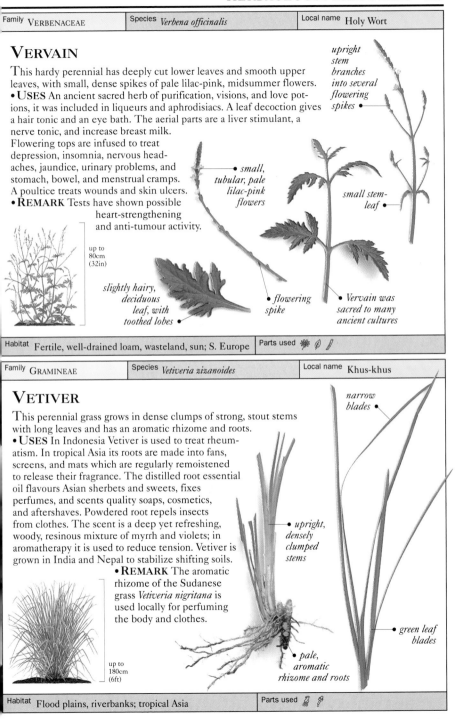

Family VERBENACEAE	Species *Verbena officinalis*	Local name Holy Wort

VERVAIN

This hardy perennial has deeply cut lower leaves and smooth upper leaves, with small, dense spikes of pale lilac-pink, midsummer flowers.
• **USES** An ancient sacred herb of purification, visions, and love potions, it was included in liqueurs and aphrodisiacs. A leaf decoction gives a hair tonic and an eye bath. The aerial parts are a liver stimulant, a nerve tonic, and increase breast milk. Flowering tops are infused to treat depression, insomnia, nervous headaches, jaundice, urinary problems, and stomach, bowel, and menstrual cramps. A poultice treats wounds and skin ulcers.
• **REMARK** Tests have shown possible heart-strengthening and anti-tumour activity.

upright stem branches into several flowering spikes

small, tubular, pale lilac-pink flowers

small stem-leaf

up to 80cm (32in)

slightly hairy, deciduous leaf, with toothed lobes

flowering spike

Vervain was sacred to many ancient cultures

Habitat Fertile, well-drained loam, wasteland, sun; S. Europe	Parts used ✹ ⌀ ∥

Family GRAMINEAE	Species *Vetiveria zizanoides*	Local name Khus-khus

VETIVER

This perennial grass grows in dense clumps of strong, stout stems with long leaves and has an aromatic rhizome and roots.
• **USES** In Indonesia Vetiver is used to treat rheumatism. In tropical Asia its roots are made into fans, screens, and mats which are regularly remoistened to release their fragrance. The distilled root essential oil flavours Asian sherbets and sweets, fixes perfumes, and scents quality soaps, cosmetics, and aftershaves. Powdered root repels insects from clothes. The scent is a deep yet refreshing, woody, resinous mixture of myrrh and violets; in aromatherapy it is used to reduce tension. Vetiver is grown in India and Nepal to stabilize shifting soils.
• **REMARK** The aromatic rhizome of the Sudanese grass *Vetiveria nigritana* is used locally for perfuming the body and clothes.

narrow blades

upright, densely clumped stems

green leaf blades

up to 180cm (6ft)

pale, aromatic rhizome and roots

Habitat Flood plains, riverbanks; tropical Asia	Parts used ⌀ ⌀

Family VIOLACEAE	Species *Viola odorata*	Local name Little Faces

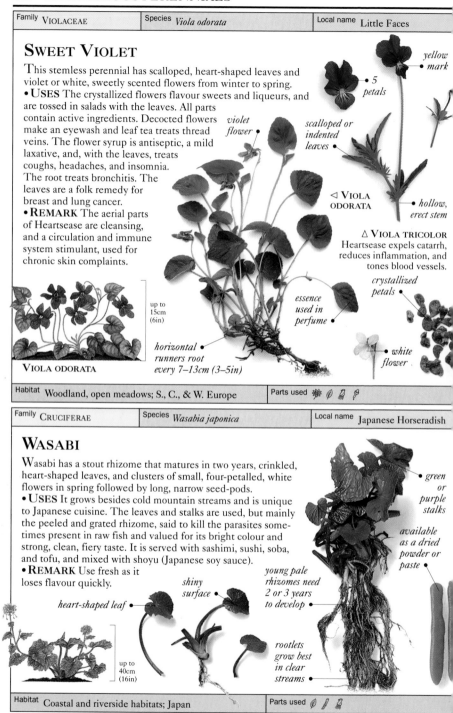

SWEET VIOLET

This stemless perennial has scalloped, heart-shaped leaves and violet or white, sweetly scented flowers from winter to spring.
• **USES** The crystallized flowers flavour sweets and liqueurs, and are tossed in salads with the leaves. All parts contain active ingredients. Decocted flowers make an eyewash and leaf tea treats thread veins. The flower syrup is antiseptic, a mild laxative, and, with the leaves, treats coughs, headaches, and insomnia. The root treats bronchitis. The leaves are a folk remedy for breast and lung cancer.
• **REMARK** The aerial parts of Heartsease are cleansing, and a circulation and immune system stimulant, used for chronic skin complaints.

yellow mark

5 petals

violet flower

scalloped or indented leaves

◁ VIOLA ODORATA

hollow, erect stem

△ VIOLA TRICOLOR Heartsease expels catarrh, reduces inflammation, and tones blood vessels.

crystallized petals

essence used in perfume

white flower

VIOLA ODORATA

up to 15cm (6in)

horizontal runners root every 7–13cm (3–5in)

Habitat Woodland, open meadows; S., C., & W. Europe	Parts used

Family CRUCIFERAE	Species *Wasabia japonica*	Local name Japanese Horseradish

WASABI

Wasabi has a stout rhizome that matures in two years, crinkled, heart-shaped leaves, and clusters of small, four-petalled, white flowers in spring followed by long, narrow seed-pods.
• **USES** It grows besides cold mountain streams and is unique to Japanese cuisine. The leaves and stalks are used, but mainly the peeled and grated rhizome, said to kill the parasites sometimes present in raw fish and valued for its bright colour and strong, clean, fiery taste. It is served with sashimi, sushi, soba, and tofu, and mixed with shoyu (Japanese soy sauce).
• **REMARK** Use fresh as it loses flavour quickly.

green or purple stalks

available as a dried powder or paste

young pale rhizomes need 2 or 3 years to develop

shiny surface

heart-shaped leaf

up to 40cm (16in)

rootlets grow best in clear streams

Habitat Coastal and riverside habitats; Japan	Parts used

Family ZINGIBERACEAE	Species *Zingiber officinale*	Local name Jiang

GINGER

Ginger has an aromatic rhizome, erect stems of two ranks, lance-shaped leaves, and spikes of white flowers.
• **USES** The rhizome is used fresh, dried, pickled, and preserved. Essential to Oriental dishes, it is used elsewhere in desserts and cordials. The shoots, leaves, and inflorescence of *Zingiber officinale*, *Z. mioga*, and *Z. zerumbet* are eaten raw or cooked. Crystallized or infused Ginger suppresses nausea. A steam inhalation treats colds and lung infections. Ginger tea eases indigestion and flatulence, and reduces fevers. One drop of the root essential oil in a massage blend helps relieve muscular pain, rheumatism, lumbago, and fatigue.
• **REMARK** Only use small doses to prevent morning sickness.

up to 1.5m (5ft)

ALPINIA ZERUMBET ▷
The inflorescence of Shell Ginger is similar to the rare "true" Ginger flower.

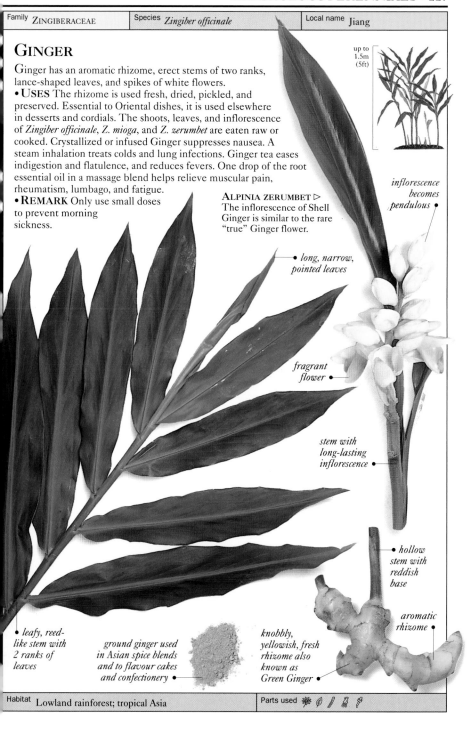

inflorescence becomes pendulous •

• long, narrow, pointed leaves

fragrant flower •

stem with long-lasting inflorescence •

• hollow stem with reddish base

aromatic rhizome •

• leafy, reed-like stem with 2 ranks of leaves

ground ginger used in Asian spice blends and to flavour cakes and confectionery •

knobbly, yellowish, fresh rhizome also known as Green Ginger •

Habitat Lowland rainforest; tropical Asia	Parts used 🌿 ✿ 🥄 📜 ✎

ANNUALS AND BIENNIALS

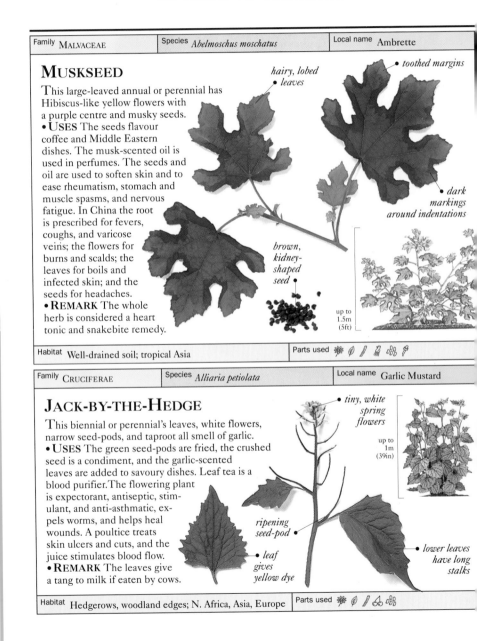

Family MALVACEAE	Species *Abelmoschus moschatus*	Local name Ambrette

MUSKSEED

This large-leaved annual or perennial has Hibiscus-like yellow flowers with a purple centre and musky seeds.
• **USES** The seeds flavour coffee and Middle Eastern dishes. The musk-scented oil is used in perfumes. The seeds and oil are used to soften skin and to ease rheumatism, stomach and muscle spasms, and nervous fatigue. In China the root is prescribed for fevers, coughs, and varicose veins; the flowers for burns and scalds; the leaves for boils and infected skin; and the seeds for headaches.
• **REMARK** The whole herb is considered a heart tonic and snakebite remedy.

hairy, lobed leaves

toothed margins

dark markings around indentations

brown, kidney-shaped seed

up to 1.5m (5ft)

Habitat Well-drained soil; tropical Asia	Parts used

Family CRUCIFERAE	Species *Alliaria petiolata*	Local name Garlic Mustard

JACK-BY-THE-HEDGE

This biennial or perennial's leaves, white flowers, narrow seed-pods, and taproot all smell of garlic.
• **USES** The green seed-pods are fried, the crushed seed is a condiment, and the garlic-scented leaves are added to savoury dishes. Leaf tea is a blood purifier. The flowering plant is expectorant, antiseptic, stimulant, and anti-asthmatic, expels worms, and helps heal wounds. A poultice treats skin ulcers and cuts, and the juice stimulates blood flow.
• **REMARK** The leaves give a tang to milk if eaten by cows.

tiny, white spring flowers

up to 1m (39in)

ripening seed-pod

leaf gives yellow dye

lower leaves have long stalks

Habitat Hedgerows, woodland edges; N. Africa, Asia, Europe	Parts used

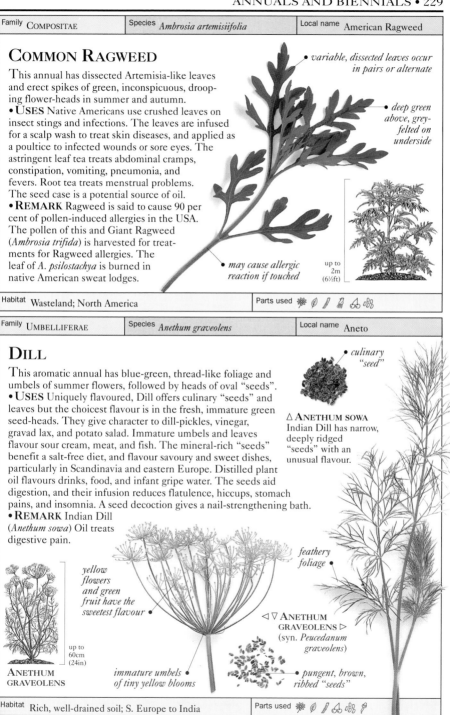

Family COMPOSITAE	Species *Ambrosia artemisiifolia*	Local name American Ragweed

COMMON RAGWEED

This annual has dissected Artemisia-like leaves and erect spikes of green, inconspicuous, drooping flower-heads in summer and autumn.

• **USES** Native Americans use crushed leaves on insect stings and infections. The leaves are infused for a scalp wash to treat skin diseases, and applied as a poultice to infected wounds or sore eyes. The astringent leaf tea treats abdominal cramps, constipation, vomiting, pneumonia, and fevers. Root tea treats menstrual problems. The seed case is a potential source of oil.

• **REMARK** Ragweed is said to cause 90 per cent of pollen-induced allergies in the USA. The pollen of this and Giant Ragweed (*Ambrosia trifida*) is harvested for treatments for Ragweed allergies. The leaf of *A. psilostachya* is burned in native American sweat lodges.

variable, dissected leaves occur in pairs or alternate

deep green above, grey-felted on underside

may cause allergic reaction if touched

up to 2m (6½ft)

Habitat Wasteland; North America	Parts used ❀ ✕ ∥ ⚏ ⚕ ⬚

Family UMBELLIFERAE	Species *Anethum graveolens*	Local name Aneto

DILL

This aromatic annual has blue-green, thread-like foliage and umbels of summer flowers, followed by heads of oval "seeds".

• **USES** Uniquely flavoured, Dill offers culinary "seeds" and leaves but the choicest flavour is in the fresh, immature green seed-heads. They give character to dill-pickles, vinegar, gravad lax, and potato salad. Immature umbels and leaves flavour sour cream, meat, and fish. The mineral-rich "seeds" benefit a salt-free diet, and flavour savoury and sweet dishes, particularly in Scandinavia and eastern Europe. Distilled plant oil flavours drinks, food, and infant gripe water. The seeds aid digestion, and their infusion reduces flatulence, hiccups, stomach pains, and insomnia. A seed decoction gives a nail-strengthening bath.

• **REMARK** Indian Dill (*Anethum sowa*) Oil treats digestive pain.

culinary "seed"

△ **ANETHUM SOWA**
Indian Dill has narrow, deeply ridged "seeds" with an unusual flavour.

feathery foliage

yellow flowers and green fruit have the sweetest flavour

◁ ▽ **ANETHUM GRAVEOLENS** ▷
(syn. *Peucedanum graveolens*)

up to 60cm (24in)

ANETHUM GRAVEOLENS

immature umbels of tiny yellow blooms

pungent, brown, ribbed "seeds"

Habitat Rich, well-drained soil; S. Europe to India	Parts used ❀ ✕ ∥ ⚕ ⬚ ⚘

Family UMBELLIFERAE	Species *Angelica archangelica*	Local name Angel's Food

ANGELICA

This three-year "biennial" has a taproot, divided leaves, and spherical umbels of green-white flowers in its third year; then it seeds and dies.
• USES All parts share the sharp flavour. The leaves are stewed with acidic fruit; the shoots used in salads; the stems and roots as vegetables; and the seeds in pastry dishes. Distilled seeds and root oil are used in gin, vermouth, and perfumes. A root incision in spring gives latex, used as a fixative. The roots, seeds, and leaves treat colds, indigestion, and rheumatism. The roots are liver and uterine stimulants. Root oil inhibits bacteria and fungus. *Angelica atropurea* is used similarly.
• REMARK Crushed leaves in car interiors reduce travel nausea.

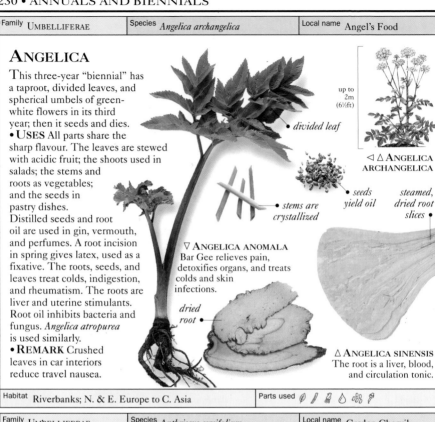

up to 2m (6½ft)

• *divided leaf*

◁ △ ANGELICA ARCHANGELICA

• *seeds yield oil*

steamed, dried root slices •

• *stems are crystallized*

▽ ANGELICA ANOMALA
Bar Gee relieves pain, detoxifies organs, and treats colds and skin infections.

dried root •

△ ANGELICA SINENSIS
The root is a liver, blood, and circulation tonic.

Habitat Riverbanks; N. & E. Europe to C. Asia	Parts used

Family UMBELLIFERAE	Species *Anthriscus cereifolium*	Local name Garden Chervil

CHERVIL

This annual has branched, hollow stems with bright green, finely divided, fern-like leaves, and umbels of white flowers.
• USES With a delicate parsley-like flavour, Chervil is part of the French *fines herbes*, and blends well with other herbs. The best flavoured foliage is grown in light shade, and used fresh as a garnish or added at the end of cooking. The leaf contains vitamin C, carotene, iron, and magnesium. Leaves and blanched stems enhance green salads, vinegar, and many subtle dishes. Leaf tea eliminates toxins and helps to purify body systems. In a face mask Chervil cleanses the skin and maintains suppleness. It is a mild digestive and circulation stimulant, reduces liver and catarrh problems, and soothes painful joints.

• *umbels of tiny white flowers appear in summer*

• *green leaf may take on pale magenta blush in late summer*

• *lacy foliage*

up to 60cm (24in)

Habitat Well-drained soil; Europe, W. Asia	Parts used

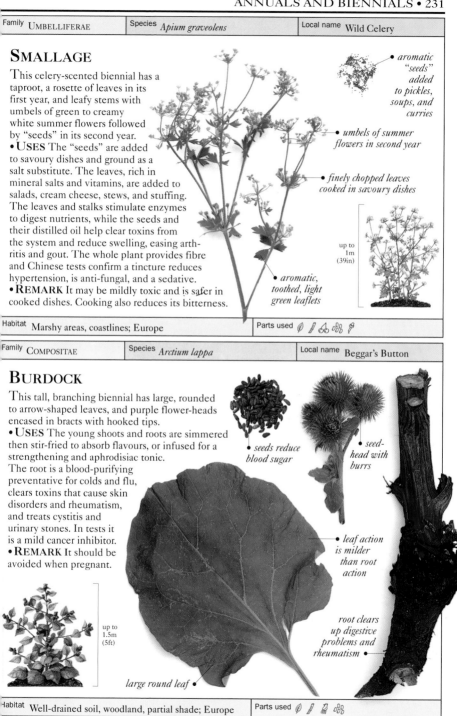

Family UMBELLIFERAE	Species *Apium graveolens*	Local name Wild Celery

SMALLAGE

This celery-scented biennial has a taproot, a rosette of leaves in its first year, and leafy stems with umbels of green to creamy white summer flowers followed by "seeds" in its second year.
• USES The "seeds" are added to savoury dishes and ground as a salt substitute. The leaves, rich in mineral salts and vitamins, are added to salads, cream cheese, stews, and stuffing. The leaves and stalks stimulate enzymes to digest nutrients, while the seeds and their distilled oil help clear toxins from the system and reduce swelling, easing arthritis and gout. The whole plant provides fibre and Chinese tests confirm a tincture reduces hypertension, is anti-fungal, and a sedative.
• REMARK It may be mildly toxic and is safer in cooked dishes. Cooking also reduces its bitterness.

• *aromatic "seeds" added to pickles, soups, and curries*

• *umbels of summer flowers in second year*

• *finely chopped leaves cooked in savoury dishes*

up to 1m (39in)

• *aromatic, toothed, light green leaflets*

Habitat Marshy areas, coastlines; Europe	Parts used

Family COMPOSITAE	Species *Arctium lappa*	Local name Beggar's Button

BURDOCK

This tall, branching biennial has large, rounded to arrow-shaped leaves, and purple flower-heads encased in bracts with hooked tips.
• USES The young shoots and roots are simmered then stir-fried to absorb flavours, or infused for a strengthening and aphrodisiac tonic. The root is a blood-purifying preventative for colds and flu, clears toxins that cause skin disorders and rheumatism, and treats cystitis and urinary stones. In tests it is a mild cancer inhibitor.
• REMARK It should be avoided when pregnant.

• *seeds reduce blood sugar*

• *seed-head with burrs*

• *leaf action is milder than root action*

up to 1.5m (5ft)

root clears up digestive problems and rheumatism •

• *large round leaf*

Habitat Well-drained soil, woodland, partial shade; Europe	Parts used

Family COMPOSITAE	Species *Artemisia annua*	Local name Quighaosu

SWEET WORMWOOD

This annual has feathery foliage, loose panicles of flower-heads from summer onwards, and red stems in autumn.
• USES In Indo-China the herb treats jaundice, dysentery, and skin complaints. Chinese herbalists recommend it to stop wound bleeding and to help new muscle growth, although they warn of possible side-effects. The Chinese army take it to prevent malaria and Chinese research has isolated an anti-malarial compound, QHS (quinghaosu), or artemisinin, which treats drug-resistant strains. The seeds treat eye disease.
• REMARK Biennial *Artemisia apiacea* is considered a beauti-fying nutriment in China as it clears toxins. It is also taken to prevent and treat malaria.

loose panicles of small, spherical, yellow-green flower-heads

vitamin A in deeply divided and toothed leaves

feathery foliage

up to 3m (10ft)

green stem, sometimes red

Habitat Wasteland; S.E. Europe, Iran, China, North America	Parts used 米 ∅ ∥ 🪰 ℘

Family CHENOPODIACEAE	Species *Atriplex hortensis* var. *rubra*	Local name Saltbush

PURPLE ORACH

Orach is an annual with arrowhead-shaped leaves and spikes of insignificant flowers producing pale seeds.
• USES The leaves and young shoots are used in salads. The leaves are cooked as spinach and in soups; the stems are stir-fried. North American settlers and native Americans used the slightly salty leaves to flavour food, and ground the seeds into a flour. Native Americans used poultices of roots, stems, and flowers of other species of *Atriplex* on insect-bites, and Europeans used them to treat sore throats, jaundice, and gout.
• REMARK Purple Orach creates a seasonal hedge.

purple-brown to crimson; gold variety also available

young leaves have a mealy surface

stem-leaves narrow with silver-green flowering spike

up to 2.5m (8ft)

mature leaf is smooth

◁ ATRIPLEX HORTENSIS ▷
Common Orach leaves are used like Purple Orach.

Habitat Saltmarsh, wasteland; W. Asia,	S. Europe	Parts used 米 ∅ ∥ 🗲

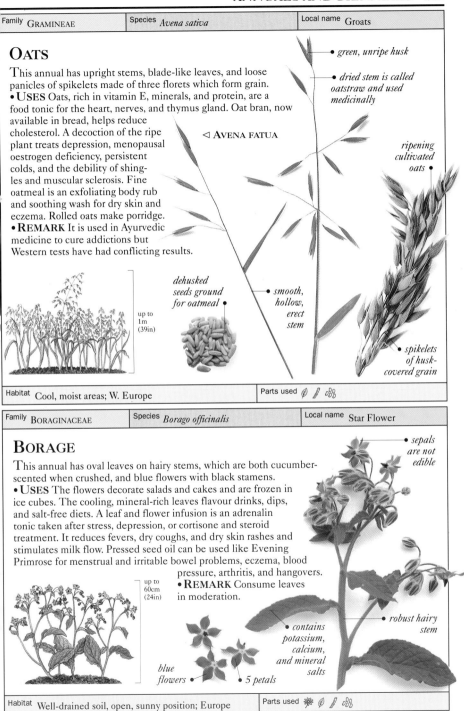

| Family GRAMINEAE | Species *Avena sativa* | Local name Groats |

OATS

This annual has upright stems, blade-like leaves, and loose panicles of spikelets made of three florets which form grain.
• **USES** Oats, rich in vitamin E, minerals, and protein, are a food tonic for the heart, nerves, and thymus gland. Oat bran, now available in bread, helps reduce cholesterol. A decoction of the ripe plant treats depression, menopausal oestrogen deficiency, persistent colds, and the debility of shingles and muscular sclerosis. Fine oatmeal is an exfoliating body rub and soothing wash for dry skin and eczema. Rolled oats make porridge.
• **REMARK** It is used in Ayurvedic medicine to cure addictions but Western tests have had conflicting results.

◁ **AVENA FATUA**

• *green, unripe husk*

• *dried stem is called oatstraw and used medicinally*

ripening cultivated oats •

dehusked seeds ground for oatmeal •

up to 1m (39in)

• *smooth, hollow, erect stem*

• *spikelets of husk-covered grain*

| Habitat Cool, moist areas; W. Europe | Parts used |

| Family BORAGINACEAE | Species *Borago officinalis* | Local name Star Flower |

BORAGE

This annual has oval leaves on hairy stems, which are both cucumber-scented when crushed, and blue flowers with black stamens.
• **USES** The flowers decorate salads and cakes and are frozen in ice cubes. The cooling, mineral-rich leaves flavour drinks, dips, and salt-free diets. A leaf and flower infusion is an adrenalin tonic taken after stress, depression, or cortisone and steroid treatment. It reduces fevers, dry coughs, and dry skin rashes and stimulates milk flow. Pressed seed oil can be used like Evening Primrose for menstrual and irritable bowel problems, eczema, blood pressure, arthritis, and hangovers.
• **REMARK** Consume leaves in moderation.

• *sepals are not edible*

up to 60cm (24in)

• *robust hairy stem*

• *contains potassium, calcium, and mineral salts*

blue flowers •

• *5 petals*

| Habitat Well-drained soil, open, sunny position; Europe | Parts used |

Family CRUCIFERAE	Species *Brassica nigra*	Local name Moutarde Noire

BLACK MUSTARD

This annual has bright green, oval leaves; clusters of four-petalled, yellow summer flowers; and dark brown seeds.

• **USES** Black Mustard seed has the strongest flavour and was used to make most mustards, but as it is difficult to harvest mechanically it has been replaced by Brown Mustard. Mustard becomes pungent only when the crushed seeds are mixed with cold water to activate the appropriate enzymes. Boiling water, applied to dormant enzymes, kills them, vinegar inhibits them, and both create a weak aroma but bitter taste. Mustard seeds stimulate circulation, which invited their use in love potions. They treat bronchitis, give a warming footbath, and, in a mustard poultice, reduce inflammation treating chilblains and rheumatism. The oil is a lubricant.

• **REMARK** In China Brown Mustard seed is used to treat colds, stomach problems, abscesses, rheumatism, lumbago, and ulcers. Leaves treat bladder inflammation.

seed-pods •

up to 2m (6½ft)

◁ ▽ △ **BRASSICA NIGRA**

flowers added to salads •

• almost scentless black seeds

• lower leaf shape is variable

• narrow stem-leaf with toothed margin

• mustard is milder if seed coat is left on

large, sand-coloured White Mustard seeds •

• Brown Mustard seed less pungent than Black Mustard seed

◁ **BRASSICA JUNCEA** Brown Mustard is a vitamin-rich annual with many Chinese varieties.

seed-pods •

• pungent leaves

• flowering stem-leaves are long, narrow, and very bitter

BRASSICA HIRTA ▷ White Mustard is a hairy annual with less flavourful seeds but with sturdy enzymes. It is a preservative used in pickles and to emulsify mayonnaise.

Habitat	Fertile, well-drained soil, sun; Europe	Parts used ❋ ∅ ⚬⚬ ♀

Family CRUCIFERAE	Species *Brassica oleracea*	Local name Colewort

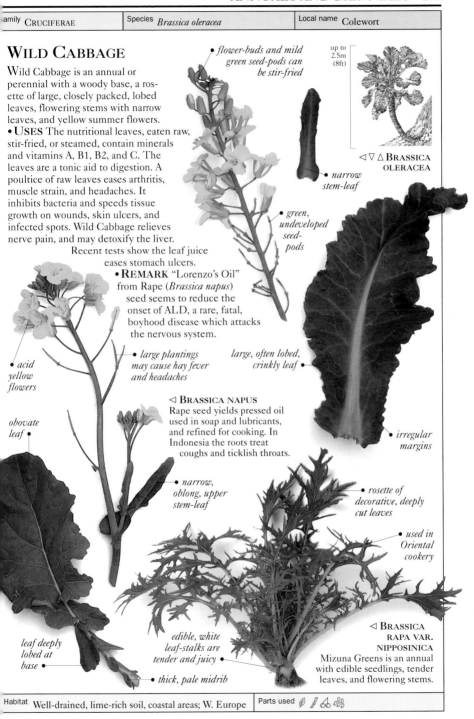

WILD CABBAGE

Wild Cabbage is an annual or perennial with a woody base, a rosette of large, closely packed, lobed leaves, flowering stems with narrow leaves, and yellow summer flowers.
• **USES** The nutritional leaves, eaten raw, stir-fried, or steamed, contain minerals and vitamins A, B1, B2, and C. The leaves are a tonic aid to digestion. A poultice of raw leaves eases arthritis, muscle strain, and headaches. It inhibits bacteria and speeds tissue growth on wounds, skin ulcers, and infected spots. Wild Cabbage relieves nerve pain, and may detoxify the liver. Recent tests show the leaf juice eases stomach ulcers.
• **REMARK** "Lorenzo's Oil" from Rape (*Brassica napus*) seed seems to reduce the onset of ALD, a rare, fatal, boyhood disease which attacks the nervous system.

flower-buds and mild green seed-pods can be stir-fried

up to 2.5m (8ft)

◁ ▽ △ **BRASSICA OLERACEA**

narrow stem-leaf

green, undeveloped seed-pods

large, often lobed, crinkly leaf

large plantings may cause hay fever and headaches

acid yellow flowers

obovate leaf

◁ **BRASSICA NAPUS**
Rape seed yields pressed oil used in soap and lubricants, and refined for cooking. In Indonesia the roots treat coughs and ticklish throats.

narrow, oblong, upper stem-leaf

irregular margins

rosette of decorative, deeply cut leaves

used in Oriental cookery

◁ **BRASSICA RAPA VAR. NIPPOSINICA**
Mizuna Greens is an annual with edible seedlings, tender leaves, and flowering stems.

leaf deeply lobed at base

edible, white leaf-stalks are tender and juicy

thick, pale midrib

Habitat Well-drained, lime-rich soil, coastal areas; W. Europe	Parts used

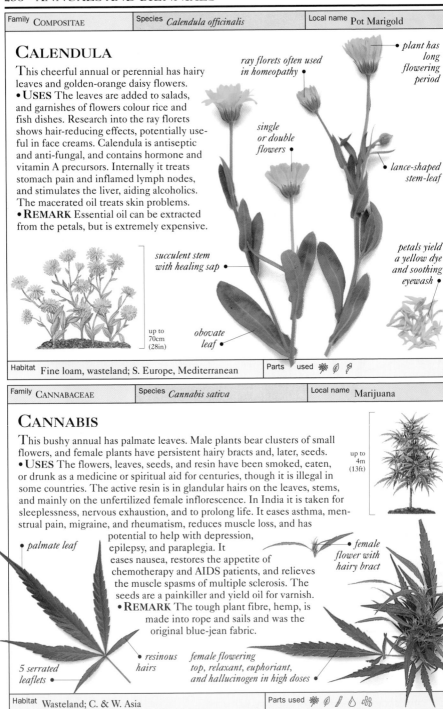

| Family COMPOSITAE | Species *Calendula officinalis* | Local name Pot Marigold |

CALENDULA

This cheerful annual or perennial has hairy leaves and golden-orange daisy flowers.
• **USES** The leaves are added to salads, and garnishes of flowers colour rice and fish dishes. Research into the ray florets shows hair-reducing effects, potentially useful in face creams. Calendula is antiseptic and anti-fungal, and contains hormone and vitamin A precursors. Internally it treats stomach pain and inflamed lymph nodes, and stimulates the liver, aiding alcoholics. The macerated oil treats skin problems.
• **REMARK** Essential oil can be extracted from the petals, but is extremely expensive.

ray florets often used in homeopathy

plant has long flowering period

single or double flowers

lance-shaped stem-leaf

succulent stem with healing sap

petals yield a yellow dye and soothing eyewash

up to 70cm (28in)

obovate leaf

| Habitat Fine loam, wasteland; S. Europe, Mediterranean | Parts used ❋ ∅ ⚘ |

| Family CANNABACEAE | Species *Cannabis sativa* | Local name Marijuana |

CANNABIS

This bushy annual has palmate leaves. Male plants bear clusters of small flowers, and female plants have persistent hairy bracts and, later, seeds.
• **USES** The flowers, leaves, seeds, and resin have been smoked, eaten, or drunk as a medicine or spiritual aid for centuries, though it is illegal in some countries. The active resin is in glandular hairs on the leaves, stems, and mainly on the unfertilized female inflorescence. In India it is taken for sleeplessness, nervous exhaustion, and to prolong life. It eases asthma, menstrual pain, migraine, and rheumatism, reduces muscle loss, and has potential to help with depression, epilepsy, and paraplegia. It eases nausea, restores the appetite of chemotherapy and AIDS patients, and relieves the muscle spasms of multiple sclerosis. The seeds are a painkiller and yield oil for varnish.
• **REMARK** The tough plant fibre, hemp, is made into rope and sails and was the original blue-jean fabric.

up to 4m (13ft)

palmate leaf

female flower with hairy bract

5 serrated leaflets

resinous hairs

female flowering top, relaxant, euphoriant, and hallucinogen in high doses

| Habitat Wasteland; C. & W. Asia | Parts used ❋ ∅ ⧸ ◊ ⸬ |

| Family SOLANACEAE | Species *Capsicum annuum* | Local name Capsicum |

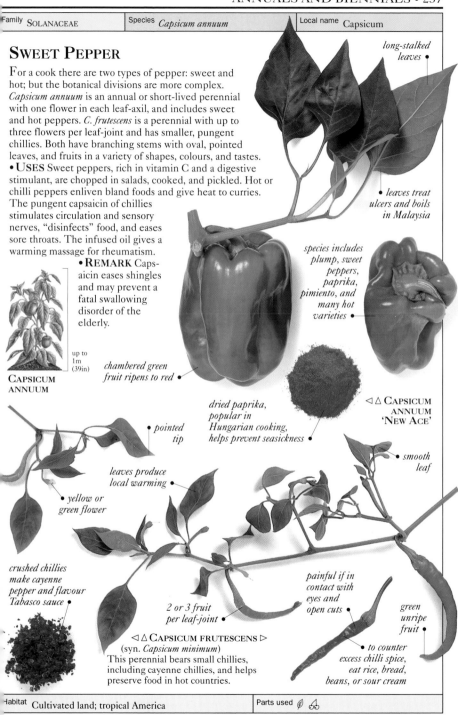

SWEET PEPPER

For a cook there are two types of pepper: sweet and hot; but the botanical divisions are more complex. *Capsicum annuum* is an annual or short-lived perennial with one flower in each leaf-axil, and includes sweet and hot peppers. *C. frutescens* is a perennial with up to three flowers per leaf-joint and has smaller, pungent chillies. Both have branching stems with oval, pointed leaves, and fruits in a variety of shapes, colours, and tastes.
• USES Sweet peppers, rich in vitamin C and a digestive stimulant, are chopped in salads, cooked, and pickled. Hot or chilli peppers enliven bland foods and give heat to curries. The pungent capsaicin of chillies stimulates circulation and sensory nerves, "disinfects" food, and eases sore throats. The infused oil gives a warming massage for rheumatism.
• REMARK Capsaicin eases shingles and may prevent a fatal swallowing disorder of the elderly.

long-stalked leaves •

• leaves treat ulcers and boils in Malaysia

species includes plump, sweet peppers, paprika, pimiento, and many hot varieties •

up to 1m (39in)

CAPSICUM ANNUUM

chambered green fruit ripens to red •

dried paprika, popular in Hungarian cooking, helps prevent seasickness •

◁ △ **CAPSICUM ANNUUM 'NEW ACE'**

• smooth leaf

• pointed tip

leaves produce local warming •

• yellow or green flower

crushed chillies make cayenne pepper and flavour Tabasco sauce •

2 or 3 fruit per leaf-joint •

painful if in contact with eyes and open cuts •

green unripe fruit •

◁ △ **CAPSICUM FRUTESCENS** ▷
(syn. *Capsicum minimum*)
This perennial bears small chillies, including cayenne chillies, and helps preserve food in hot countries.

• to counter excess chilli spice, eat rice, bread, beans, or sour cream

| Habitat Cultivated land; tropical America | Parts used 🌿 |

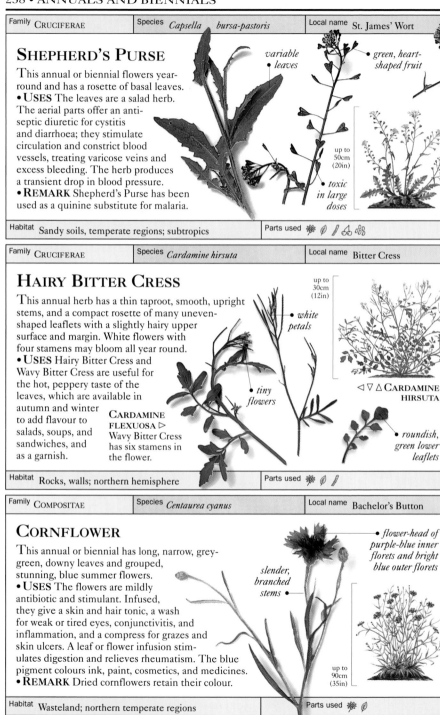

| Family CRUCIFERAE | Species *Capsella bursa-pastoris* | Local name St. James' Wort |

SHEPHERD'S PURSE

This annual or biennial flowers year-round and has a rosette of basal leaves.
• **USES** The leaves are a salad herb.
The aerial parts offer an anti-septic diuretic for cystitis
and diarrhoea; they stimulate
circulation and constrict blood
vessels, treating varicose veins and
excess bleeding. The herb produces
a transient drop in blood pressure.
• **REMARK** Shepherd's Purse has been
used as a quinine substitute for malaria.

variable leaves

green, heart-shaped fruit

up to
50cm
(20in)

toxic in large doses

| Habitat Sandy soils, temperate regions; subtropics | Parts used |

| Family CRUCIFERAE | Species *Cardamine hirsuta* | Local name Bitter Cress |

HAIRY BITTER CRESS

This annual herb has a thin taproot, smooth, upright
stems, and a compact rosette of many uneven-shaped leaflets with a slightly hairy upper
surface and margin. White flowers with
four stamens may bloom all year round.
• **USES** Hairy Bitter Cress and
Wavy Bitter Cress are useful for
the hot, peppery taste of the
leaves, which are available in
autumn and winter
to add flavour to
salads, soups, and
sandwiches, and
as a garnish.

**CARDAMINE
FLEXUOSA** ▷
Wavy Bitter Cress
has six stamens in
the flower.

up to
30cm
(12in)

white petals

tiny flowers

◁ ▽ △ **CARDAMINE
HIRSUTA**

roundish, green lower leaflets

| Habitat Rocks, walls; northern hemisphere | Parts used |

| Family COMPOSITAE | Species *Centaurea cyanus* | Local name Bachelor's Button |

CORNFLOWER

This annual or biennial has long, narrow, grey-green, downy leaves and grouped,
stunning, blue summer flowers.
• **USES** The flowers are mildly
antibiotic and stimulant. Infused,
they give a skin and hair tonic, a wash
for weak or tired eyes, conjunctivitis, and
inflammation, and a compress for grazes and
skin ulcers. A leaf or flower infusion stim-ulates digestion and relieves rheumatism. The blue
pigment colours ink, paint, cosmetics, and medicines.
• **REMARK** Dried cornflowers retain their colour.

flower-head of purple-blue inner florets and bright blue outer florets

slender, branched stems

up to
90cm
(35in)

| Habitat Wasteland; northern temperate regions | Parts used |

| Family UMBELLIFERAE | Species *Carum carvi* | Local name Karawya |

CARAWAY

Caraway is a hardy biennial with finely
cut, feathery leaves, umbels of small
flower-heads in midsummer, and capsules
containing two curved, narrow seeds.
• USES The seeds are a popular spice,
especially in central Europe. They enhance
pork, goulash, sauerkraut, cheese, and pickles,
and are added to cooking cabbage to reduce the
smell. They flavour breads and cakes, and are
eaten raw or sugar-coated as Caraway comfits
after a spicy meal. They sweeten
the breath, aid digestion, and relieve
flatulence. Chopped leaves are added
to soups and salads, and the root is
cooked as a vegetable. Essential oil,
distilled from the seeds, flavours
confectionery, gin, the liqueur
Kümmel, and mouthwashes, and
scents soaps and aftershaves. The
seeds are antiseptic and a vermifuge.
• REMARK Caraway seeds have been
used in cooking since the Stone Age.

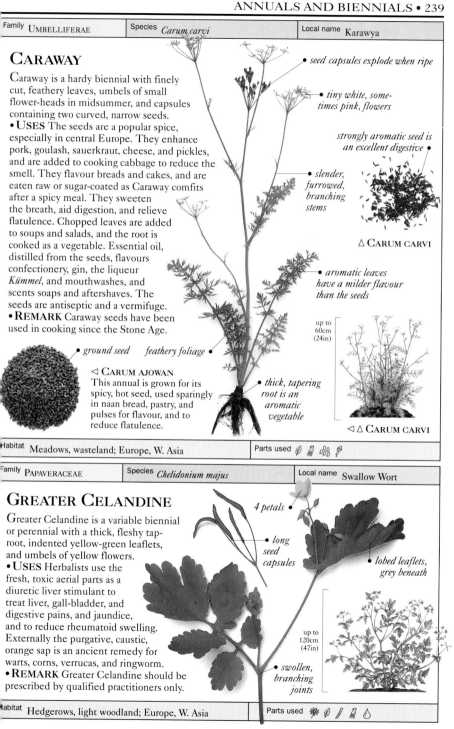

• seed capsules explode when ripe

• tiny white, some-
times pink, flowers

strongly aromatic seed is
an excellent digestive •

• slender,
furrowed,
branching
stems

△ CARUM CARVI

• aromatic leaves
have a milder flavour
than the seeds

up to
60cm
(24in)

• ground seed   feathery foliage •

◁ CARUM AJOWAN
This annual is grown for its
spicy, hot seed, used sparingly
in naan bread, pastry, and
pulses for flavour, and to
reduce flatulence.

• thick, tapering
root is an
aromatic
vegetable

◁ △ CARUM CARVI

| Habitat Meadows, wasteland; Europe, W. Asia | Parts used |

| Family PAPAVERACEAE | Species *Chelidonium majus* | Local name Swallow Wort |

GREATER CELANDINE

Greater Celandine is a variable biennial
or perennial with a thick, fleshy taproot, indented yellow-green leaflets,
and umbels of yellow flowers.
• USES Herbalists use the
fresh, toxic aerial parts as a
diuretic liver stimulant to
treat liver, gall-bladder, and
digestive pains, and jaundice,
and to reduce rheumatoid swelling.
Externally the purgative, caustic,
orange sap is an ancient remedy for
warts, corns, verrucas, and ringworm.
• REMARK Greater Celandine should be
prescribed by qualified practitioners only.

4 petals •

• long
seed
capsules

• lobed leaflets,
grey beneath

up to
120cm
(47in)

• swollen,
branching
joints

| Habitat Hedgerows, light woodland; Europe, W. Asia | Parts used |

Family CHENOPODIACEAE	Species *Chenopodium ambrosioides*	Local name Fragrant Tiger Bones

AMERICAN WORMSEED

This annual, or short-lived perennial, has large and small spear-shaped, deeply toothed leaves, green summer flowers, and small, dry fruit.
• **USES** The pungent leaves season soup, corn, black beans, and shellfish in Mexico and are brewed for "Jesuit Tea", but the herb's main use is to expel intestinal roundworms, hook worms, and small tapeworms from humans and animals. All parts contain a worm-repelling compound, ascaridole, but the fruit, and chenopodium oil distilled from it, are most potent and toxic. Locally called "Herba Sancti Mariæ", the leaf is used to expel catarrh and treat asthma. Some Amazon tribes take it to encourage milk-flow.
• **REMARK** American Wormseed is poisonous and should be used by qualified practitioners only.

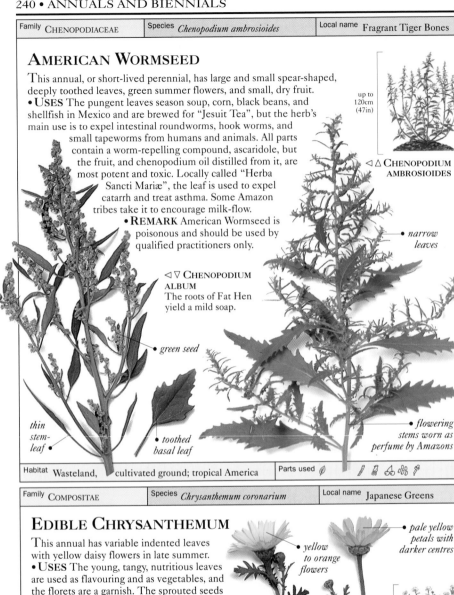

up to 120cm (47in)

◁ △ CHENOPODIUM AMBROSIOIDES

• *narrow leaves*

◁ ▽ CHENOPODIUM ALBUM
The roots of Fat Hen yield a mild soap.

• *green seed*

thin stem-leaf •

• *toothed basal leaf*

• *flowering stems worn as perfume by Amazons*

Habitat Wasteland, cultivated ground; tropical America	Parts used

Family COMPOSITAE	Species *Chrysanthemum coronarium*	Local name Japanese Greens

EDIBLE CHRYSANTHEMUM

This annual has variable indented leaves with yellow daisy flowers in late summer.
• **USES** The young, tangy, nutritious leaves are used as flavouring and as vegetables, and the florets are a garnish. The sprouted seeds are a winter snack. Flower-heads of the variety *spatiosum* have a unique flavour.
• **REMARK** The flower-heads of Wild Chrysanthemum, (*Dendranthema indicum* syn. *Chrysanthemum indicum*) were part of the Taoist elixir of immortality.

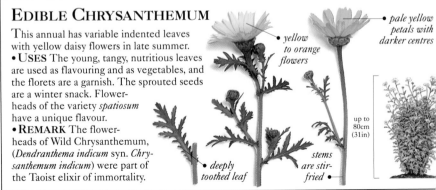

• *pale yellow petals with darker centres*

• *yellow to orange flowers*

up to 80cm (31in)

stems are stir-fried •

• *deeply toothed leaf*

Habitat Moisture-retentive, fertile soil, sun; Mediterranean	Parts used

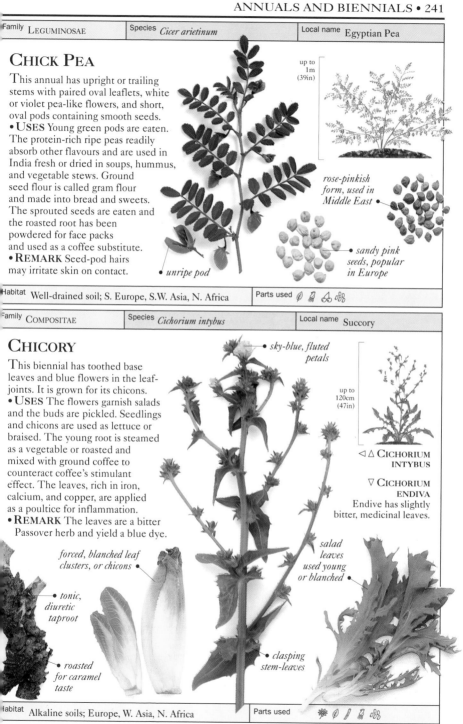

| Family | LEGUMINOSAE | Species | *Cicer arietinum* | Local name | Egyptian Pea |

CHICK PEA

This annual has upright or trailing
stems with paired oval leaflets, white
or violet pea-like flowers, and short,
oval pods containing smooth seeds.
• **USES** Young green pods are eaten.
The protein-rich ripe peas readily
absorb other flavours and are used in
India fresh or dried in soups, hummus,
and vegetable stews. Ground
seed flour is called gram flour
and made into bread and sweets.
The sprouted seeds are eaten and
the roasted root has been
powdered for face packs
and used as a coffee substitute.
• **REMARK** Seed-pod hairs
may irritate skin on contact.

up to
1m
(39in)

*rose-pinkish
form, used in
Middle East* •

• *unripe pod*

• *sandy pink
seeds, popular
in Europe*

| Habitat | Well-drained soil; S. Europe, S.W. Asia, N. Africa | Parts used | |

| Family | COMPOSITAE | Species | *Cichorium intybus* | Local name | Succory |

CHICORY

This biennial has toothed base
leaves and blue flowers in the leaf-
joints. It is grown for its chicons.
• **USES** The flowers garnish salads
and the buds are pickled. Seedlings
and chicons are used as lettuce or
braised. The young root is steamed
as a vegetable or roasted and
mixed with ground coffee to
counteract coffee's stimulant
effect. The leaves, rich in iron,
calcium, and copper, are applied
as a poultice for inflammation.
• **REMARK** The leaves are a bitter
   Passover herb and yield a blue dye.

• *sky-blue, fluted
petals*

up to
120cm
(47in)

◁ △ CICHORIUM
INTYBUS

▽ CICHORIUM
ENDIVA
Endive has slightly
bitter, medicinal leaves.

*salad
leaves
used young
or blanched* •

*forced, blanched leaf
clusters, or chicons* •

• *tonic,
diuretic
taproot*

• *roasted
for caramel
taste*

• *clasping
stem-leaves*

| Habitat | Alkaline soils; Europe, W. Asia, N. Africa | Parts used | |

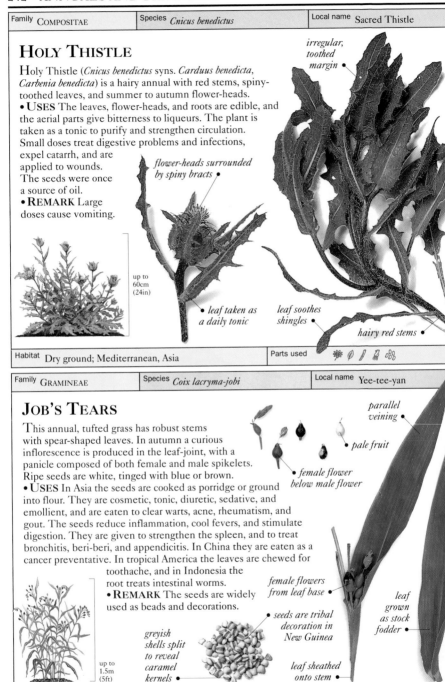

| Family COMPOSITAE | Species *Cnicus benedictus* | Local name Sacred Thistle |

HOLY THISTLE

Holy Thistle (*Cnicus benedictus* syns. *Carduus benedicta, Carbenia benedicta*) is a hairy annual with red stems, spiny-toothed leaves, and summer to autumn flower-heads.
• **USES** The leaves, flower-heads, and roots are edible, and the aerial parts give bitterness to liqueurs. The plant is taken as a tonic to purify and strengthen circulation. Small doses treat digestive problems and infections, expel catarrh, and are applied to wounds. The seeds were once a source of oil.
• **REMARK** Large doses cause vomiting.

irregular, toothed margin

flower-heads surrounded by spiny bracts

up to 60cm (24in)

leaf taken as a daily tonic

leaf soothes shingles

hairy red stems

| Habitat Dry ground; Mediterranean, Asia | Parts used |

| Family GRAMINEAE | Species *Coix lacryma-jobi* | Local name Yee-tee-yan |

JOB'S TEARS

This annual, tufted grass has robust stems with spear-shaped leaves. In autumn a curious inflorescence is produced in the leaf-joint, with a panicle composed of both female and male spikelets. Ripe seeds are white, tinged with blue or brown.
• **USES** In Asia the seeds are cooked as porridge or ground into flour. They are cosmetic, tonic, diuretic, sedative, and emollient, and are eaten to clear warts, acne, rheumatism, and gout. The seeds reduce inflammation, cool fevers, and stimulate digestion. They are given to strengthen the spleen, and to treat bronchitis, beri-beri, and appendicitis. In China they are eaten as a cancer preventative. In tropical America the leaves are chewed for toothache, and in Indonesia the root treats intestinal worms.
• **REMARK** The seeds are widely used as beads and decorations.

parallel veining

pale fruit

female flower below male flower

female flowers from leaf base

leaf grown as stock fodder

seeds are tribal decoration in New Guinea

greyish shells split to reveal caramel kernels

up to 1.5m (5ft)

leaf sheathed onto stem

| Habitat Moist soils; S.E. Asia | Parts used |

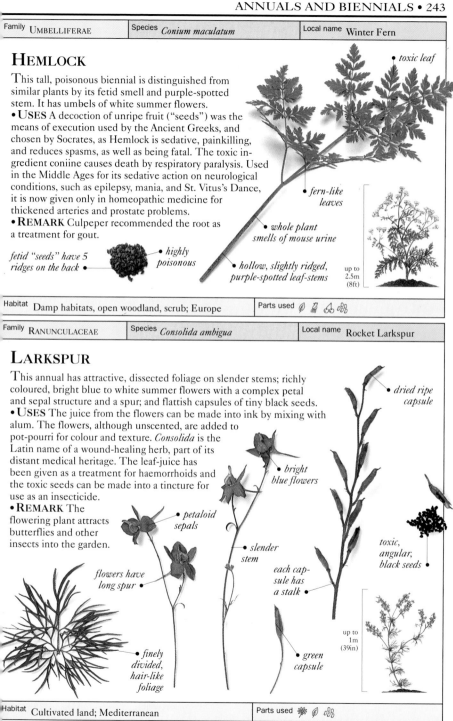

Family UMBELLIFERAE	Species *Conium maculatum*	Local name Winter Fern

HEMLOCK

This tall, poisonous biennial is distinguished from similar plants by its fetid smell and purple-spotted stem. It has umbels of white summer flowers.

• **USES** A decoction of unripe fruit ("seeds") was the means of execution used by the Ancient Greeks, and chosen by Socrates, as Hemlock is sedative, painkilling, and reduces spasms, as well as being fatal. The toxic ingredient coniine causes death by respiratory paralysis. Used in the Middle Ages for its sedative action on neurological conditions, such as epilepsy, mania, and St. Vitus's Dance, it is now given only in homeopathic medicine for thickened arteries and prostate problems.

• **REMARK** Culpeper recommended the root as a treatment for gout.

• *toxic leaf*

• *fern-like leaves*

• *whole plant smells of mouse urine*

fetid "seeds" have 5 ridges on the back •

• *highly poisonous*

• *hollow, slightly ridged, purple-spotted leaf-stems*

up to 2.5m (8ft)

Habitat Damp habitats, open woodland, scrub; Europe	Parts used

Family RANUNCULACEAE	Species *Consolida ambigua*	Local name Rocket Larkspur

LARKSPUR

This annual has attractive, dissected foliage on slender stems; richly coloured, bright blue to white summer flowers with a complex petal and sepal structure and a spur; and flattish capsules of tiny black seeds.

• **USES** The juice from the flowers can be made into ink by mixing with alum. The flowers, although unscented, are added to pot-pourri for colour and texture. *Consolida* is the Latin name of a wound-healing herb, part of its distant medical heritage. The leaf-juice has been given as a treatment for haemorrhoids and the toxic seeds can be made into a tincture for use as an insecticide.

• **REMARK** The flowering plant attracts butterflies and other insects into the garden.

• *dried ripe capsule*

• *bright blue flowers*

• *petaloid sepals*

• *slender stem*

toxic, angular, black seeds •

flowers have long spur •

each capsule has a stalk •

up to 1m (39in)

• *finely divided, hair-like foliage*

• *green capsule*

Habitat Cultivated land; Mediterranean	Parts used

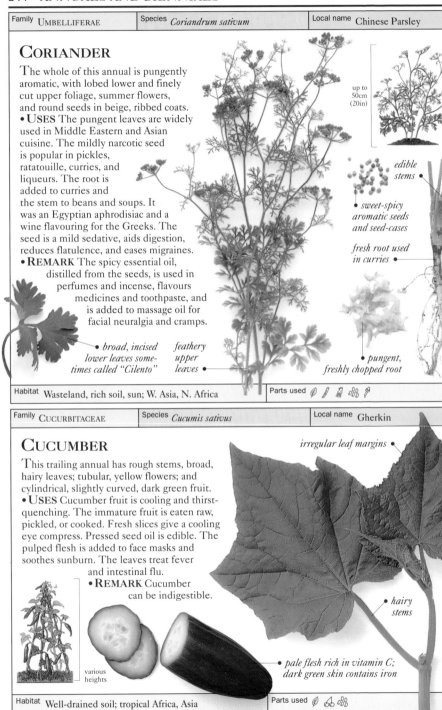

Family UMBELLIFERAE	Species *Coriandrum sativum*	Local name Chinese Parsley

CORIANDER

The whole of this annual is pungently aromatic, with lobed lower and finely cut upper foliage, summer flowers, and round seeds in beige, ribbed coats.
• USES The pungent leaves are widely used in Middle Eastern and Asian cuisine. The mildly narcotic seed is popular in pickles, ratatouille, curries, and liqueurs. The root is added to curries and the stem to beans and soups. It was an Egyptian aphrodisiac and a wine flavouring for the Greeks. The seed is a mild sedative, aids digestion, reduces flatulence, and eases migraines.
• REMARK The spicy essential oil, distilled from the seeds, is used in perfumes and incense, flavours medicines and toothpaste, and is added to massage oil for facial neuralgia and cramps.

up to 50cm (20in)

edible stems

sweet-spicy aromatic seeds and seed-cases

fresh root used in curries

broad, incised lower leaves sometimes called "Cilento"

feathery upper leaves

pungent, freshly chopped root

Habitat Wasteland, rich soil, sun; W. Asia, N. Africa	Parts used

Family CUCURBITACEAE	Species *Cucumis sativus*	Local name Gherkin

CUCUMBER

This trailing annual has rough stems, broad, hairy leaves; tubular, yellow flowers; and cylindrical, slightly curved, dark green fruit.
• USES Cucumber fruit is cooling and thirst-quenching. The immature fruit is eaten raw, pickled, or cooked. Fresh slices give a cooling eye compress. Pressed seed oil is edible. The pulped flesh is added to face masks and soothes sunburn. The leaves treat fever and intestinal flu.
• REMARK Cucumber can be indigestible.

irregular leaf margins

hairy stems

various heights

pale flesh rich in vitamin C; dark green skin contains iron

Habitat Well-drained soil; tropical Africa, Asia	Parts used

Family CUCURBITACEAE	Species *Cucurbita pepo*	Local name Squash

PUMPKIN

This trailing annual has sprawling, prickly stems, tendrils opposite large leaves, large, orange-yellow male flowers in leaf-axils, female flowers on stalks, and green to orange fruit.

• **USES** The species contains pumpkins, squashes, marrows, and courgettes, whose flowers are stuffed or battered and the flesh cooked in sweet and savoury dishes. Nutritious pumpkin seeds are roasted for snacks and considered a longevity food in China. The seeds yield a culinary oil and help expel intestinal worms.

• **REMARK** Seeds of *Cucurbita moschata* var. *toonas*, *C. pepo*, and *C. maxima* expel worms and prevent prostate trouble.

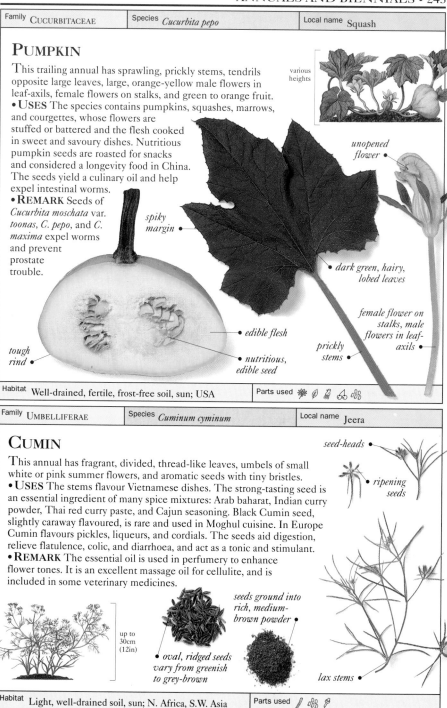

various heights

unopened flower •

spiky margin •

• dark green, hairy, lobed leaves

female flower on stalks, male flowers in leaf-axils •

tough rind •

• edible flesh

prickly stems •

• nutritious, edible seed

Habitat Well-drained, fertile, frost-free soil, sun; USA	Parts used ✻ 🍋 🌿 🍃 ⚬

Family UMBELLIFERAE	Species *Cuminum cyminum*	Local name Jeera

CUMIN

This annual has fragrant, divided, thread-like leaves, umbels of small white or pink summer flowers, and aromatic seeds with tiny bristles.

• **USES** The stems flavour Vietnamese dishes. The strong-tasting seed is an essential ingredient of many spice mixtures: Arab baharat, Indian curry powder, Thai red curry paste, and Cajun seasoning. Black Cumin seed, slightly caraway flavoured, is rare and used in Moghul cuisine. In Europe Cumin flavours pickles, liqueurs, and cordials. The seeds aid digestion, relieve flatulence, colic, and diarrhoea, and act as a tonic and stimulant.

• **REMARK** The essential oil is used in perfumery to enhance flower tones. It is an excellent massage oil for cellulite, and is included in some veterinary medicines.

seed-heads •

• ripening seeds

up to 30cm (12in)

seeds ground into rich, medium-brown powder •

• oval, ridged seeds vary from greenish to grey-brown

lax stems •

Habitat Light, well-drained soil, sun; N. Africa, S.W. Asia	Parts used 🌿 ⚬ 🍋

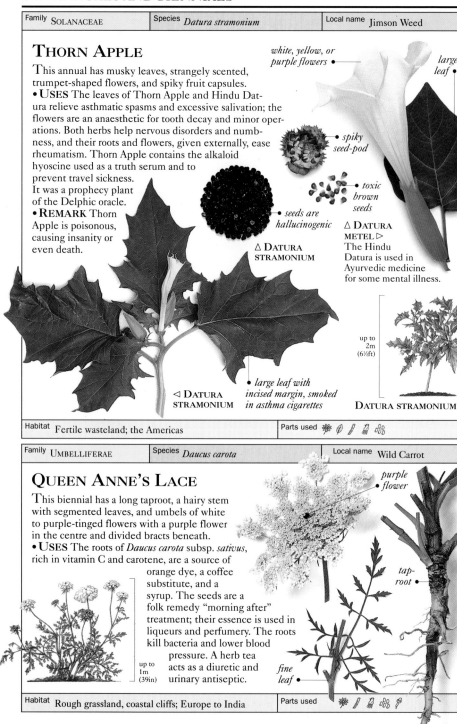

| Family SOLANACEAE | Species *Datura stramonium* | Local name Jimson Weed |

THORN APPLE

This annual has musky leaves, strangely scented, trumpet-shaped flowers, and spiky fruit capsules.
• **USES** The leaves of Thorn Apple and Hindu Datura relieve asthmatic spasms and excessive salivation; the flowers are an anaesthetic for tooth decay and minor operations. Both herbs help nervous disorders and numbness, and their roots and flowers, given externally, ease rheumatism. Thorn Apple contains the alkaloid hyoscine used as a truth serum and to prevent travel sickness. It was a prophecy plant of the Delphic oracle.
• **REMARK** Thorn Apple is poisonous, causing insanity or even death.

white, yellow, or purple flowers

large leaf

spiky seed-pod

toxic brown seeds

seeds are hallucinogenic

△ **DATURA STRAMONIUM**

△ **DATURA METEL** ▷
The Hindu Datura is used in Ayurvedic medicine for some mental illness.

up to 2m (6¼ft)

◁ **DATURA STRAMONIUM**

• *large leaf with incised margin, smoked in asthma cigarettes*

DATURA STRAMONIUM

| Habitat Fertile wasteland; the Americas | Parts used ✿ ◖ ▮ ▨ ⬚ |

| Family UMBELLIFERAE | Species *Daucus carota* | Local name Wild Carrot |

QUEEN ANNE'S LACE

This biennial has a long taproot, a hairy stem with segmented leaves, and umbels of white to purple-tinged flowers with a purple flower in the centre and divided bracts beneath.
• **USES** The roots of *Daucus carota* subsp. *sativus*, rich in vitamin C and carotene, are a source of orange dye, a coffee substitute, and a syrup. The seeds are a folk remedy "morning after" treatment; their essence is used in liqueurs and perfumery. The roots kill bacteria and lower blood pressure. A herb tea acts as a diuretic and urinary antiseptic.

purple flower

taproot

up to 1m (39in)

fine leaf

| Habitat Rough grassland, coastal cliffs; Europe to India | Parts used ✿ ▮ ▨ ⬚ ◖ |

Family SCROPHULARIACEAE	Species *Digitalis lanata*	Local name Witches' Gloves

GRECIAN FOXGLOVE

This biennial or perennial has purple-tinged stems with narrow leaves, terminating in a raceme of pinky beige, tubular flowers in summer.
• **USES** The drugs digitoxin and digoxin are prepared from the leaves of this species and used in orthodox medicine for heart disease; they increase the strength of heart contractions without increasing oxygen consumption (acting as stimulants), and regulate the heartbeat. The compounds were discovered in the Common Foxglove, but compounds in Grecian Foxglove are up to four times as potent. The leaves of Straw Foxglove are less dangerous as their effects are not accumulative. The leaves have been prescribed for epilepsy and tumours.
• **REMARK** The plant is poisonous and should be used by qualified personnel only.

DIGITALIS PURPUREA ▷
Common Foxglove is the other main species from which orthodox drugs are prepared.

unopened flower •

purple to white flowers •

flowers attract bees •

• *pale flower with pinky brown veining and pink-flushed white lip*

• *flowers open up the stem*

• *leafy bracts mostly shorter than the flowers*

◁ **DIGITALIS LANATA**

• *green leaves with reddish vein*

◁ **DIGITALIS LUTEA**
Straw Foxglove is a perennial with pale yellow to white flowers. The leaf glycosides are used in heart drugs.

spotted interior •

• *pale yellow or white flowers*

• *narrow, pointed leaf with finely serrated edge*

DIGITALIS PURPUREA ▽▷

up to 1m (39in)

DIGITALIS LANATA

smooth, bright green stem and leaves •

DIGITALIS LUTEA ▷

oval, pointed, textured, basal leaf with finely serrated margin •

Habitat Woodland clearings; Balkans, Hungary, Romania	Parts used 🖋

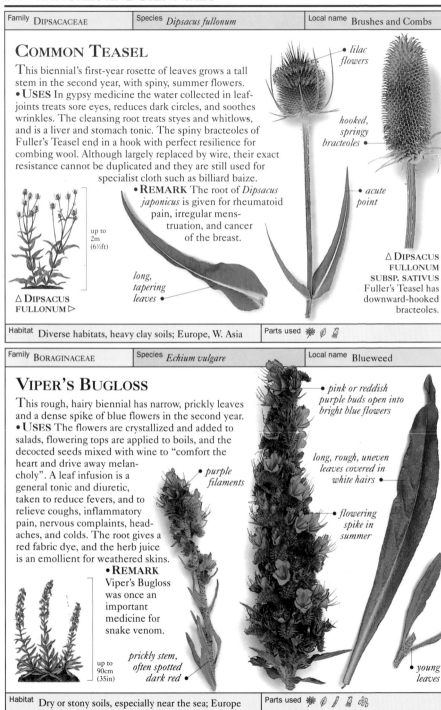

| Family DIPSACACEAE | Species *Dipsacus fullonum* | Local name Brushes and Combs |

COMMON TEASEL

This biennial's first-year rosette of leaves grows a tall stem in the second year, with spiny, summer flowers.
• USES In gypsy medicine the water collected in leaf-joints treats sore eyes, reduces dark circles, and soothes wrinkles. The cleansing root treats styes and whitlows, and is a liver and stomach tonic. The spiny bracteoles of Fuller's Teasel end in a hook with perfect resilience for combing wool. Although largely replaced by wire, their exact resistance cannot be duplicated and they are still used for specialist cloth such as billiard baize.
• REMARK The root of *Dipsacus japonicus* is given for rheumatoid pain, irregular menstruation, and cancer of the breast.

lilac flowers

hooked, springy bracteoles

acute point

up to 2m (6½ft)

long, tapering leaves

△ DIPSACUS FULLONUM ▷

△ DIPSACUS FULLONUM SUBSP. SATIVUS Fuller's Teasel has downward-hooked bracteoles.

| Habitat Diverse habitats, heavy clay soils; Europe, W. Asia | Parts used ❀ ⬯ ☊ |

| Family BORAGINACEAE | Species *Echium vulgare* | Local name Blueweed |

VIPER'S BUGLOSS

This rough, hairy biennial has narrow, prickly leaves and a dense spike of blue flowers in the second year.
• USES The flowers are crystallized and added to salads, flowering tops are applied to boils, and the decocted seeds mixed with wine to "comfort the heart and drive away melancholy". A leaf infusion is a general tonic and diuretic, taken to reduce fevers, and to relieve coughs, inflammatory pain, nervous complaints, headaches, and colds. The root gives a red fabric dye, and the herb juice is an emollient for weathered skins.
• REMARK Viper's Bugloss was once an important medicine for snake venom.

pink or reddish purple buds open into bright blue flowers

long, rough, uneven leaves covered in white hairs

purple filaments

flowering spike in summer

up to 90cm (35in)

prickly stem, often spotted dark red

young leaves

| Habitat Dry or stony soils, especially near the sea; Europe | Parts used ❀ ⬯ ❘ ☊ ✿ |

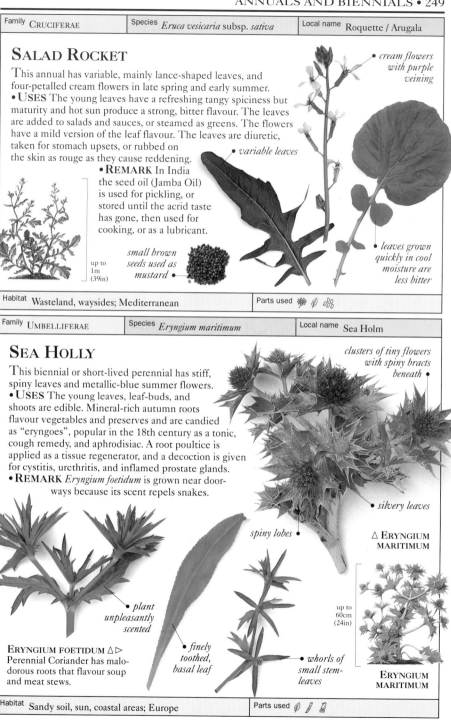

| Family CRUCIFERAE | Species *Eruca vesicaria* subsp. *sativa* | Local name Roquette / Arugala |

SALAD ROCKET

This annual has variable, mainly lance-shaped leaves, and four-petalled cream flowers in late spring and early summer.
• USES The young leaves have a refreshing tangy spiciness but maturity and hot sun produce a strong, bitter flavour. The leaves are added to salads and sauces, or steamed as greens. The flowers have a mild version of the leaf flavour. The leaves are diuretic, taken for stomach upsets, or rubbed on the skin as rouge as they cause reddening.
• REMARK In India the seed oil (Jamba Oil) is used for pickling, or stored until the acrid taste has gone, then used for cooking, or as a lubricant.

cream flowers with purple veining

variable leaves

leaves grown quickly in cool moisture are less bitter

up to 1m (39in)

small brown seeds used as mustard

| Habitat Wasteland, waysides; Mediterranean | Parts used |

| Family UMBELLIFERAE | Species *Eryngium maritimum* | Local name Sea Holm |

SEA HOLLY

This biennial or short-lived perennial has stiff, spiny leaves and metallic-blue summer flowers.
• USES The young leaves, leaf-buds, and shoots are edible. Mineral-rich autumn roots flavour vegetables and preserves and are candied as "eryngoes", popular in the 18th century as a tonic, cough remedy, and aphrodisiac. A root poultice is applied as a tissue regenerator, and a decoction is given for cystitis, urethritis, and inflamed prostate glands.
• REMARK *Eryngium foetidum* is grown near doorways because its scent repels snakes.

clusters of tiny flowers with spiny bracts beneath

silvery leaves

△ ERYNGIUM MARITIMUM

spiny lobes

plant unpleasantly scented

ERYNGIUM FOETIDUM △▷
Perennial Coriander has malodorous roots that flavour soup and meat stews.

finely toothed, basal leaf

whorls of small stem-leaves

up to 60cm (24in)

ERYNGIUM MARITIMUM

| Habitat Sandy soil, sun, coastal areas; Europe | Parts used |

Family PAPAVERACEAE	Species *Eschscholzia californica*	Local name Cup of Gold

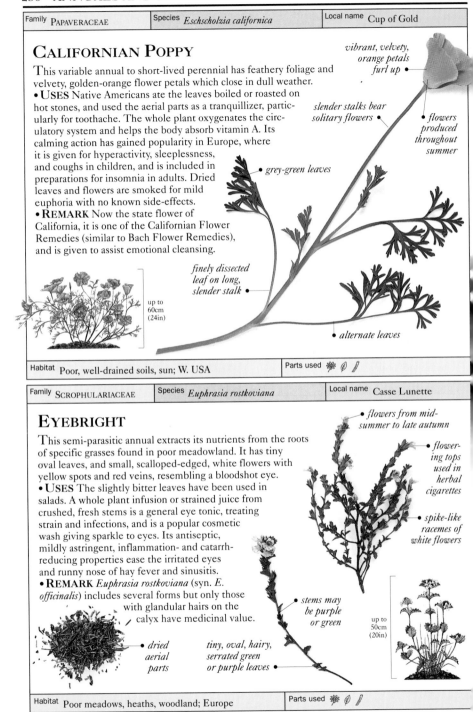

CALIFORNIAN POPPY

This variable annual to short-lived perennial has feathery foliage and velvety, golden-orange flower petals which close in dull weather.
• **USES** Native Americans ate the leaves boiled or roasted on hot stones, and used the aerial parts as a tranquillizer, particularly for toothache. The whole plant oxygenates the circulatory system and helps the body absorb vitamin A. Its calming action has gained popularity in Europe, where it is given for hyperactivity, sleeplessness, and coughs in children, and is included in preparations for insomnia in adults. Dried leaves and flowers are smoked for mild euphoria with no known side-effects.
• **REMARK** Now the state flower of California, it is one of the Californian Flower Remedies (similar to Bach Flower Remedies), and is given to assist emotional cleansing.

vibrant, velvety, orange petals furl up •

slender stalks bear solitary flowers •

• flowers produced throughout summer

• grey-green leaves

finely dissected leaf on long, slender stalk •

up to 60cm (24in)

• alternate leaves

Habitat Poor, well-drained soils, sun; W. USA	Parts used ✻ ∅ ⫽

Family SCROPHULARIACEAE	Species *Euphrasia rostkoviana*	Local name Casse Lunette

EYEBRIGHT

This semi-parasitic annual extracts its nutrients from the roots of specific grasses found in poor meadowland. It has tiny oval leaves, and small, scalloped-edged, white flowers with yellow spots and red veins, resembling a bloodshot eye.
• **USES** The slightly bitter leaves have been used in salads. A whole plant infusion or strained juice from crushed, fresh stems is a general eye tonic, treating strain and infections, and is a popular cosmetic wash giving sparkle to eyes. Its antiseptic, mildly astringent, inflammation- and catarrh-reducing properties ease the irritated eyes and runny nose of hay fever and sinusitis.
• **REMARK** *Euphrasia rostkoviana* (syn. *E. officinalis*) includes several forms but only those with glandular hairs on the calyx have medicinal value.

• flowers from mid-summer to late autumn

• flowering tops used in herbal cigarettes

• spike-like racemes of white flowers

• stems may be purple or green

up to 50cm (20in)

• dried aerial parts

tiny, oval, hairy, serrated green or purple leaves •

Habitat Poor meadows, heaths, woodland; Europe	Parts used ✻ ∅ ⫽

| Family PAPAVERACEAE | Species *Fumaria officinalis* | Local name Earth Smoke |

FUMITORY

This toxic annual has erect or trailing stems of finely segmented, blue-green foliage and racemes of small, tubular, pink flowers.
• **USES** The cleansing aerial parts are taken internally, with supervision, to improve skin conditions as they clear blood toxins and are mildly diuretic and laxative. Externally they are applied as an antiseptic, anti-inflammatory lotion for spots and eczema, and to fade freckles. Fumitory stimulates the liver and gall-bladder and regulates the bile system.
• **REMARK** Large doses can cause diarrhoea and respiratory failure.

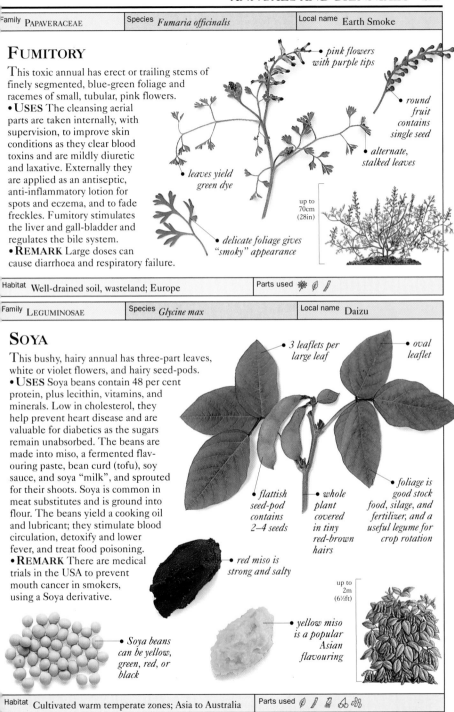

• *pink flowers with purple tips*

• *round fruit contains single seed*

• *alternate, stalked leaves*

• *leaves yield green dye*

up to 70cm (28in)

• *delicate foliage gives "smoky" appearance*

| Habitat Well-drained soil, wasteland; Europe | Parts used ❀ ✇ ⌇ |

| Family LEGUMINOSAE | Species *Glycine max* | Local name Daizu |

SOYA

This bushy, hairy annual has three-part leaves, white or violet flowers, and hairy seed-pods.
• **USES** Soya beans contain 48 per cent protein, plus lecithin, vitamins, and minerals. Low in cholesterol, they help prevent heart disease and are valuable for diabetics as the sugars remain unabsorbed. The beans are made into miso, a fermented flavouring paste, bean curd (tofu), soy sauce, and soya "milk", and sprouted for their shoots. Soya is common in meat substitutes and is ground into flour. The beans yield a cooking oil and lubricant; they stimulate blood circulation, detoxify and lower fever, and treat food poisoning.
• **REMARK** There are medical trials in the USA to prevent mouth cancer in smokers, using a Soya derivative.

• *3 leaflets per large leaf*

• *oval leaflet*

• *flattish seed-pod contains 2–4 seeds*

• *whole plant covered in tiny red-brown hairs*

• *foliage is good stock food, silage, and fertilizer, and a useful legume for crop rotation*

• *red miso is strong and salty*

up to 2m (6½ft)

• *yellow miso is a popular Asian flavouring*

• *Soya beans can be yellow, green, red, or black*

| Habitat Cultivated warm temperate zones; Asia to Australia | Parts used ✇ ⌇ ⧉ ⚬ ⚘ |

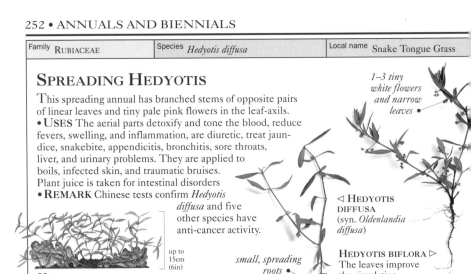

Family RUBIACEAE	Species *Hedyotis diffusa*	Local name Snake Tongue Grass

SPREADING HEDYOTIS

This spreading annual has branched stems of opposite pairs of linear leaves and tiny pale pink flowers in the leaf-axils.
• **USES** The aerial parts detoxify and tone the blood, reduce fevers, swelling, and inflammation, are diuretic, treat jaundice, snakebite, appendicitis, bronchitis, sore throats, liver, and urinary problems. They are applied to boils, infected skin, and traumatic bruises. Plant juice is taken for intestinal disorders
• **REMARK** Chinese tests confirm *Hedyotis diffusa* and five other species have anti-cancer activity.

1–3 tiny white flowers and narrow leaves

◁ **HEDYOTIS DIFFUSA**
(syn. *Oldenlandia diffusa*)

HEDYOTIS DIFFUSA

up to 15cm (6in)

small, spreading roots

HEDYOTIS BIFLORA ▷
The leaves improve the circulation.

Habitat Damp edges of fields, ditches, roadsides; Asia	Parts used ❋ ◐ ∥ ⧠ ⚬ ░

Family COMPOSITAE	Species *Helianthus annuus*	Local name Chimalati

SUNFLOWER

This fast-growing annual has a thick, tall, hairy stem, heart-shaped leaves, and large yellow flower-heads in late summer.
• **USES** The nutritious seeds are eaten raw, roasted, and ground into meal or nut butter, and were used by native American warriors as "energy cakes". The flower-buds give a yellow dye and are cooked like artichokes. The pressed seeds yield an all-purpose oil with culinary, cosmetic, and industrial uses. Medicinally the seeds are used as a diuretic and expectorant, and treat coughs, dysentery, and kidney inflammation. The root is a laxative and treats stomach pain. The stem pith yields potash and fibres for textiles and paper, and its cellular lightness is used for microscope slide mounts.
• **REMARK** Seed-heads provide food for birds in winter.

gold ray florets

edible seeds in geometric patterns

up to 5m (16½ft)

alternate leaves with prominent veins

kernels contain vitamins, phosphorus, potassium, and proteins

brown seed-shell with grey-white stripes

Habitat Fertile, well-drained soil, sun; USA	Parts used ❋ ◐ ∥ ⧠ ░

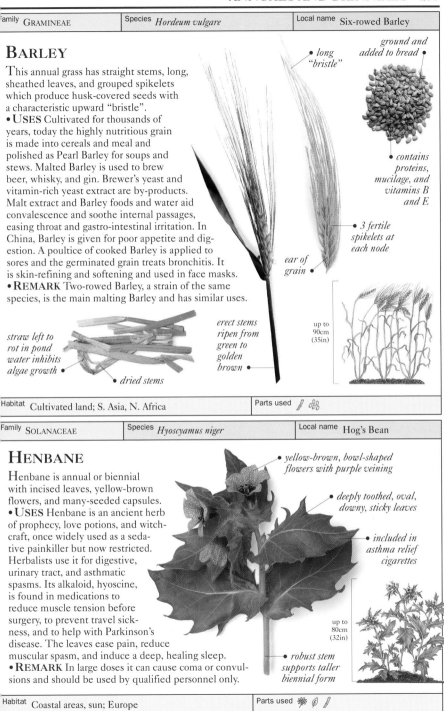

| Family GRAMINEAE | Species *Hordeum vulgare* | Local name Six-rowed Barley |

BARLEY

This annual grass has straight stems, long, sheathed leaves, and grouped spikelets which produce husk-covered seeds with a characteristic upward "bristle".

• **USES** Cultivated for thousands of years, today the highly nutritious grain is made into cereals and meal and polished as Pearl Barley for soups and stews. Malted Barley is used to brew beer, whisky, and gin. Brewer's yeast and vitamin-rich yeast extract are by-products. Malt extract and Barley foods and water aid convalescence and soothe internal passages, easing throat and gastro-intestinal irritation. In China, Barley is given for poor appetite and digestion. A poultice of cooked Barley is applied to sores and the germinated grain treats bronchitis. It is skin-refining and softening and used in face masks.

• **REMARK** Two-rowed Barley, a strain of the same species, is the main malting Barley and has similar uses.

long "bristle"

ground and added to bread

contains proteins, mucilage, and vitamins B and E

3 fertile spikelets at each node

ear of grain

straw left to rot in pond water inhibits algae growth

dried stems

erect stems ripen from green to golden brown

up to 90cm (35in)

| Habitat Cultivated land; S. Asia, N. Africa | Parts used |

| Family SOLANACEAE | Species *Hyoscyamus niger* | Local name Hog's Bean |

HENBANE

Henbane is annual or biennial with incised leaves, yellow-brown flowers, and many-seeded capsules.

• **USES** Henbane is an ancient herb of prophecy, love potions, and witchcraft, once widely used as a sedative painkiller but now restricted. Herbalists use it for digestive, urinary tract, and asthmatic spasms. Its alkaloid, hyoscine, is found in medications to reduce muscle tension before surgery, to prevent travel sickness, and to help with Parkinson's disease. The leaves ease pain, reduce muscular spasm, and induce a deep, healing sleep.

• **REMARK** In large doses it can cause coma or convulsions and should be used by qualified personnel only.

yellow-brown, bowl-shaped flowers with purple veining

deeply toothed, oval, downy, sticky leaves

included in asthma relief cigarettes

up to 80cm (32in)

robust stem supports taller biennial form

| Habitat Coastal areas, sun; Europe | Parts used |

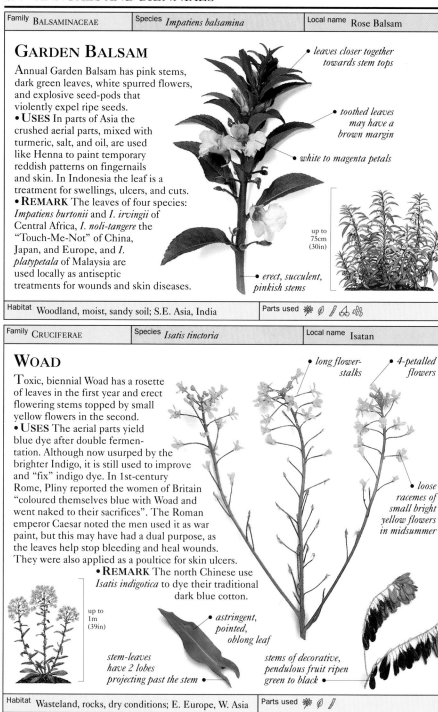

| Family BALSAMINACEAE | Species *Impatiens balsamina* | Local name Rose Balsam |

GARDEN BALSAM

Annual Garden Balsam has pink stems, dark green leaves, white spurred flowers, and explosive seed-pods that violently expel ripe seeds.
• USES In parts of Asia the crushed aerial parts, mixed with turmeric, salt, and oil, are used like Henna to paint temporary reddish patterns on fingernails and skin. In Indonesia the leaf is a treatment for swellings, ulcers, and cuts.
• REMARK The leaves of four species: *Impatiens burtonii* and *I. irvingii* of Central Africa, *I. noli-tangere* the "Touch-Me-Not" of China, Japan, and Europe, and *I. platypetala* of Malaysia are used locally as antiseptic treatments for wounds and skin diseases.

leaves closer together towards stem tops

toothed leaves may have a brown margin

white to magenta petals

up to 75cm (30in)

erect, succulent, pinkish stems

| Habitat Woodland, moist, sandy soil; S.E. Asia, India | Parts used |

| Family CRUCIFERAE | Species *Isatis tinctoria* | Local name Isatan |

WOAD

Toxic, biennial Woad has a rosette of leaves in the first year and erect flowering stems topped by small yellow flowers in the second.
• USES The aerial parts yield blue dye after double fermen-tation. Although now usurped by the brighter Indigo, it is still used to improve and "fix" indigo dye. In 1st-century Rome, Pliny reported the women of Britain "coloured themselves blue with Woad and went naked to their sacrifices". The Roman emperor Caesar noted the men used it as war paint, but this may have had a dual purpose, as the leaves help stop bleeding and heal wounds. They were also applied as a poultice for skin ulcers.
• REMARK The north Chinese use *Isatis indigotica* to dye their traditional dark blue cotton.

long flower-stalks

4-petalled flowers

loose racemes of small bright yellow flowers in midsummer

up to 1m (39in)

astringent, pointed, oblong leaf

stem-leaves have 2 lobes projecting past the stem

stems of decorative, pendulous fruit ripen green to black

| Habitat Wasteland, rocks, dry conditions; E. Europe, W. Asia | Parts used |

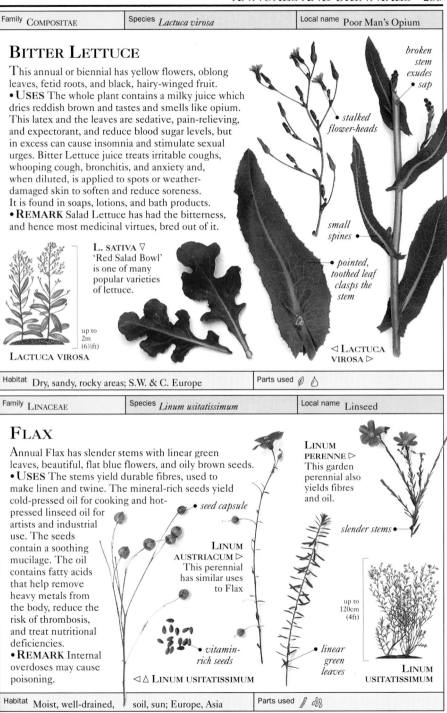

| Family COMPOSITAE | Species *Lactuca virosa* | Local name Poor Man's Opium |

BITTER LETTUCE

This annual or biennial has yellow flowers, oblong leaves, fetid roots, and black, hairy-winged fruit.
• USES The whole plant contains a milky juice which dries reddish brown and tastes and smells like opium. This latex and the leaves are sedative, pain-relieving, and expectorant, and reduce blood sugar levels, but in excess can cause insomnia and stimulate sexual urges. Bitter Lettuce juice treats irritable coughs, whooping cough, bronchitis, and anxiety and, when diluted, is applied to spots or weather-damaged skin to soften and reduce soreness. It is found in soaps, lotions, and bath products.
• REMARK Salad Lettuce has had the bitterness, and hence most medicinal virtues, bred out of it.

broken stem exudes sap

stalked flower-heads

small spines

pointed, toothed leaf clasps the stem

L. SATIVA ▽
'Red Salad Bowl' is one of many popular varieties of lettuce.

up to 2m (6½ft)

LACTUCA VIROSA

◁ LACTUCA VIROSA ▷

| Habitat Dry, sandy, rocky areas; S.W. & C. Europe | Parts used |

| Family LINACEAE | Species *Linum usitatissimum* | Local name Linseed |

FLAX

Annual Flax has slender stems with linear green leaves, beautiful, flat blue flowers, and oily brown seeds.
• USES The stems yield durable fibres, used to make linen and twine. The mineral-rich seeds yield cold-pressed oil for cooking and hot-pressed linseed oil for artists and industrial use. The seeds contain a soothing mucilage. The oil contains fatty acids that help remove heavy metals from the body, reduce the risk of thrombosis, and treat nutritional deficiencies.
• REMARK Internal overdoses may cause poisoning.

LINUM PERENNE ▷
This garden perennial also yields fibres and oil.

seed capsule

slender stems

LINUM AUSTRIACUM ▷
This perennial has similar uses to Flax

up to 120cm (4ft)

vitamin-rich seeds

linear green leaves

◁ △ LINUM USITATISSIMUM

LINUM USITATISSIMUM

| Habitat Moist, well-drained, | soil, sun; Europe, Asia | Parts used |

Family SOLANACEAE	Species *Lycopersicon esculentum*	Local name Love Apple

TOMATO

This short-lived perennial, usually grown as an annual, has distinctly aromatic, glandular leaves, weak stems, greeny yellow flowers, and trusses of round red fruit.
• USES Tomatoes are used raw or cooked and are a major flavouring. They are digestive, and rich in minerals and vitamins needed for vitality and to prevent premature ageing. The acidic fruit pulp cleanses spots, refines pores, and restores the skin's pH level. In homeopathy it treats head-aches and rheumatism. In Mexico the toxic green parts are hung up as their odour deters cockroaches.

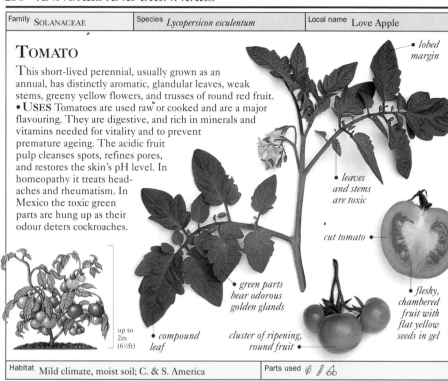

• lobed margin

• leaves and stems are toxic

cut tomato •

• fleshy, chambered fruit with flat yellow seeds in gel

• green parts bear odorous golden glands

cluster of ripening, round fruit •

up to 2m (6½ft)

• compound leaf

Habitat Mild climate, moist soil; C. & S. America	Parts used

Family COMPOSITAE	Species *Matricaria recutita*	Local name German Chamomile

ANNUAL CHAMOMILE

This annual has finely cut foliage and honey-scented daisy flowers with white "petals" and conical, yellow centres.
• USES The flowers share the cosmetic and medicinal properties of the flowers of Perennial Chamomile (see p.159), except for its anti-tumour activity. Extracts soothe nervous stress, digestive problems, and ulcerated or inflamed bowels. Excess intake can weaken stomach muscles.
• REMARK The essential oils of both chamomiles share some compounds but in differing amounts, and Perennial Chamomile's oil may cause skin irritation. Blue azulenes, their most valued compounds, are formed under acid conditions, during distillation, and possibly when the flowers are dried. Both oils prevent allergic seizures, inhibit inflammation, bacteria, ulcers, viruses, and fungi. On wounds, herpes, eczema, and infections, the diluted, cooling, analgesic oils aid cell-renewal. They also help irradiated skin. The oil of Annual Chamomile aids liver regeneration.

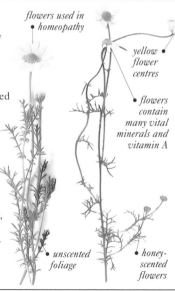

flowers used in • homeopathy

yellow • flower centres

• flowers contain many vital minerals and vitamin A

• unscented foliage

• honey-scented flowers

up to 60cm (24in)

Habitat Well-drained soil, sun; Europe, W. Asia to India	Parts used

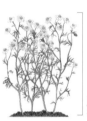

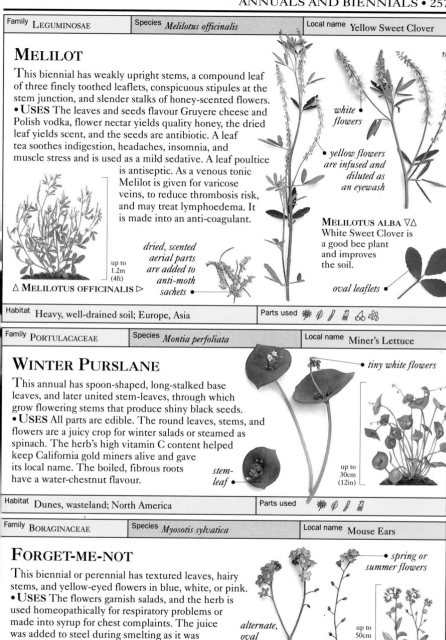

| Family LEGUMINOSAE | Species *Melilotus officinalis* | Local name Yellow Sweet Clover |

MELILOT

This biennial has weakly upright stems, a compound leaf of three finely toothed leaflets, conspicuous stipules at the stem junction, and slender stalks of honey-scented flowers.
• **USES** The leaves and seeds flavour Gruyere cheese and Polish vodka, flower nectar yields quality honey, the dried leaf yields scent, and the seeds are antibiotic. A leaf tea soothes indigestion, headaches, insomnia, and muscle stress and is used as a mild sedative. A leaf poultice is antiseptic. As a venous tonic Melilot is given for varicose veins, to reduce thrombosis risk, and may treat lymphoedema. It is made into an anti-coagulant.

white flowers

yellow flowers are infused and diluted as an eyewash

MELILOTUS ALBA ▽△
White Sweet Clover is a good bee plant and improves the soil.

up to 1.2m (4ft)

△ **MELILOTUS OFFICINALIS** ▷

dried, scented aerial parts are added to anti-moth sachets

oval leaflets

| Habitat Heavy, well-drained soil; Europe, Asia | Parts used |

| Family PORTULACACEAE | Species *Montia perfoliata* | Local name Miner's Lettuce |

WINTER PURSLANE

This annual has spoon-shaped, long-stalked base leaves, and later united stem-leaves, through which grow flowering stems that produce shiny black seeds.
• **USES** All parts are edible. The round leaves, stems, and flowers are a juicy crop for winter salads or steamed as spinach. The herb's high vitamin C content helped keep California gold miners alive and gave its local name. The boiled, fibrous roots have a water-chestnut flavour.

tiny white flowers

stem-leaf

up to 30cm (12in)

| Habitat Dunes, wasteland; North America | Parts used |

| Family BORAGINACEAE | Species *Myosotis sylvatica* | Local name Mouse Ears |

FORGET-ME-NOT

This biennial or perennial has textured leaves, hairy stems, and yellow-eyed flowers in blue, white, or pink.
• **USES** The flowers garnish salads, and the herb is used homeopathically for respiratory problems or made into syrup for chest complaints. The juice was added to steel during smelting as it was believed to increase tensile strength.
• **REMARK** The smaller perennial Alpine Forget-me-not (*Myosotis alpestris*) treats eye diseases and helps heal wounds and nose bleeds.

spring or summer flowers

alternate, oval leaves

up to 50cm (20in)

| Habitat Damp woodland; N. Africa, Europe, W. Asia | Parts used |

Family SOLANACEAE	Species *Nicandra physaloides*	Local name Apple of Peru

SHOO-FLY

This free-branching annual has large, oval leaves with wavy or toothed margins. The bell-shaped, lilac-blue flowers become papery pods, each containing a berry, with seeds capable of dormancy for decades.

• **USES** Shoo-Fly is grown for its decorative flowers and seed-pods, and because it may repel flies when growing in confined spaces. More successfully the leaf is applied as an insecticide to kill flies.

• **REMARK** The leaves of the Shoo-Fly are used to eradicate head-lice.

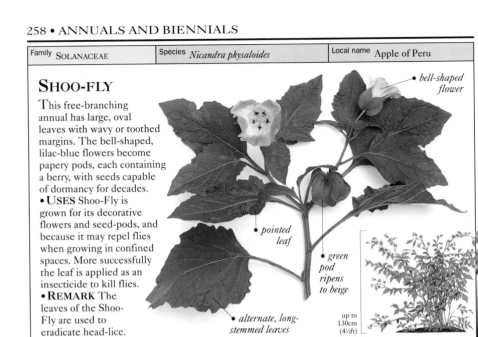

• *bell-shaped flower*

• *pointed leaf*

• *green pod ripens to beige*

• *alternate, long-stemmed leaves*

up to 130cm (4½ft)

Habitat Wasteland, rich, well-drained soil; Peru	Parts used

Family SOLANACEAE	Species *Nicotiana tabacum*	Local name Common Tobacco

TOBACCO

This annual or biennial has large, long leaves and green-white to rose, tubular flowers.

• **USES** The cured, dried leaves are smoked as a narcotic, but the poisonous nicotine they contain causes heart and lung disease and cancer. North and South American tribes smoke the leaves in ceremonies and apply poultices to sprains, to infected cuts and bites, and to problem skin. The juice is applied externally to relieve facial neuralgia, and wet leaves offer a quick cure for haemorrhoids. Research has revealed a chemical in the leaves that inhibits tumours.

• **REMARK** Aztec Tobacco (*Nicotiana rustica*) yields a coarser leaf, grown for smoking and for use in insecticides.

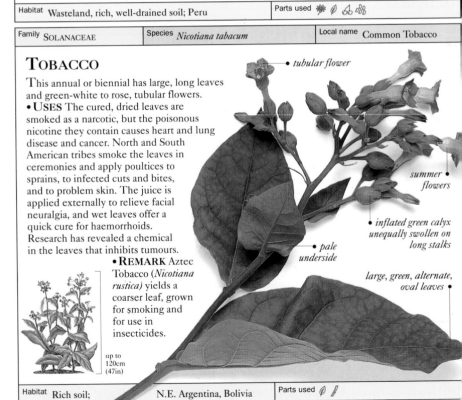

• *tubular flower*

summer flowers

• *inflated green calyx unequally swollen on long stalks*

• *pale underside*

large, green, alternate, oval leaves •

up to 120cm (47in)

Habitat Rich soil;	N.E. Argentina, Bolivia	Parts used

Family RANUNCULACEAE	Species *Nigella sativa*	Local name Kalonji

NIGELLA

This hardy annual has feathery foliage, grey-blue flowers, and inflated pods of black seeds.
• **USES** The strawberry-scented seeds have a peppery, nutmeg taste popular in India, Egypt, Greece, and Turkey. Fresh or dry roasted Nigella seeds flavour curries, vegetables, and pulses. In India they are used to repel insects from clothes and are given to treat intestinal worms and nerve defects, to reduce flatulence, induce sweating, and stimulate milk flow.
• **REMARK** The warm, ground seed was once used in sweet powders and sniffed to restore a lost sense of smell.

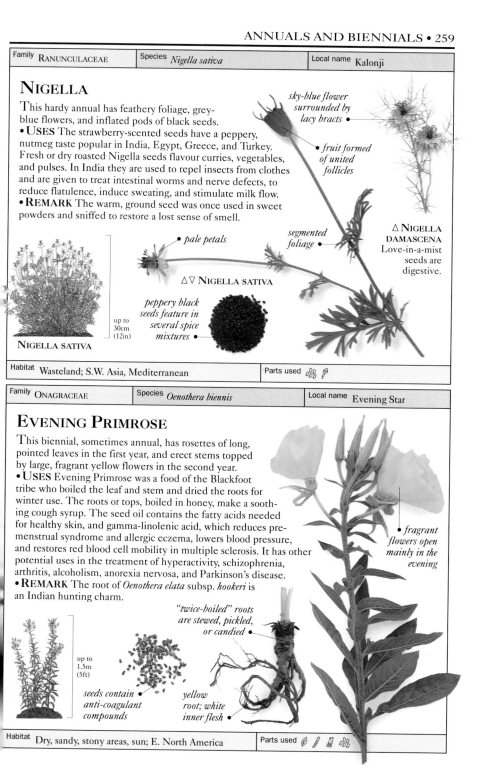

sky-blue flower surrounded by lacy bracts

fruit formed of united follicles

△ **NIGELLA DAMASCENA**
Love-in-a-mist seeds are digestive.

pale petals

segmented foliage

△▽ **NIGELLA SATIVA**

peppery black seeds feature in several spice mixtures

up to 30cm (12in)

NIGELLA SATIVA

Habitat Wasteland; S.W. Asia, Mediterranean	Parts used

Family ONAGRACEAE	Species *Oenothera biennis*	Local name Evening Star

EVENING PRIMROSE

This biennial, sometimes annual, has rosettes of long, pointed leaves in the first year, and erect stems topped by large, fragrant yellow flowers in the second year.
• **USES** Evening Primrose was a food of the Blackfoot tribe who boiled the leaf and stem and dried the roots for winter use. The roots or tops, boiled in honey, make a sooth-ing cough syrup. The seed oil contains the fatty acids needed for healthy skin, and gamma-linolenic acid, which reduces pre-menstrual syndrome and allergic eczema, lowers blood pressure, and restores red blood cell mobility in multiple sclerosis. It has other potential uses in the treatment of hyperactivity, schizophrenia, arthritis, alcoholism, anorexia nervosa, and Parkinson's disease.
• **REMARK** The root of *Oenothera elata* subsp. *hookeri* is an Indian hunting charm.

fragrant flowers open mainly in the evening

"twice-boiled" roots are stewed, pickled, or candied

up to 1.5m (5ft)

seeds contain anti-coagulant compounds

yellow root; white inner flesh

Habitat Dry, sandy, stony areas, sun; E. North America	Parts used

Family LABIATAE	Species *Ocimum basilicum*	Local name Garden Basil / Tulsi

SWEET BASIL

This annual or short-lived perennial has square stems with strong, fresh, clove-scented, toothed leaves and small, white, scented flowers in late summer.

up to 60cm (24in)

• USES The warm, spicy taste of this popular herb's leaf combines well with garlic, tomatoes, aubergines, and Italian dishes; basil flavours vinegar, oil, and pesto sauce. The gelatinous seeds of the variety *comosum* make *Cherbet Tokhum* – a Mediterranean drink. The essential oil flavours condiments, liqueurs, perfumes, and soap. The leaf wine is tonic and aphrodisiac, as Basil stimulates the adrenal cortex. The leaves are mosquito-repellent, expel worms, and treat ringworm, snakebite, insect bites, and acne. An infusion aids digestion and is anti-bacterial.

△ OCIMUM
BASILICUM ▽

• REMARK Inhaling the essential oil refreshes the mind and stimulates a sense of smell dulled by viral infection.

In massage oils, it is a nerve tonic and eases over-worked muscles. Basil should be avoided on sensitive skin and during pregnancy.

shredded leaf a popular tomato and soup garnish •

puckered leaf surface •

• *whorls of 6 white flowers with clove-flavoured nectar*

◁ OCIMUM
BASILICUM ▷

• *oval, pointed leaf with warm, spicy, clove scent*

• *leaf soothes insect bites*

• *long-stemmed leaf*

fresh leaves are best torn, not cut, and release a better taste than dried •

lemon scent •

tiny ovate leaves •

OCIMUM BASILICUM VAR. CITRIODORUM ▷
Lemon Basil is annual, with white flowers and green leaves, delicious in sauces and with chicken.

pink or white flowers •

◁ **OCIMUM SANCTUM**
The woody-based Holy Basil, sacred to Hindus, is planted around temples. I discourages mosquitoes.

• *strong basil scent*

◁ **OCIMUM BASILICUM VAR. MINIMUM**
Bush or Greek Basil is a compact, rounded bush with a good medium flavour. It tolerates a cooler climate better than Sweet Basil.

spicy aroma •

• *hairy, serrated le*

Habitat Well-drained soil, sun; tropical Asia	Parts used 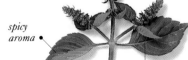

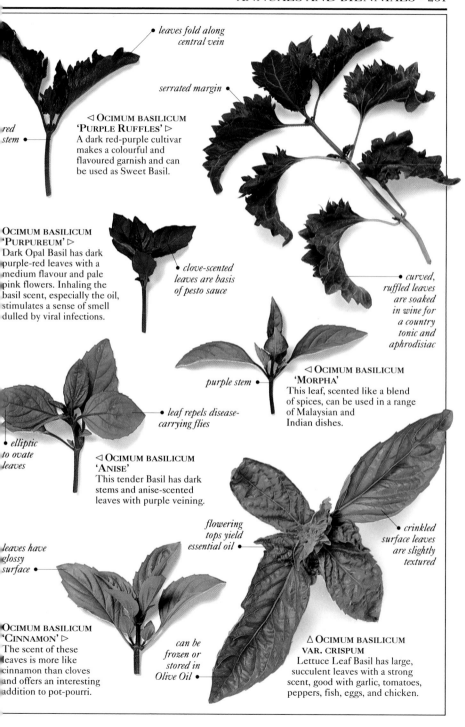

leaves fold along central vein

serrated margin

red stem

◁ **OCIMUM BASILICUM 'PURPLE RUFFLES'** ▷
A dark red-purple cultivar makes a colourful and flavoured garnish and can be used as Sweet Basil.

OCIMUM BASILICUM 'PURPUREUM' ▷
Dark Opal Basil has dark purple-red leaves with a medium flavour and pale pink flowers. Inhaling the basil scent, especially the oil, stimulates a sense of smell dulled by viral infections.

clove-scented leaves are basis of pesto sauce

curved, ruffled leaves are soaked in wine for a country tonic and aphrodisiac

purple stem

◁ **OCIMUM BASILICUM 'MORPHA'**
This leaf, scented like a blend of spices, can be used in a range of Malaysian and Indian dishes.

leaf repels disease-carrying flies

elliptic to ovate leaves

◁ **OCIMUM BASILICUM 'ANISE'**
This tender Basil has dark stems and anise-scented leaves with purple veining.

flowering tops yield essential oil

crinkled surface leaves are slightly textured

leaves have glossy surface

OCIMUM BASILICUM 'CINNAMON' ▷
The scent of these leaves is more like cinnamon than cloves and offers an interesting addition to pot-pourri.

can be frozen or stored in Olive Oil

△ **OCIMUM BASILICUM VAR. CRISPUM**
Lettuce Leaf Basil has large, succulent leaves with a strong scent, good with garlic, tomatoes, peppers, fish, eggs, and chicken.

Family COMPOSITAE	Species *Onopordum acanthium*	Local name Cotton Thistle

SCOTS THISTLE

This tall, imposing biennial has spiny, winged stems, toothed, spiny leaves covered in fine, white down, and thistle flower-heads with purple-pink or white florets.
• USES The large flower-discs can be boiled or steamed and served with butter, after removing the outer bracts. The young stems are blanched and peeled, eaten raw with oil and vinegar, or steamed. The seeds once produced oil for cooking and lamps, and the leaf- and stem-down was collected as pillow stuffing. The leaf juice was taken for cancerous complaints and applied to skin ulcers, and a root decoction used to reduce mucus discharges.
• REMARK The Thistle became the emblem of Scotland, in the ancient Order of the Thistle.

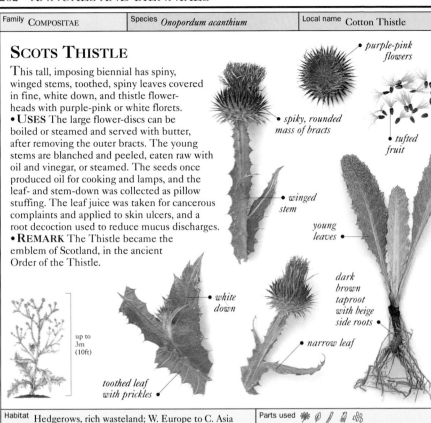

• *purple-pink flowers*

• *spiky, rounded mass of bracts*

• *tufted fruit*

• *winged stem*

young leaves •

• *white down*

dark brown taproot with beige side roots

up to 3m (10ft)

• *narrow leaf*

toothed leaf with prickles •

Habitat Hedgerows, rich wasteland; W. Europe to C. Asia	Parts used

Family OROBANCHACEAE	Species *Orobanche alba*	Local name Ghost Plant

THYME BROOMRAPE

The genus lacks chlorophyll, and hence green colouring, as the plants are parasitic on the roots of Labiatae, Leguminosae, Solanaceae, and other plant families. This species has purple-brown stems, small leaves, and clove-scented flowers.
• USES The whole plant is used medicinally but the root is most potent. Externally it offers a strong, astringent poultice; internally it is a sedative and mild laxative, given to restore muscle tone after debilitating illness or mild stroke. It is prescribed for impotence, and is now being researched as a treatment for the menopause and uterine bleeding. In China *Orobanche* species (So yang) are considered aphrodisiac.
• REMARK All *Orobanche* species are believed to have potent medicinal properties.

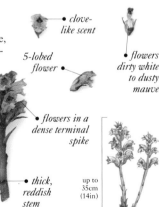

• *clove-like scent*

5-lobed flower •

• *flowers dirty white to dusty mauve*

• *flowers in a dense terminal spike*

host Thyme plant from whose roots the Broomrape extracts nutrients •

• *thick, reddish stem*

up to 35cm (14in)

Habitat Temperate, rocky regions on shrubs; Europe, China	Parts used

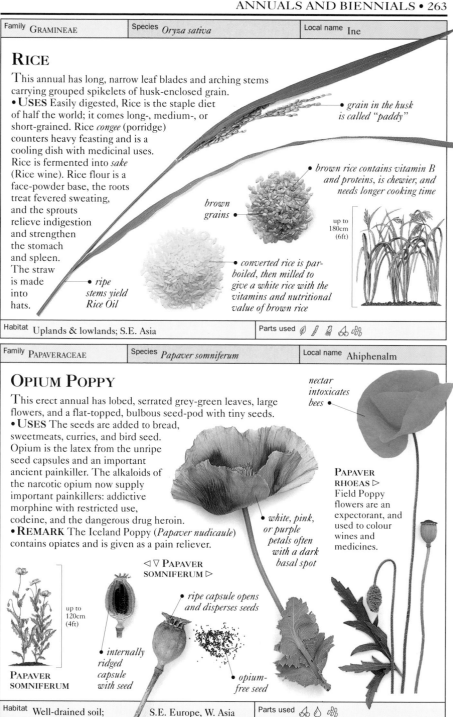

| Family GRAMINEAE | Species *Oryza sativa* | Local name Ine |

RICE

This annual has long, narrow leaf blades and arching stems
carrying grouped spikelets of husk-enclosed grain.
• **USES** Easily digested, Rice is the staple diet
of half the world; it comes long-, medium-, or
short-grained. Rice *congee* (porridge)
counters heavy feasting and is a
cooling dish with medicinal uses.
Rice is fermented into *sake*
(Rice wine). Rice flour is a
face-powder base, the roots
treat fevered sweating,
and the sprouts
relieve indigestion
and strengthen
the stomach
and spleen.
The straw
is made
into
hats.

• *grain in the husk
is called "paddy"*

• *brown rice contains vitamin B
and proteins, is chewier, and
needs longer cooking time*

*brown
grains* •

up to
180cm
(6ft)

• *ripe
stems yield
Rice Oil*

• *converted rice is par-
boiled, then milled to
give a white rice with the
vitamins and nutritional
value of brown rice*

| Habitat Uplands & lowlands; S.E. Asia | Parts used |

| Family PAPAVERACEAE | Species *Papaver somniferum* | Local name Ahiphenalm |

OPIUM POPPY

This erect annual has lobed, serrated grey-green leaves, large
flowers, and a flat-topped, bulbous seed-pod with tiny seeds.
• **USES** The seeds are added to bread,
sweetmeats, curries, and bird seed.
Opium is the latex from the unripe
seed capsules and an important
ancient painkiller. The alkaloids of
the narcotic opium now supply
important painkillers: addictive
morphine with restricted use,
codeine, and the dangerous drug heroin.
• **REMARK** The Iceland Poppy (*Papaver nudicaule*)
contains opiates and is given as a pain reliever.

*nectar
intoxicates
bees* •

**PAPAVER
RHOEAS** ▷
Field Poppy
flowers are an
expectorant, and
used to colour
wines and
medicines.

• *white, pink,
or purple
petals often
with a dark
basal spot*

◁ ▽ **PAPAVER
SOMNIFERUM** ▷

• *ripe capsule opens
and disperses seeds*

up to
120cm
(4ft)

**PAPAVER
SOMNIFERUM**

• *internally
ridged
capsule
with seed*

• *opium-
free seed*

| Habitat Well-drained soil; | S.E. Europe, W. Asia | Parts used |

Family UMBELLIFERAE	Species *Petroselinium crispum*	Local name Persil

PARSLEY

Parsley is a taprooted biennial with solid stems of triangular, toothed, and curled leaves divided into three segments, umbels of tiny creamy summer flowers, and aromatic "seeds".
• **USES** Vitamin- and mineral-rich leaves and stems are added to salads and savoury dishes. Parsley is used in *bouquet garni* and eaten to freshen breath. Leaf infusions are a tonic for hair, skin, and eyes. The leaves are eaten as a vegetable in the Middle East. The root is used in soups and stews. The leaves, root, and seeds are diuretic, scavenge skin-ageing free radicals, and reduce the release of histamine. They relieve rheumatism, aid digestion, and tone uterine muscles after birth. Leaf poultices soothe sprains and cuts.
• **REMARK** Grown near roses, it improves their health and scent.

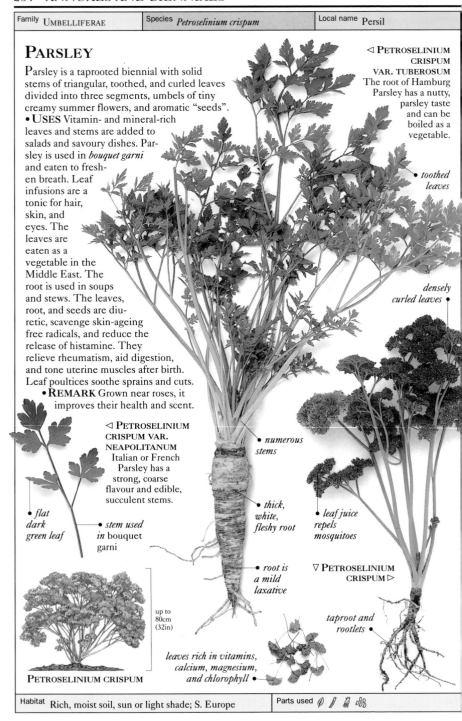

◁ **PETROSELINIUM CRISPUM VAR. TUBEROSUM** The root of Hamburg Parsley has a nutty, parsley taste and can be boiled as a vegetable.

• *toothed leaves*

• *densely curled leaves*

◁ **PETROSELINIUM CRISPUM VAR. NEAPOLITANUM** Italian or French Parsley has a strong, coarse flavour and edible, succulent stems.

• *flat dark green leaf*

• *stem used in bouquet garni*

• *numerous stems*

• *thick, white, fleshy root*

• *leaf juice repels mosquitoes*

▽ **PETROSELINIUM CRISPUM** ▷

up to 80cm (32in)

• *root is a mild laxative*

taproot and rootlets •

PETROSELINIUM CRISPUM

leaves rich in vitamins, calcium, magnesium, and chlorophyll •

Habitat Rich, moist soil, sun or light shade; S. Europe	Parts used 🌿 ⫽ 🥕 ⚬⚬⚬

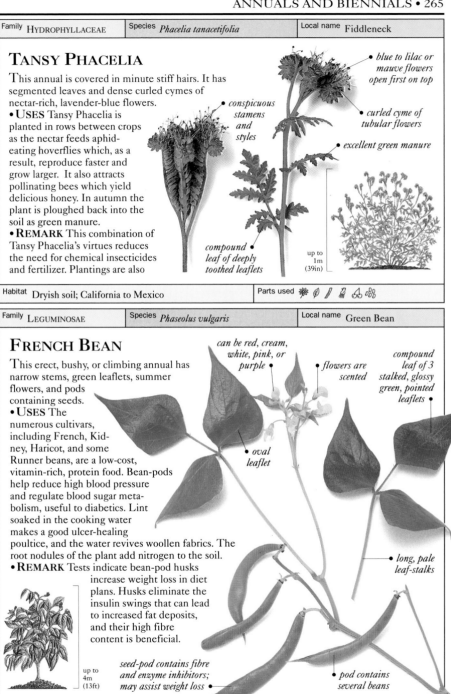

| Family HYDROPHYLLACEAE | Species *Phacelia tanacetifolia* | Local name Fiddleneck |

TANSY PHACELIA

This annual is covered in minute stiff hairs. It has
segmented leaves and dense curled cymes of
nectar-rich, lavender-blue flowers.
• **USES** Tansy Phacelia is
planted in rows between crops
as the nectar feeds aphid-
eating hoverflies which, as a
result, reproduce faster and
grow larger. It also attracts
pollinating bees which yield
delicious honey. In autumn the
plant is ploughed back into the
soil as green manure.
• **REMARK** This combination of
Tansy Phacelia's virtues reduces
the need for chemical insecticides
and fertilizer. Plantings are also

*blue to lilac or
mauve flowers
open first on top*

*conspicuous
stamens
and
styles*

*curled cyme of
tubular flowers*

excellent green manure

*compound
leaf of deeply
toothed leaflets*

up to
1m
(39in)

| Habitat Dryish soil; California to Mexico | Parts used |

| Family LEGUMINOSAE | Species *Phaseolus vulgaris* | Local name Green Bean |

FRENCH BEAN

This erect, bushy, or climbing annual has
narrow stems, green leaflets, summer
flowers, and pods
containing seeds.
• **USES** The
numerous cultivars,
including French, Kid-
ney, Haricot, and some
Runner beans, are a low-cost,
vitamin-rich, protein food. Bean-pods
help reduce high blood pressure
and regulate blood sugar metabolism, useful to diabetics. Lint
soaked in the cooking water
makes a good ulcer-healing
poultice, and the water revives woollen fabrics. The
root nodules of the plant add nitrogen to the soil.
• **REMARK** Tests indicate bean-pod husks
increase weight loss in diet
plans. Husks eliminate the
insulin swings that can lead
to increased fat deposits,
and their high fibre
content is beneficial.

*can be red, cream,
white, pink, or
purple*

*flowers are
scented*

*compound
leaf of 3
stalked, glossy
green, pointed
leaflets*

*oval
leaflet*

*long, pale
leaf-stalks*

up to
4m
(13ft)

*seed-pod contains fibre
and enzyme inhibitors;
may assist weight loss*

*pod contains
several beans*

| Habitat Sun, reasonable soil; tropical America | Parts used |

Family UMBELLIFERAE	Species *Pimpinella anisum*	Local name Anise

ANISEED

Aniseed has sweetly aromatic leaves, rounded at the base and narrower on the stem, with umbels of flowers followed by aromatic fruit.

• **USES** Popular in European, Arabic, and Indian cooking, whole or crushed seeds add sweet, spicy flavour to desserts, confectionery, pickles, curries, and spirits such as *Pernod, Anisette, Ricard, ouzo,* and *arrak.* The flowers and leaves are used in fruit salads, the stem and roots in sweet soups. In cooking or infused as a tea, the seeds aid digestion, quell nausea, and ease flatulence and colic. Aniseed is used in cough mixtures as it is expectorant and soothes spasms for irritant coughs and bronchial problems. It has a mild oestrogenic effect, and is used to encourage breast milk, ease childbirth, and stimulate libido. In tests it has significantly increased liver regeneration in rats.

• **REMARK** Minute amounts of the essential oil, produced from the seeds, are added to toothpastes, perfumes, and mouthwashes, and used to mask bitter medicines, but in large amounts it is highly toxic.

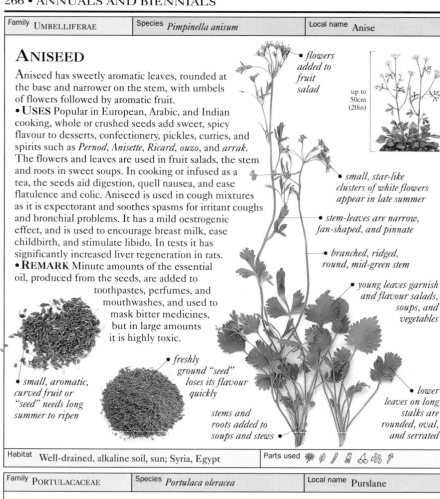

• *flowers added to fruit salad*

up to 50cm (20in)

• *small, star-like clusters of white flowers appear in late summer*

• *stem-leaves are narrow, fan-shaped, and pinnate*

• *branched, ridged, round, mid-green stem*

• *young leaves garnish and flavour salads, soups, and vegetables*

• *freshly ground "seed" loses its flavour quickly*

• *small, aromatic, curved fruit or "seed" needs long summer to ripen*

stems and roots added to soups and stews •

• *lower leaves on long stalks are rounded, oval, and serrated*

Habitat Well-drained, alkaline soil, sun; Syria, Egypt	Parts used 🌸 🖉 ⫰ 🗒 🔗 🕸 ⚘

Family PORTULACACEAE	Species *Portulaca oleracea*	Local name Purslane

SUMMER PURSLANE

This annual has thick, fleshy pink to green stems, succulent leaves, and bright yellow midsummer flowers with sensitive stamens.

• **USES** Rich in iron and vitamin C, the crunchy, cooling leaves and stems blend well with hotter salad herbs. They make a succulent pickle and are cooked as a vegetable and are added to soups. The dried seed is ground and added to flour. In China the whole plant is given for diarrhoea, urinary infections, and to reduce fevers. In Indonesia it is prescribed for cardiac weakness, and the seed and fruit for laboured breathing. The juice treats skin diseases.

rounded, succulent leaves •

leaves make a soothing, cooling poultice •

up to 30cm (12in)

small, easily spreading roots make the plant mat-forming •

Habitat Well-drained light soil, shelter, sun; India, Eurasia	Parts used

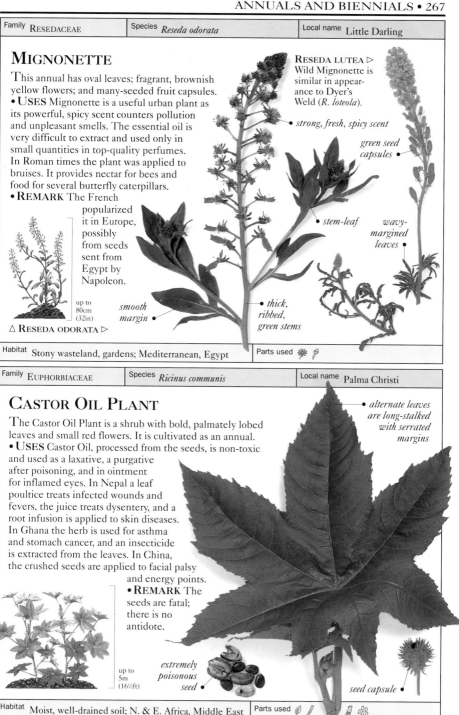

Family RESEDACEAE	Species *Reseda odorata*	Local name Little Darling

MIGNONETTE

This annual has oval leaves; fragrant, brownish yellow flowers; and many-seeded fruit capsules.
• USES Mignonette is a useful urban plant as its powerful, spicy scent counters pollution and unpleasant smells. The essential oil is very difficult to extract and used only in small quantities in top-quality perfumes. In Roman times the plant was applied to bruises. It provides nectar for bees and food for several butterfly caterpillars.
• REMARK The French popularized it in Europe, possibly from seeds sent from Egypt by Napoleon.

RESEDA LUTEA ▷
Wild Mignonette is similar in appearance to Dyer's Weld (*R. loteola*).

• *strong, fresh, spicy scent*

green seed capsules •

• *stem-leaf*

wavy-margined leaves •

up to 80cm (32in)

smooth margin •

△ RESEDA ODORATA ▷

• *thick, ribbed, green stems*

Habitat Stony wasteland, gardens; Mediterranean, Egypt	Parts used ❋ ✐

Family EUPHORBIACEAE	Species *Ricinus communis*	Local name Palma Christi

CASTOR OIL PLANT

The Castor Oil Plant is a shrub with bold, palmately lobed leaves and small red flowers. It is cultivated as an annual.
• USES Castor Oil, processed from the seeds, is non-toxic and used as a laxative, a purgative after poisoning, and in ointment for inflamed eyes. In Nepal a leaf poultice treats infected wounds and fevers, the juice treats dysentery, and a root infusion is applied to skin diseases. In Ghana the herb is used for asthma and stomach cancer, and an insecticide is extracted from the leaves. In China, the crushed seeds are applied to facial palsy and energy points.
• REMARK The seeds are fatal; there is no antidote.

• *alternate leaves are long-stalked with serrated margins*

up to 5m (16½ft)

extremely poisonous seed •

seed capsule •

Habitat Moist, well-drained soil; N. & E. Africa, Middle East	Parts used ✐ ✐ 🍃 ✿

Family CHENOPODIACEAE	Species *Salicornia europaea*	Local name Marsh Samphire

GLASSWORT

This upright annual has woody brown stems and succulent, jointed branches. Minute green flowers appear in autumn.
• **USES** The juicy, salty, mineral-rich stems are like Samphire and are eaten during their ripe green season. They can be pickled or eaten like asparagus: boiled and served hot with butter or cold with vinegar. Seeds were once ground into flour and the whole plant burned for its ash, Barilla, and used in glass- and soap-making.
• **REMARK** Cattle relish its high salt content.

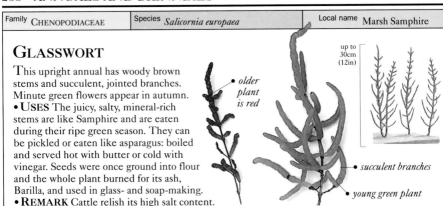

up to 30cm (12in)

• *older plant is red*

• *succulent branches*

• *young green plant*

Habitat Saltmarshes, estuaries; Europe, Asia, North America	Parts used 🌿

Family CHENOPODIACEAE	Species *Salsola kali*	Local name Tumble-weed

SALTWORT

Saltwort has stiff, ribbed branches with fleshy, spine-tipped leaves and single, late-summer flowers at the leaf-axils.
• **USES** The young, mineral-rich shoots are boiled and served with butter or a vinegar dressing. It has a Biblical history of being harvested and burned for the sodium carbonate (Barilla) in its ash and used in glass- and soap-making. It was taken as a diuretic.
• **REMARK** In polluted areas Saltwort can contain toxic levels of nitrates and oxalates.

• *waxy, succulent leaves*

up to 1m (39in)

• *oval to oblong leaves*

• *tiny late-summer flowers in leaf-axils*

Habitat Sandy, alkaline soils, saline conditions; Europe, USA	Parts used 🌿

Family CRUCIFERAE	Species *Sisymbrium officinale*	Local name Singer's Plant

HEDGE MUSTARD

This taprooted annual has a rosette of pinnately-lobed basal leaves, small, mustard-yellow summer flowers, and downy seed-pods pressed to the erect stem.
• **USES** The mustard-flavoured plant is used in sauces and is rich in vitamin C. Fresh, it is often gargled with Watercress and Horseradish juice, and treats congestion and irritation of the larynx, hoarseness, throat disease, and weak lungs. It is a stimulant tonic, expels catarrh, and soothes coughs and asthma.
• **REMARK** As it can revive a failing voice, it is also known as the Singer's Plant.

• *seed-pods pressed against the stem*

• *sharply lobed basal leaves retain dust*

• *4-petalled flowers*

up to 50cm (20in)

• *narrow, arrow-shaped leaves with irregular margins*

Habitat Wasteland; temperate Europe	Parts used ✳ 🌿

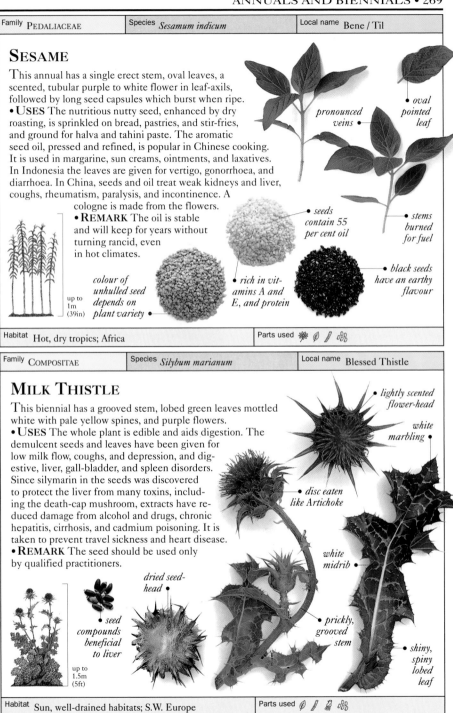

Family PEDALIACEAE	Species *Sesamum indicum*	Local name Bene / Til

SESAME

This annual has a single erect stem, oval leaves, a scented, tubular purple to white flower in leaf-axils, followed by long seed capsules which burst when ripe.
• **USES** The nutritious nutty seed, enhanced by dry roasting, is sprinkled on bread, pastries, and stir-fries, and ground for halva and tahini paste. The aromatic seed oil, pressed and refined, is popular in Chinese cooking. It is used in margarine, sun creams, ointments, and laxatives. In Indonesia the leaves are given for vertigo, gonorrhoea, and diarrhoea. In China, seeds and oil treat weak kidneys and liver, coughs, rheumatism, paralysis, and incontinence. A cologne is made from the flowers.
• **REMARK** The oil is stable and will keep for years without turning rancid, even in hot climates.

oval pointed leaf

pronounced veins

seeds contain 55 per cent oil

stems burned for fuel

black seeds have an earthy flavour

rich in vitamins A and E, and protein

colour of unhulled seed depends on plant variety

up to 1m (39in)

Habitat Hot, dry tropics; Africa	Parts used

Family COMPOSITAE	Species *Silybum marianum*	Local name Blessed Thistle

MILK THISTLE

This biennial has a grooved stem, lobed green leaves mottled white with pale yellow spines, and purple flowers.
• **USES** The whole plant is edible and aids digestion. The demulcent seeds and leaves have been given for low milk flow, coughs, and depression, and digestive, liver, gall-bladder, and spleen disorders. Since silymarin in the seeds was discovered to protect the liver from many toxins, including the death-cap mushroom, extracts have reduced damage from alcohol and drugs, chronic hepatitis, cirrhosis, and cadmium poisoning. It is taken to prevent travel sickness and heart disease.
• **REMARK** The seed should be used only by qualified practitioners.

lightly scented flower-head

white marbling

disc eaten like Artichoke

white midrib

seed compounds beneficial to liver

dried seed-head

prickly, grooved stem

shiny, spiny lobed leaf

up to 1.5m (5ft)

Habitat Sun, well-drained habitats; S.W. Europe	Parts used

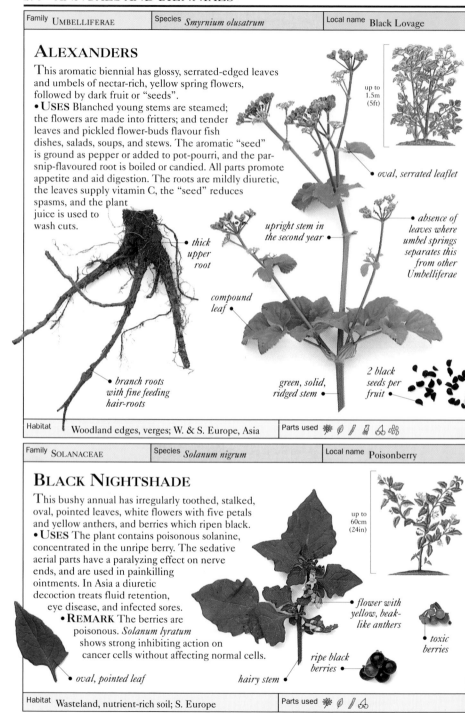

| Family UMBELLIFERAE | Species *Smyrnium olusatrum* | Local name Black Lovage |

ALEXANDERS

This aromatic biennial has glossy, serrated-edged leaves and umbels of nectar-rich, yellow spring flowers, followed by dark fruit or "seeds".
• **USES** Blanched young stems are steamed; the flowers are made into fritters; and tender leaves and pickled flower-buds flavour fish dishes, salads, soups, and stews. The aromatic "seed" is ground as pepper or added to pot-pourri, and the parsnip-flavoured root is boiled or candied. All parts promote appetite and aid digestion. The roots are mildly diuretic, the leaves supply vitamin C, the "seed" reduces spasms, and the plant juice is used to wash cuts.

up to 1.5m (5ft)

oval, serrated leaflet

thick upper root

upright stem in the second year

absence of leaves where umbel springs separates this from other Umbelliferae

compound leaf

branch roots with fine feeding hair-roots

green, solid, ridged stem

2 black seeds per fruit

| Habitat Woodland edges, verges; W. & S. Europe, Asia | Parts used |

| Family SOLANACEAE | Species *Solanum nigrum* | Local name Poisonberry |

BLACK NIGHTSHADE

This bushy annual has irregularly toothed, stalked, oval, pointed leaves, white flowers with five petals and yellow anthers, and berries which ripen black.
• **USES** The plant contains poisonous solanine, concentrated in the unripe berry. The sedative aerial parts have a paralyzing effect on nerve ends, and are used in painkilling ointments. In Asia a diuretic decoction treats fluid retention, eye disease, and infected sores.
• **REMARK** The berries are poisonous. *Solanum lyratum* shows strong inhibiting action on cancer cells without affecting normal cells.

up to 60cm (24in)

flower with yellow, beak-like anthers

toxic berries

ripe black berries

oval, pointed leaf

hairy stem

| Habitat Wasteland, nutrient-rich soil; S. Europe | Parts used |

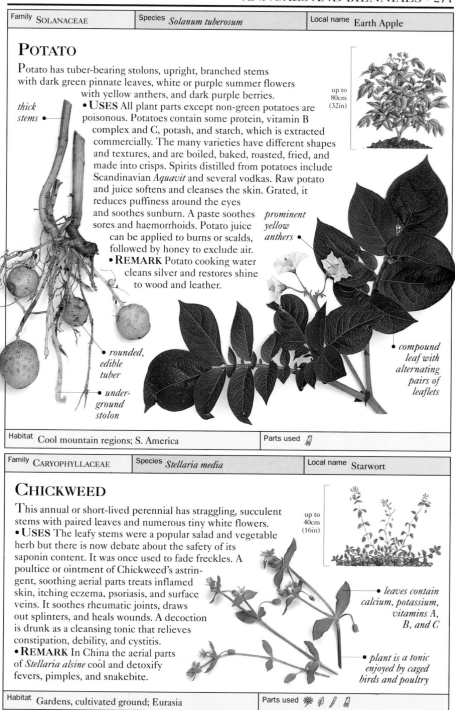

| Family SOLANACEAE | Species *Solanum tuberosum* | Local name Earth Apple |

POTATO

Potato has tuber-bearing stolons, upright, branched stems
with dark green pinnate leaves, white or purple summer flowers
with yellow anthers, and dark purple berries.

up to
80cm
(32in)

*thick
stems*

• USES All plant parts except non-green potatoes are
poisonous. Potatoes contain some protein, vitamin B
complex and C, potash, and starch, which is extracted
commercially. The many varieties have different shapes
and textures, and are boiled, baked, roasted, fried, and
made into crisps. Spirits distilled from potatoes include
Scandinavian *Aquavit* and several vodkas. Raw potato
and juice softens and cleanses the skin. Grated, it
reduces puffiness around the eyes
and soothes sunburn. A paste soothes
sores and haemorrhoids. Potato juice
can be applied to burns or scalds,
followed by honey to exclude air.
• REMARK Potato cooking water
cleans silver and restores shine
to wood and leather.

*prominent
yellow
anthers*

*rounded,
edible
tuber*

*under-
ground
stolon*

*compound
leaf with
alternating
pairs of
leaflets*

| Habitat Cool mountain regions; S. America | Parts used |

| Family CARYOPHYLLACEAE | Species *Stellaria media* | Local name Starwort |

CHICKWEED

This annual or short-lived perennial has straggling, succulent
stems with paired leaves and numerous tiny white flowers.
• USES The leafy stems were a popular salad and vegetable
herb but there is now debate about the safety of its
saponin content. It was once used to fade freckles. A
poultice or ointment of Chickweed's astringent, soothing aerial parts treats inflamed
skin, itching eczema, psoriasis, and surface
veins. It soothes rheumatic joints, draws
out splinters, and heals wounds. A decoction
is drunk as a cleansing tonic that relieves
constipation, debility, and cystitis.
• REMARK In China the aerial parts
of *Stellaria alsine* cool and detoxify
fevers, pimples, and snakebite.

up to
40cm
(16in)

*leaves contain
calcium, potassium,
vitamins A,
B, and C*

*plant is a tonic
enjoyed by caged
birds and poultry*

| Habitat Gardens, cultivated ground; Eurasia | Parts used |

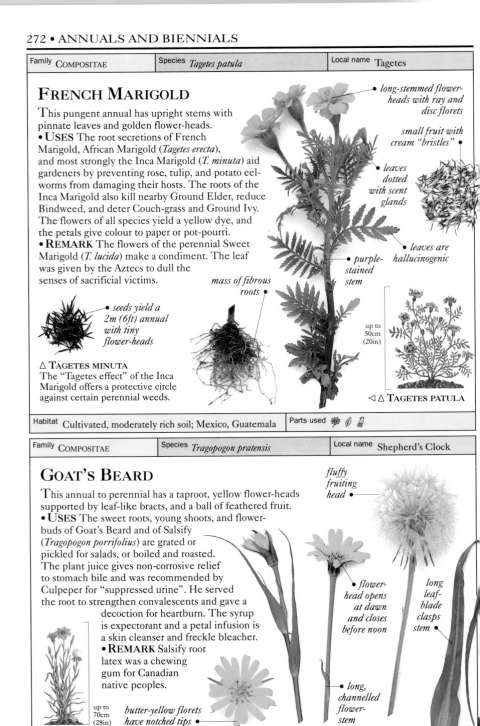

Family COMPOSITAE	Species *Tagetes patula*	Local name Tagetes

FRENCH MARIGOLD

This pungent annual has upright stems with pinnate leaves and golden flower-heads.
• **USES** The root secretions of French Marigold, African Marigold (*Tagetes erecta*), and most strongly the Inca Marigold (*T. minuta*) aid gardeners by preventing rose, tulip, and potato eel-worms from damaging their hosts. The roots of the Inca Marigold also kill nearby Ground Elder, reduce Bindweed, and deter Couch-grass and Ground Ivy. The flowers of all species yield a yellow dye, and the petals give colour to paper or pot-pourri.
• **REMARK** The flowers of the perennial Sweet Marigold (*T. lucida*) make a condiment. The leaf was given by the Aztecs to dull the senses of sacrificial victims.

• long-stemmed flower-heads with ray and disc florets

small fruit with cream "bristles" •

• leaves dotted with scent glands

• leaves are hallucinogenic

• purple-stained stem

mass of fibrous roots •

• seeds yield a 2m (6ft) annual with tiny flower-heads

up to 50cm (20in)

△ **TAGETES MINUTA**
The "Tagetes effect" of the Inca Marigold offers a protective circle against certain perennial weeds.

◁ △ **TAGETES PATULA**

Habitat Cultivated, moderately rich soil; Mexico, Guatemala	Parts used ❀ ∅ 🜎

Family COMPOSITAE	Species *Tragopogon pratensis*	Local name Shepherd's Clock

GOAT'S BEARD

This annual to perennial has a taproot, yellow flower-heads supported by leaf-like bracts, and a ball of feathered fruit.
• **USES** The sweet roots, young shoots, and flower-buds of Goat's Beard and of Salsify (*Tragopogon porrifolius*) are grated or pickled for salads, or boiled and roasted. The plant juice gives non-corrosive relief to stomach bile and was recommended by Culpeper for "suppressed urine". He served the root to strengthen convalescents and gave a decoction for heartburn. The syrup is expectorant and a petal infusion is a skin cleanser and freckle bleacher.
• **REMARK** Salsify root latex was a chewing gum for Canadian native peoples.

fluffy fruiting head •

• flower-head opens at dawn and closes before noon

long leaf-blade clasps stem •

• long, channelled flower-stem

up to 70cm (28in)

butter-yellow florets have notched tips •

Habitat Grassland, wasteland; Europe, USA	Parts used ❀ ∅ 🌿 🜎

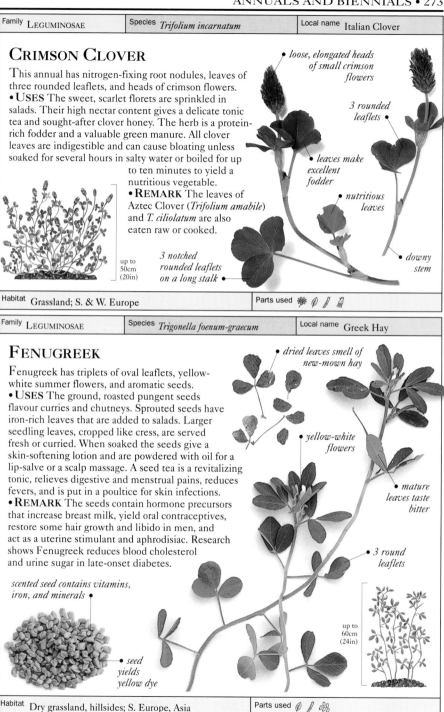

Family LEGUMINOSAE	Species *Trifolium incarnatum*	Local name Italian Clover

CRIMSON CLOVER

This annual has nitrogen-fixing root nodules, leaves of three rounded leaflets, and heads of crimson flowers.
• USES The sweet, scarlet florets are sprinkled in salads. Their high nectar content gives a delicate tonic tea and sought-after clover honey. The herb is a protein-rich fodder and a valuable green manure. All clover leaves are indigestible and can cause bloating unless soaked for several hours in salty water or boiled for up to ten minutes to yield a nutritious vegetable.
• REMARK The leaves of Aztec Clover (*Trifolium amabile*) and *T. ciliolatum* are also eaten raw or cooked.

loose, elongated heads of small crimson flowers

3 rounded leaflets

leaves make excellent fodder

nutritious leaves

downy stem

up to 50cm (20in)

3 notched rounded leaflets on a long stalk

Habitat Grassland; S. & W. Europe	Parts used

Family LEGUMINOSAE	Species *Trigonella foenum-graecum*	Local name Greek Hay

FENUGREEK

Fenugreek has triplets of oval leaflets, yellow-white summer flowers, and aromatic seeds.
• USES The ground, roasted pungent seeds flavour curries and chutneys. Sprouted seeds have iron-rich leaves that are added to salads. Larger seedling leaves, cropped like cress, are served fresh or curried. When soaked the seeds give a skin-softening lotion and are powdered with oil for a lip-salve or a scalp massage. A seed tea is a revitalizing tonic, relieves digestive and menstrual pains, reduces fevers, and is put in a poultice for skin infections.
• REMARK The seeds contain hormone precursors that increase breast milk, yield oral contraceptives, restore some hair growth and libido in men, and act as a uterine stimulant and aphrodisiac. Research shows Fenugreek reduces blood cholesterol and urine sugar in late-onset diabetes.

dried leaves smell of new-mown hay

yellow-white flowers

mature leaves taste bitter

3 round leaflets

scented seed contains vitamins, iron, and minerals

up to 60cm (24in)

seed yields yellow dye

Habitat Dry grassland, hillsides; S. Europe, Asia	Parts used

Family TROPAEOLACEAE	Species *Tropaeolum majus*	Local name Indian Cress

NASTURTIUM

This annual has climbing and dwarf forms, with wavy-margined leaves, spurred flowers, and large seeds.
• **USES** The fresh leaves and flowers give bite to savoury foods, and green seed-pods are pickled. The whole plant, a reputed rejuvenator and aphrodisiac, is used in hair and scalp tonics. The seeds contain an antibiotic and, with the leaves and flowers, fight respiratory bacteria without destroying intestinal flora. An infusion treats coughs, colds, and genito-urinary infections.
• **REMARK** Mashua (*Tropaeoleum tuberosum*) has been grown in the Andes for 8,000 years. It has edible tubers that are anaphrodisiac, lowering testosterone levels in tests.

leaves variegated in this 'Alaska' hybrid

brightly coloured flowers

fresh leaves used in salads

vitamin-rich flowers attract hoverflies which eat aphids

up to 60m (24in)

seed-pod divides into 3 seeds

Habitat Well-drained, poor soil, sun; Colombia to Bolivia	Parts used ✿ ◖ ⚭ ❀

Family SCROPHULARIACEAE	Species *Verbascum thapsus*	Verbascum / Torches

MULLEIN

This biennial has a rosette of woolly leaves and a tall, thick, downy, resinous stem of bright yellow flowers, followed by many-seeded capsules.
• **USES** The honey-scented flowers flavour liqueurs and yield skin-softening mucilage. The expectorant, soothing, and spasm-sedating properties of the leaf and flowers are used to treat raspy coughs, and in herbal tobacco. Research has confirmed anti-tubercular activity in plant extracts. Leaf smoke was used by native Americans to revive the unconscious. The flowers reduce eczema inflammation and help heal wounds; the seed oil soothes chilblains and chapped skin; the root is diuretic; and a homeopathic leaf tincture treats migraine and earache. Woolly leaf-wraps preserve figs, and are used as tinder and emergency bandages.

stems dipped in suet or tallow make long-lasting torches

flower-buds open midsummer to mid-autumn

5-petalled yellow flowers open randomly around the stem

flowers have faint honey scent

crushed capsules and tiny seeds are used to stupefy fish

up to 2m (6½ft)

leaf hairs can cause irritation; strain infusion before drinking

infused flowers will highlight fair hair

Habitat Dry, gravelly hillsides, woodland; Europe, Asia	Parts used ✿ ◖ ✄ ▨ ❀

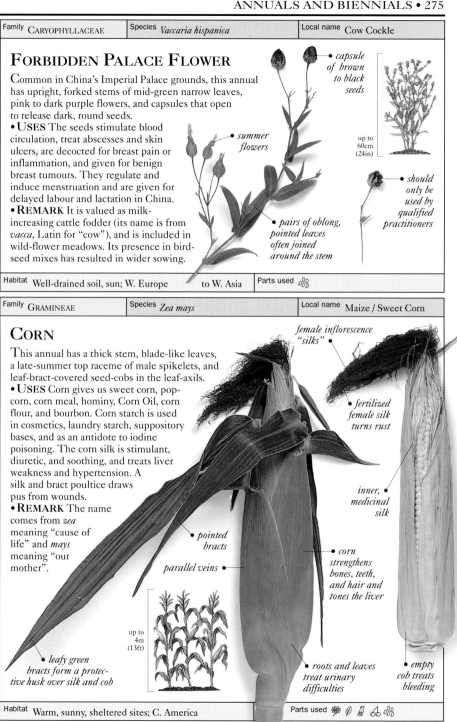

Family CARYOPHYLLACEAE	Species *Vaccaria hispanica*	Local name Cow Cockle

FORBIDDEN PALACE FLOWER

Common in China's Imperial Palace grounds, this annual
has upright, forked stems of mid-green narrow leaves,
pink to dark purple flowers, and capsules that open
to release dark, round seeds.
• **USES** The seeds stimulate blood
circulation, treat abscesses and skin
ulcers, are decocted for breast pain or
inflammation, and given for benign
breast tumours. They regulate and
induce menstruation and are given for
delayed labour and lactation in China.
• **REMARK** It is valued as milk-
increasing cattle fodder (its name is from
vacca, Latin for "cow"), and is included in
wild-flower meadows. Its presence in bird-
seed mixes has resulted in wider sowing.

*capsule
of brown
to black
seeds*

*summer
flowers*

up to
60cm
(24in)

*should
only be
used by
qualified
practitioners*

*pairs of oblong,
pointed leaves
often joined
around the stem*

Habitat Well-drained soil, sun; W. Europe	to W. Asia	Parts used

Family GRAMINEAE	Species *Zea mays*	Local name Maize / Sweet Corn

CORN

This annual has a thick stem, blade-like leaves,
a late-summer top raceme of male spikelets, and
leaf-bract-covered seed-cobs in the leaf-axils.
• **USES** Corn gives us sweet corn, pop-
corn, corn meal, hominy, Corn Oil, corn
flour, and bourbon. Corn starch is used
in cosmetics, laundry starch, suppository
bases, and as an antidote to iodine
poisoning. The corn silk is stimulant,
diuretic, and soothing, and treats liver
weakness and hypertension. A
silk and bract poultice draws
pus from wounds.
• **REMARK** The name
comes from *zea*
meaning "cause of
life" and *mays*
meaning "our
mother".

*female inflorescence
"silks"*

*fertilized
female silk
turns rust*

*inner,
medicinal
silk*

*pointed
bracts*

parallel veins

*corn
strengthens
bones, teeth,
and hair and
tones the liver*

up to
4m
(13ft)

*leafy green
bracts form a protec-
tive husk over silk and cob*

*roots and leaves
treat urinary
difficulties*

*empty
cob treats
bleeding*

Habitat Warm, sunny, sheltered sites; C. America	Parts used

CLIMBERS

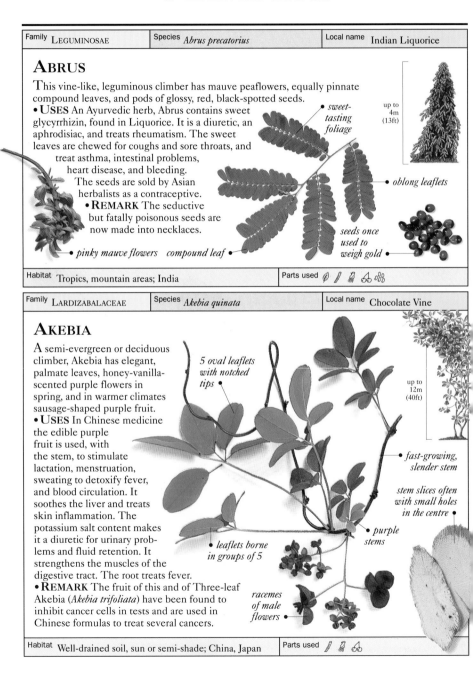

Family LEGUMINOSAE	Species *Abrus precatorius*	Local name Indian Liquorice

ABRUS

This vine-like, leguminous climber has mauve peaflowers, equally pinnate compound leaves, and pods of glossy, red, black-spotted seeds.
• **USES** An Ayurvedic herb, Abrus contains sweet glycyrrhizin, found in Liquorice. It is a diuretic, an aphrodisiac, and treats rheumatism. The sweet leaves are chewed for coughs and sore throats, and treat asthma, intestinal problems, heart disease, and bleeding. The seeds are sold by Asian herbalists as a contraceptive.
• **REMARK** The seductive but fatally poisonous seeds are now made into necklaces.

sweet-tasting foliage

up to 4m (13ft)

oblong leaflets

seeds once used to weigh gold

pinky mauve flowers   compound leaf

Habitat Tropics, mountain areas; India	Parts used

Family LARDIZABALACEAE	Species *Akebia quinata*	Local name Chocolate Vine

AKEBIA

A semi-evergreen or deciduous climber, Akebia has elegant, palmate leaves, honey-vanilla-scented purple flowers in spring, and in warmer climates sausage-shaped purple fruit.
• **USES** In Chinese medicine the edible purple fruit is used, with the stem, to stimulate lactation, menstruation, sweating to detoxify fever, and blood circulation. It soothes the liver and treats skin inflammation. The potassium salt content makes it a diuretic for urinary prob-lems and fluid retention. It strengthens the muscles of the digestive tract. The root treats fever.
• **REMARK** The fruit of this and of Three-leaf Akebia (*Akebia trifoliata*) have been found to inhibit cancer cells in tests and are used in Chinese formulas to treat several cancers.

5 oval leaflets with notched tips

up to 12m (40ft)

fast-growing, slender stem

stem slices often with small holes in the centre

purple stems

leaflets borne in groups of 5

racemes of male flowers

Habitat Well-drained soil, sun or semi-shade; China, Japan	Parts used

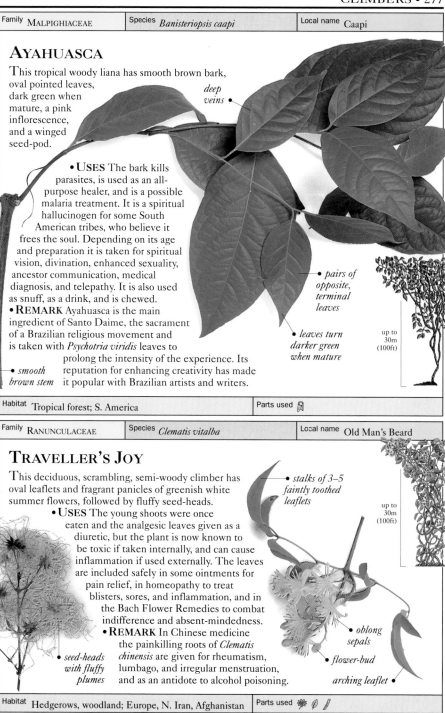

Family MALPIGHIACEAE	Species *Banisteriopsis caapi*	Local name Caapi

AYAHUASCA

This tropical woody liana has smooth brown bark, oval pointed leaves, dark green when mature, a pink inflorescence, and a winged seed-pod.

deep veins •

• **USES** The bark kills parasites, is used as an all-purpose healer, and is a possible malaria treatment. It is a spiritual hallucinogen for some South American tribes, who believe it frees the soul. Depending on its age and preparation it is taken for spiritual vision, divination, enhanced sexuality, ancestor communication, medical diagnosis, and telepathy. It is also used as snuff, as a drink, and is chewed.
• **REMARK** Ayahuasca is the main ingredient of Santo Daime, the sacrament of a Brazilian religious movement and is taken with *Psychotria viridis* leaves to prolong the intensity of the experience. Its reputation for enhancing creativity has made it popular with Brazilian artists and writers.

• pairs of opposite, terminal leaves

• leaves turn darker green when mature

• smooth brown stem

up to 30m (100ft)

Habitat Tropical forest; S. America	Parts used

Family RANUNCULACEAE	Species *Clematis vitalba*	Local name Old Man's Beard

TRAVELLER'S JOY

This deciduous, scrambling, semi-woody climber has oval leaflets and fragrant panicles of greenish white summer flowers, followed by fluffy seed-heads.

• stalks of 3–5 faintly toothed leaflets

up to 30m (100ft)

• **USES** The young shoots were once eaten and the analgesic leaves given as a diuretic, but the plant is now known to be toxic if taken internally, and can cause inflammation if used externally. The leaves are included safely in some ointments for pain relief, in homeopathy to treat blisters, sores, and inflammation, and in the Bach Flower Remedies to combat indifference and absent-mindedness.
• **REMARK** In Chinese medicine the painkilling roots of *Clematis chinensis* are given for rheumatism, lumbago, and irregular menstruation, and as an antidote to alcohol poisoning.

• seed-heads with fluffy plumes

• oblong sepals

• flower-bud

arching leaflet •

Habitat Hedgerows, woodland; Europe, N. Iran, Afghanistan	Parts used

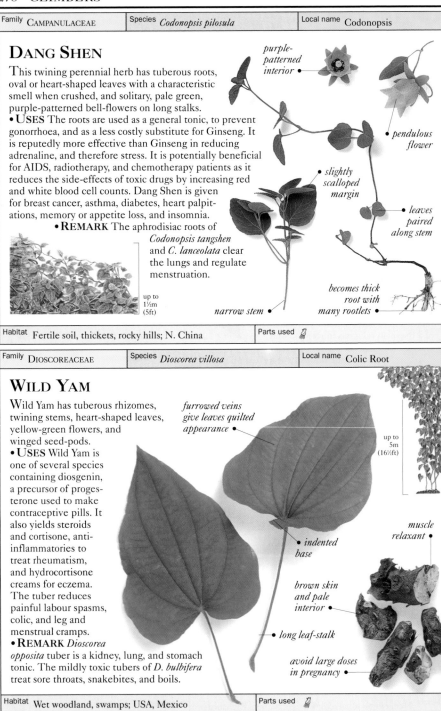

Family CAMPANULACEAE	Species *Codonopsis pilosula*	Local name Codonopsis

DANG SHEN

This twining perennial herb has tuberous roots, oval or heart-shaped leaves with a characteristic smell when crushed, and solitary, pale green, purple-patterned bell-flowers on long stalks.
• USES The roots are used as a general tonic, to prevent gonorrhoea, and as a less costly substitute for Ginseng. It is reputedly more effective than Ginseng in reducing adrenaline, and therefore stress. It is potentially beneficial for AIDS, radiotherapy, and chemotherapy patients as it reduces the side-effects of toxic drugs by increasing red and white blood cell counts. Dang Shen is given for breast cancer, asthma, diabetes, heart palpitations, memory or appetite loss, and insomnia.
• REMARK The aphrodisiac roots of *Codonopsis tangshen* and *C. lanceolata* clear the lungs and regulate menstruation.

purple-patterned interior •

• pendulous flower

• slightly scalloped margin

• leaves paired along stem

up to 1⅓m (5ft)

narrow stem •

becomes thick root with many rootlets •

Habitat Fertile soil, thickets, rocky hills; N. China	Parts used

Family DIOSCOREACEAE	Species *Dioscorea villosa*	Local name Colic Root

WILD YAM

Wild Yam has tuberous rhizomes, twining stems, heart-shaped leaves, yellow-green flowers, and winged seed-pods.
• USES Wild Yam is one of several species containing diosgenin, a precursor of progesterone used to make contraceptive pills. It also yields steroids and cortisone, anti-inflammatories to treat rheumatism, and hydrocortisone creams for eczema. The tuber reduces painful labour spasms, colic, and leg and menstrual cramps.
• REMARK *Dioscorea opposita* tuber is a kidney, lung, and stomach tonic. The mildly toxic tubers of *D. bulbifera* treat sore throats, snakebites, and boils.

furrowed veins give leaves quilted appearance •

up to 5m (16½ft)

muscle relaxant •

• indented base

brown skin and pale interior •

• long leaf-stalk

avoid large doses in pregnancy •

Habitat Wet woodland, swamps; USA, Mexico	Parts used

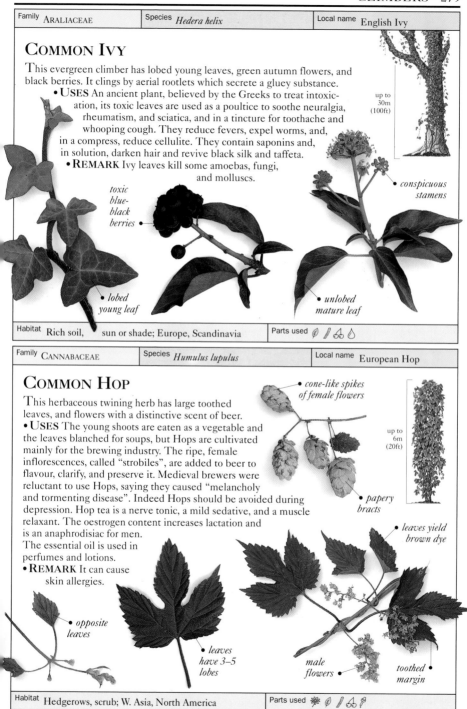

Family ARALIACEAE	Species *Hedera helix*	Local name English Ivy

COMMON IVY

This evergreen climber has lobed young leaves, green autumn flowers, and black berries. It clings by aerial rootlets which secrete a gluey substance.
• **USES** An ancient plant, believed by the Greeks to treat intoxication, its toxic leaves are used as a poultice to soothe neuralgia, rheumatism, and sciatica, and in a tincture for toothache and whooping cough. They reduce fevers, expel worms, and, in a compress, reduce cellulite. They contain saponins and, in solution, darken hair and revive black silk and taffeta.
• **REMARK** Ivy leaves kill some amoebas, fungi, and molluscs.

up to 30m (100ft)

conspicuous stamens

toxic blue-black berries

lobed young leaf

unlobed mature leaf

Habitat Rich soil, sun or shade; Europe, Scandinavia	Parts used

Family CANNABACEAE	Species *Humulus lupulus*	Local name European Hop

COMMON HOP

This herbaceous twining herb has large toothed leaves, and flowers with a distinctive scent of beer.
• **USES** The young shoots are eaten as a vegetable and the leaves blanched for soups, but Hops are cultivated mainly for the brewing industry. The ripe, female inflorescences, called "strobiles", are added to beer to flavour, clarify, and preserve it. Medieval brewers were reluctant to use Hops, saying they caused "melancholy and tormenting disease". Indeed Hops should be avoided during depression. Hop tea is a nerve tonic, a mild sedative, and a muscle relaxant. The oestrogen content increases lactation and is an anaphrodisiac for men. The essential oil is used in perfumes and lotions.
• **REMARK** It can cause skin allergies.

cone-like spikes of female flowers

up to 6m (20ft)

papery bracts

leaves yield brown dye

opposite leaves

leaves have 3–5 lobes

male flowers

toothed margin

Habitat Hedgerows, scrub; W. Asia, North America	Parts used

Family CONVOLVULACEAE	Species *Ipomoea hederacea*	Local name Tlililtzin / Piule

MORNING GLORY

This usually hairy, annual climber has three or five lobed, long-stalked leaves and trumpet-shaped flowers.
• **USES** The whole plant, especially the roots, are purgative. The dried, ripe seeds are hallucinogenic and toxic, and are used in Asia to expel worms, treat constipation, as a diuretic, and to promote menstruation.

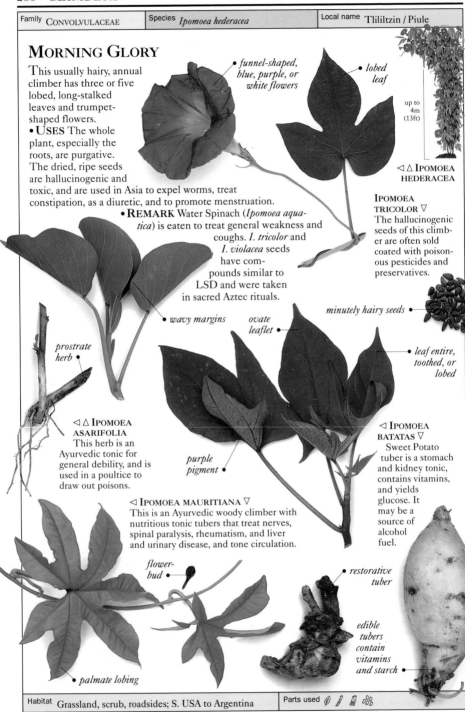

• *funnel-shaped, blue, purple, or white flowers*

• *lobed leaf*

up to 4m (13ft)

◁ △ **IPOMOEA HEDERACEA**

IPOMOEA TRICOLOR ▽
The hallucinogenic seeds of this climber are often sold coated with poisonous pesticides and preservatives.

• **REMARK** Water Spinach (*Ipomoea aquatica*) is eaten to treat general weakness and coughs. *I. tricolor* and *I. violacea* seeds have compounds similar to LSD and were taken in sacred Aztec rituals.

• *wavy margins*

ovate leaflet •

minutely hairy seeds •

• *leaf entire, toothed, or lobed*

prostrate herb •

◁ △ **IPOMOEA ASARIFOLIA**
This herb is an Ayurvedic tonic for general debility, and is used in a poultice to draw out poisons.

purple pigment •

◁ **IPOMOEA BATATAS** ▽
Sweet Potato tuber is a stomach and kidney tonic, contains vitamins, and yields glucose. It may be a source of alcohol fuel.

◁ **IPOMOEA MAURITIANA** ▽
This is an Ayurvedic woody climber with nutritious tonic tubers that treat nerves, spinal paralysis, rheumatism, and liver and urinary disease, and tone circulation.

flower-bud •

• *restorative tuber*

edible tubers contain vitamins and starch •

• *palmate lobing*

Habitat Grassland, scrub, roadsides; S. USA to Argentina	Parts used

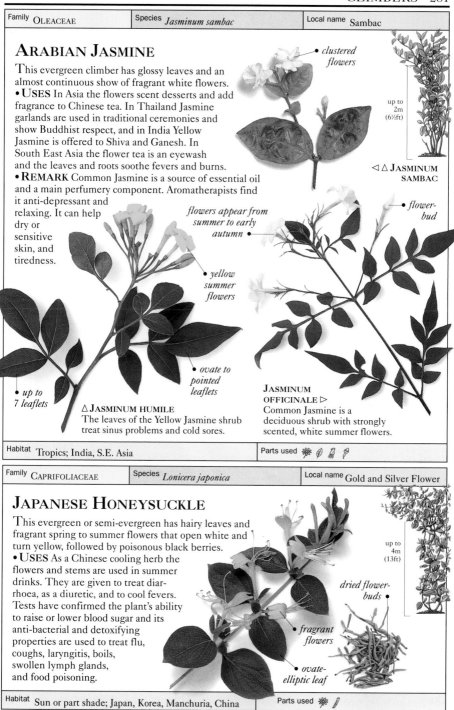

| Family OLEACEAE | Species *Jasminum sambac* | Local name Sambac |

ARABIAN JASMINE

This evergreen climber has glossy leaves and an almost continuous show of fragrant white flowers.
• **USES** In Asia the flowers scent desserts and add fragrance to Chinese tea. In Thailand Jasmine garlands are used in traditional ceremonies and show Buddhist respect, and in India Yellow Jasmine is offered to Shiva and Ganesh. In South East Asia the flower tea is an eyewash and the leaves and roots soothe fevers and burns.
• **REMARK** Common Jasmine is a source of essential oil and a main perfumery component. Aromatherapists find it anti-depressant and relaxing. It can help dry or sensitive skin, and tiredness.

clustered flowers

up to 2m (6½ft)

◁ △ **JASMINUM SAMBAC**

flower-bud

flowers appear from summer to early autumn

yellow summer flowers

ovate to pointed leaflets

up to 7 leaflets

△ **JASMINUM HUMILE**
The leaves of the Yellow Jasmine shrub treat sinus problems and cold sores.

JASMINUM OFFICINALE ▷
Common Jasmine is a deciduous shrub with strongly scented, white summer flowers.

| Habitat Tropics; India, S.E. Asia | Parts used |

| Family CAPRIFOLIACEAE | Species *Lonicera japonica* | Local name Gold and Silver Flower |

JAPANESE HONEYSUCKLE

This evergreen or semi-evergreen has hairy leaves and fragrant spring to summer flowers that open white and turn yellow, followed by poisonous black berries.
• **USES** As a Chinese cooling herb the flowers and stems are used in summer drinks. They are given to treat diarrhoea, as a diuretic, and to cool fevers. Tests have confirmed the plant's ability to raise or lower blood sugar and its anti-bacterial and detoxifying properties are used to treat flu, coughs, laryngitis, boils, swollen lymph glands, and food poisoning.

up to 4m (13ft)

dried flower-buds

fragrant flowers

ovate-elliptic leaf

| Habitat Sun or part shade; Japan, Korea, Manchuria, China | Parts used |

Family CUCURBITACEAE	Species *Luffa cylindrica*	Local name Vegetable Sponge

SMOOTH LOOFAH

This annual vine has conspicuous
female flowers, yellow male flowers,
and smooth, cylindrical fruit.
• **USES** The flower-buds, shoots,
young leaves, and fruit are eaten; the
seeds yield edible oil. Leaf juice is applied
to prickly heat, and the steeped flowers and
gourds are drunk for throat and lung problems.
The painkilling fruit fibre treats uterine
bleeding, piles, and dysentery.
• **REMARK** When dried, soaked, and
bleached the fruit reveals the fibrous
loofah, used for scrubbing the skin
and cleaning pans, and
as a shock absorber.

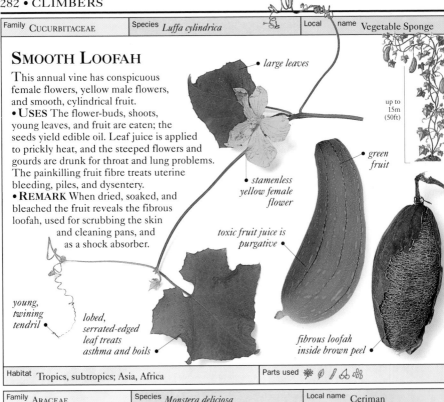

• large leaves

up to
15m
(50ft)

• green
fruit

• stamenless
yellow female
flower

toxic fruit juice is
purgative •

young,
twining
tendril •

lobed,
serrated-edged
leaf treats
asthma and boils •

fibrous loofah
inside brown peel •

Habitat Tropics, subtropics; Asia, Africa	Parts used ❋ ⌀ ∦ ⚶ ⸚

Family ARACEAE	Species *Monstera deliciosa*	Local name Ceriman

SWISS-CHEESE PLANT

This vine has large, segmented adult leaves,
aerial roots, and bracted inflorescences
which swell into cream fruit.
• **USES** The Aztecs toasted the
seeds as a strong purgative,
while Chinese medicine
uses the leaves to treat
some cancers. In the
Caribbean the
compound, cone-
shaped, ripe fruit,
with a pineapple
and banana flavour,
is eaten or pulped
for ices and drinks.
• **REMARK** Tiny
crystals in the
fruit can
spike the
mouth.

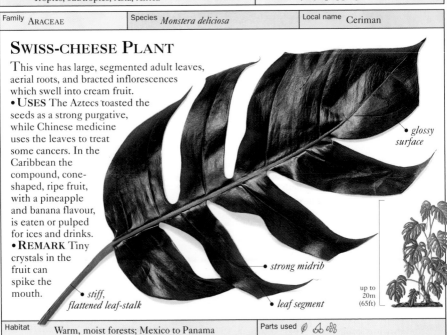

• glossy
surface

strong midrib •

• stiff,
flattened leaf-stalk

• leaf segment

up to
20m
(65ft)

Habitat Warm, moist forests; Mexico to Panama	Parts used ⌀ ⚶ ⸚

Family PIPERACEAE	Species *Piper nigrum*	Local name Vine Pepper

BLACK PEPPER

This perennial vine has stout stems, white flowering spikes, and green to dark red fruit.
• **USES** Black, green, and white pepper are all made from the berries, taken at different stages of maturity and processed differently. Now a worldwide spice, its value was an incentive to early trade voyagers. The alkaloid piperine in pepper stimulates saliva and gastric juices, aiding digestion and killing bacteria. The diuretic fruit treats flatulence, colic, rheumatism, headaches, and diarrhoea.
• **REMARK** The essential oil gives commercial foods pepper flavour without the pungency, and adds spicy notes to perfumes. In massage oils it is stimulating and toning.

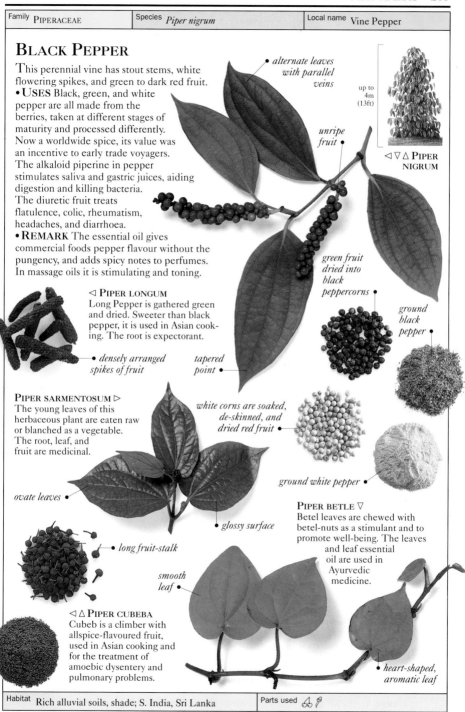

alternate leaves with parallel veins

unripe fruit

up to 4m (13ft)

◁ ▽ △ **PIPER NIGRUM**

green fruit dried into black peppercorns

ground black pepper

◁ **PIPER LONGUM**
Long Pepper is gathered green and dried. Sweeter than black pepper, it is used in Asian cooking. The root is expectorant.

densely arranged spikes of fruit

tapered point

PIPER SARMENTOSUM ▷
The young leaves of this herbaceous plant are eaten raw or blanched as a vegetable. The root, leaf, and fruit are medicinal.

white corns are soaked, de-skinned, and dried red fruit

ovate leaves

ground white pepper

PIPER BETLE ▽
Betel leaves are chewed with betel-nuts as a stimulant and to promote well-being. The leaves and leaf essential oil are used in Ayurvedic medicine.

glossy surface

long fruit-stalk

smooth leaf

◁ △ **PIPER CUBEBA**
Cubeb is a climber with allspice-flavoured fruit, used in Asian cooking and for the treatment of amoebic dysentery and pulmonary problems.

heart-shaped, aromatic leaf

Habitat Rich alluvial soils, shade; S. India, Sri Lanka	Parts used 🍃🌶

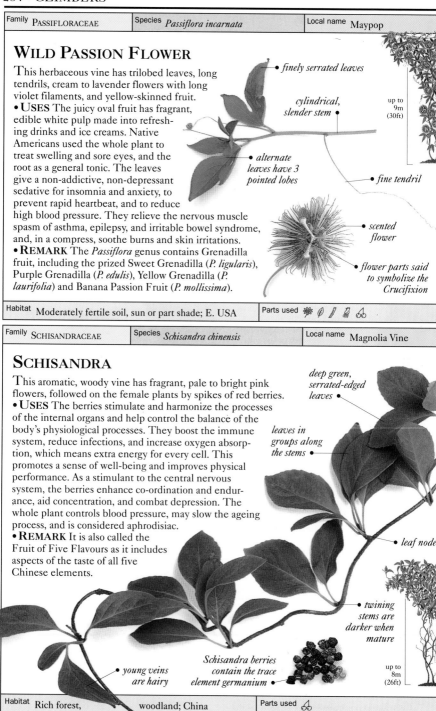

| Family PASSIFLORACEAE | Species *Passiflora incarnata* | Local name Maypop |

WILD PASSION FLOWER

This herbaceous vine has trilobed leaves, long tendrils, cream to lavender flowers with long violet filaments, and yellow-skinned fruit.
• **USES** The juicy oval fruit has fragrant, edible white pulp made into refreshing drinks and ice creams. Native Americans used the whole plant to treat swelling and sore eyes, and the root as a general tonic. The leaves give a non-addictive, non-depressant sedative for insomnia and anxiety, to prevent rapid heartbeat, and to reduce high blood pressure. They relieve the nervous muscle spasm of asthma, epilepsy, and irritable bowel syndrome, and, in a compress, soothe burns and skin irritations.
• **REMARK** The *Passiflora* genus contains Grenadilla fruit, including the prized Sweet Grenadilla (*P. ligularis*), Purple Grenadilla (*P. edulis*), Yellow Grenadilla (*P. laurifolia*) and Banana Passion Fruit (*P. mollissima*).

• finely serrated leaves

cylindrical, slender stem •

up to 9m (30ft)

• alternate leaves have 3 pointed lobes

• fine tendril

• scented flower

• flower parts said to symbolize the Crucifixion

| Habitat Moderately fertile soil, sun or part shade; E. USA | Parts used |

| Family SCHISANDRACEAE | Species *Schisandra chinensis* | Local name Magnolia Vine |

SCHISANDRA

This aromatic, woody vine has fragrant, pale to bright pink flowers, followed on the female plants by spikes of red berries.
• **USES** The berries stimulate and harmonize the processes of the internal organs and help control the balance of the body's physiological processes. They boost the immune system, reduce infections, and increase oxygen absorption, which means extra energy for every cell. This promotes a sense of well-being and improves physical performance. As a stimulant to the central nervous system, the berries enhance co-ordination and endurance, aid concentration, and combat depression. The whole plant controls blood pressure, may slow the ageing process, and is considered aphrodisiac.
• **REMARK** It is also called the Fruit of Five Flavours as it includes aspects of the taste of all five Chinese elements.

deep green, serrated-edged leaves •

leaves in groups along the stems •

• leaf node

• twining stems are darker when mature

up to 8m (26ft)

young veins are hairy •

Schisandra berries contain the trace element germanium •

| Habitat Rich forest, woodland; China | Parts used |

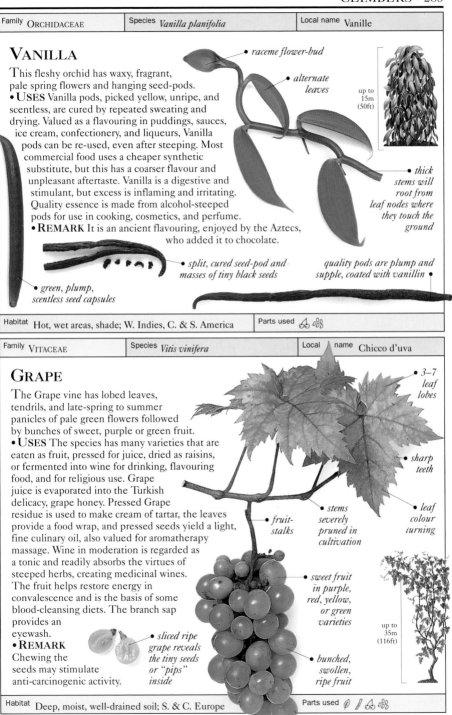

| Family ORCHIDACEAE | Species *Vanilla planifolia* | Local name Vanille |

VANILLA

This fleshy orchid has waxy, fragrant,
pale spring flowers and hanging seed-pods.
• USES Vanilla pods, picked yellow, unripe, and
scentless, are cured by repeated sweating and
drying. Valued as a flavouring in puddings, sauces,
ice cream, confectionery, and liqueurs, Vanilla
pods can be re-used, even after steeping. Most
commercial food uses a cheaper synthetic
substitute, but this has a coarser flavour and
unpleasant aftertaste. Vanilla is a digestive and
stimulant, but excess is inflaming and irritating.
Quality essence is made from alcohol-steeped
pods for use in cooking, cosmetics, and perfume.
• REMARK It is an ancient flavouring, enjoyed by the Aztecs,
who added it to chocolate.

• *raceme flower-bud*

• *alternate leaves*

up to
15m
(50ft)

• *thick stems will root from leaf nodes where they touch the ground*

• *split, cured seed-pod and masses of tiny black seeds*

quality pods are plump and supple, coated with vanillin •

• *green, plump, scentless seed capsules*

| Habitat Hot, wet areas, shade; W. Indies, C. & S. America | Parts used |

| Family VITACEAE | Species *Vitis vinifera* | Local name Chicco d'uva |

GRAPE

The Grape vine has lobed leaves,
tendrils, and late-spring to summer
panicles of pale green flowers followed
by bunches of sweet, purple or green fruit.
• USES The species has many varieties that are
eaten as fruit, pressed for juice, dried as raisins,
or fermented into wine for drinking, flavouring
food, and for religious use. Grape
juice is evaporated into the Turkish
delicacy, grape honey. Pressed Grape
residue is used to make cream of tartar, the leaves
provide a food wrap, and pressed seeds yield a light,
fine culinary oil, also valued for aromatherapy
massage. Wine in moderation is regarded as
a tonic and readily absorbs the virtues of
steeped herbs, creating medicinal wines.
The fruit helps restore energy in
convalescence and is the basis of some
blood-cleansing diets. The branch sap
provides an
eyewash.
• REMARK
Chewing the
seeds may stimulate
anti-carcinogenic activity.

• *3–7 leaf lobes*

• *sharp teeth*

• *leaf colour turning*

• *stems severely pruned in cultivation*

• *fruit-stalks*

• *sweet fruit in purple, red, yellow, or green varieties*

up to
35m
(116ft)

• *sliced ripe grape reveals the tiny seeds or "pips" inside*

• *bunched, swollen, ripe fruit*

| Habitat Deep, moist, well-drained soil; S. & C. Europe | Parts used |

OTHER HERBS

Family	Species	Local name
PTERIDACEAE	*Adiantum capillus-veneris*	Venus's Hair

MAIDENHAIR FERN

◁ **ADIANTUM CAPILLUS-VENERIS**

This elegant, creeping fern has arched fronds with dark stalks and lobed, fan-shaped leaflets.
• **USES** A frond tea soothes sore throats and asthma, and expels chest catarrh. With *Adiantum caudatum* it was included in Capillaire, a famous 19th-century cough syrup. Reputedly detoxifying, the fronds have potential for treating alcoholism.
The Navajo used a frond wash for bee-stings, centipede bites and snakebites, to expel worms, and ease fevers.
• **REMARK** The expectorant *A. pedatum* was used by Canadian native peoples for chest catarrh, and the stems for a hair wash.

fan-shaped leaflets •

toothed leaflets •

up to 70cm (28in)

ADIANTUM CAPILLUS-VENERIS

ADIANTUM CAUDATUM ▷
The Trailing Maidenhair has large fronds.

Habitat	Parts used
Forest, stream edges, rock crevices; widespread	

Family	Species	Local name
AMANITACEAE	*Amanita muscaria*	Deadly Amanita

FLY AGARIC

This storybook "toadstool" is an autumn fruiting body with a stem ringed with remnants of veil, and a red cap usually with pale warts.
• **USES** Perhaps the world's oldest hallucinogen, this mushroom may be India's legendary *soma*. It is a popular reindeer food, and was used by Siberians to induce elation, and by Siberian Shamans in vision quests and healing ceremonies. The effects can include a sense of flying, visions, nausea, mood swings, convulsions, gastroenteritis, and deep sleep. It is a homeopathic remedy for scabies and neurological problems. It is broken into milk as a fly killer.
• **REMARK** Lapland Shamans eat it for enlightenment. This practice may have given rise to the flying reindeer and red-and white-costumed "Santa" legends.

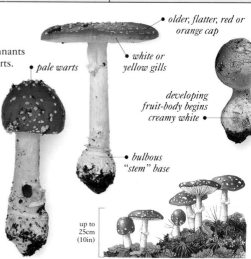

• *older, flatter, red or orange cap*

• *white or yellow gills*

• *pale warts*

developing fruit-body begins creamy white •

• *bulbous "stem" base*

up to 25cm (10in)

Habitat	Parts used
Thin forests with Birch; Europe, North America	Fruit-body

Family CLAVICIPITACEAE	Species *Claviceps purpurea*	Local name Secale Cornuti

ERGOT

A parasitic fungus, Ergot produces an over-wintering sclerotium with a violet crust and unpleasant scent.
• **USES** A fungus found on rye and other cereals, Ergot was given by midwives in medieval times to stimulate contractions during childbirth. Doctors still use extracts for this purpose, as a vaso-constrictor to relieve migraines, and as a basis for psychiatric drugs; LSD was first isolated from Ergot.
• **REMARK** It was probably used in rituals of the Ancient Greek Eleusinian Mysteries. The milling of Ergot-infected grain in Medieval times caused mass poisoning, with epileptic or gangrenous symptoms. The outbreaks were called St. Anthony's Fire, after his own fiery spiritual trials.

• parasitic fungus replaces the kernel

• dark colouring

• curved spur

up to 6cm (2⅓in)

• rye stalk

Habitat Parasitic on cereals & grasses; worldwide	Parts used Fruit-body

Family DRYOPTERIDACEAE	Species *Dryopteris filix-mas*	Local name Sweet Brake

MALE FERN

This fern has broad, deciduous, and elegantly divided green fronds, which unroll from the crown of the rhizome.
• **USES** The young, curled fronds of Male Fern can be boiled as a vegetable, and during Norwegian famines were mixed with bread and brewed for beer. For centuries the rhizome was used to expel tapeworms and other intestinal parasites. The rhizome, the dark green oil extracted from it, and the frond bases (called Male Fern Fingers) are still used by medical practitioners and vets for this purpose, with care for their toxicity. The fronds are a source of potash.
• **REMARK** The mysterious regeneration of ferns led to the ancient belief that their seed could confer invisibility. The root was added to love potions, and the fronds eaten by those embarking on love quests – until later associations involved evil spirits.

spore-bearing clusters in round masses along veins •

• young frond, one of many that uncurl from base

• thick, short, creeping, reddish brown, scaled rhizome

• fibrous roots

up to 90cm (35in)

• leaflets divided into serrated-edged segments

• stalk covered with scaly, brown hairs

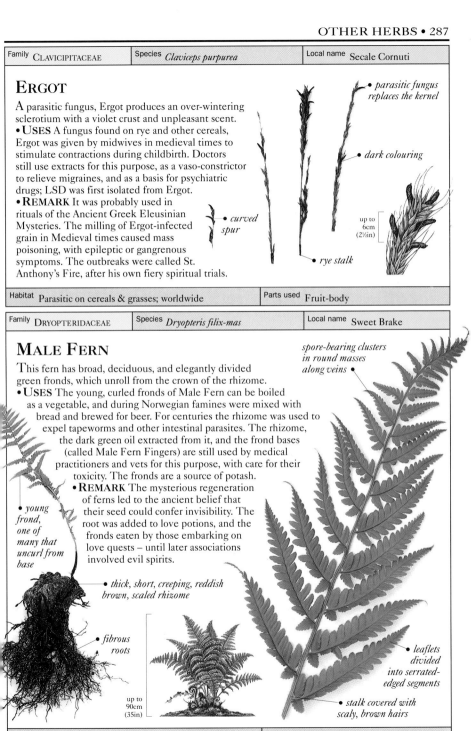

Habitat Damp woods, hedgerows; North America, Eurasia	Parts used

Family EQUISETACEAE	Species *Equisetum arvense*	Local name Shave Brush

HORSETAIL

This ancient, primitive, non-flowering herb grows both brown, fertile stems, ending in upright cones containing spores, and green, sterile stems.
• **USES** The young heads are eaten boiled, and in Japan are pickled. The stems staunch bleeding, are astringent and diuretic, given for genito-urinary disorders and bed-wetting, and are homeostatic, balancing the body's physiological processes. Horsetail's minerals and salts enrich the blood, and strengthen hair and nails. The silica content promotes the re-growth, strength, and elasticity of connective tissues, and treats arthritis, ulcers, and eczema.
• **REMARK** Horsetail provides a yellow dye. In China the stems of *Equisetum hyemale* treat "cloudy" eyes and cool fevers.

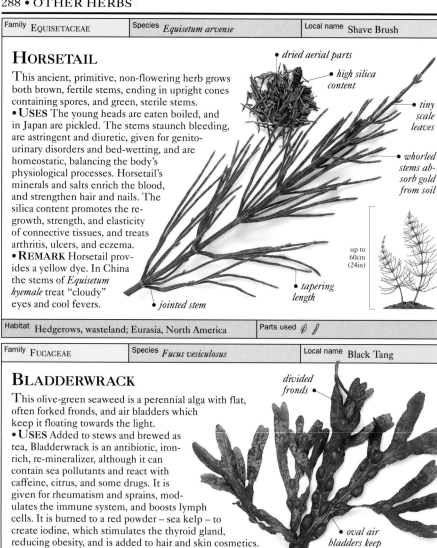

dried aerial parts

high silica content

tiny scale leaves

whorled stems absorb gold from soil

up to 60cm (24in)

tapering length

jointed stem

Habitat Hedgerows, wasteland; Eurasia, North America	Parts used

Family FUCACEAE	Species *Fucus vesiculosus*	Local name Black Tang

BLADDERWRACK

This olive-green seaweed is a perennial alga with flat, often forked fronds, and air bladders which keep it floating towards the light.
• **USES** Added to stews and brewed as tea, Bladderwrack is an antibiotic, iron-rich, re-mineralizer, although it can contain sea pollutants and react with caffeine, citrus, and some drugs. It is given for rheumatism and sprains, mod-ulates the immune system, and boosts lymph cells. It is burned to a red powder – sea kelp – to create iodine, which stimulates the thyroid gland, reducing obesity, and is added to hair and skin cosmetics.
• **REMARK** In harsh coastal areas Bladderwrack provides sheep and cattle winter fodder and is an organic fertilizer.

divided fronds

oval air bladders keep fronds afloat

fronds absorb heavy metals and other sea pollutants

up to 90cm (35in)

dried fronds, source of trace elements, used in slimming products

holdfast clasps rock

Habitat Rocks & stones at middle tide; Europe, N. Atlantic	Parts used Fronds

Family GANODERMATACEAE	Species *Ganoderma lucidum*	Local name Ling Zhi

REISHI MUSHROOM

This fungus has a long-stalked, shiny, chestnut-brown fruit-body. The laterally attached, hard-crusted cap is kidney- to fan-shaped, with concentric furrows, rusty spores, and off-white to dull brown pores, through which the spores are released.

• **USES** A Taoist "Elixir of Life", the legendary "Mushroom of Deathlessness", and once reserved for the Emperor, Reishi has a long association with longevity and increased spiritual energy. It is said to improve circulation and reduce heart strain, while lowering blood pressure. It is calming and pain-relieving, given to ease arthritis, asthma, bronchitis, allergies, and insomnia. It boosts the immune system and reduces ageing free radicals by fifty per cent.

• **REMARK** In Chinese medicine Reishi is prescribed for various forms of cancer and it is being researched in Japan.

laterally attached, grooved cap

angled cap

almost shiny surface

long fruit-body stalk

bumpy and irregular

stout stem

up to 30cm (12in)

Habitat Stumps or roots of broadleaf trees; Europe, China	Parts used Fruit-body

Family LYCOPERDACEAE	Species *Langermannia gigantea*	Local name Dusty Star

GIANT PUFFBALL

Puffballs appear in late summer like white footballs. Later the skin browns and cracks and spores are dispersed.

• **USES** Young fruit-bodies last several days after picking and can be boiled, fried, or roasted. The ripe flesh staunches bleeding and was used by the Blackfoot tribes for wounds, haemorrhages, and to soothe babies by rubbing the spores on their cheeks. In China the spores are given with honey for sore throats.

• **REMARK** Puffball flesh contains tiny amounts of calvacin, a cancer cell inhibitor.

grey-white and downy, then cream and smooth, becomes brown and dry

fruit-body base

up to 30cm (12in)

Habitat Grassy areas, wood edges; Europe, North America	Parts used Fruit-body

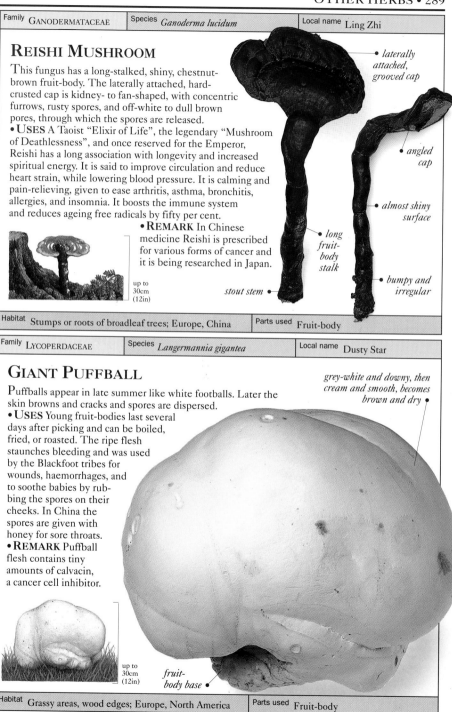

| Family LAMINARIACEAE | Species *Laminaria saccharina* | Local name Sugar Kelp |

SWEET WRACK

Sweet Wrack has long, single, undulating brown
fronds with round stalks and a strong hold-fast.
• **USES** This vitamin- and mineral-rich seaweed, an
important source of kelp, which contains iodine, exudes a sugary
liquid which dries as crystals. This is dusted on chewing gum and unpleasantly
flavoured pills, and used in the manufacture of paper, polish, and explosives.
Young plants are eaten raw or cooked and provide alginates used to stabilize ice
cream, dehydrated and prepared foods, cosmetic creams, hairspray, water softeners,
and dental plates. Kelp fertilizers are popular with organic
gardeners because of their micro-nutrients.
• **REMARK** In traditional Chinese
medicine it is given to disperse
hard lumps, such as swollen
lymph nodes and tumours.

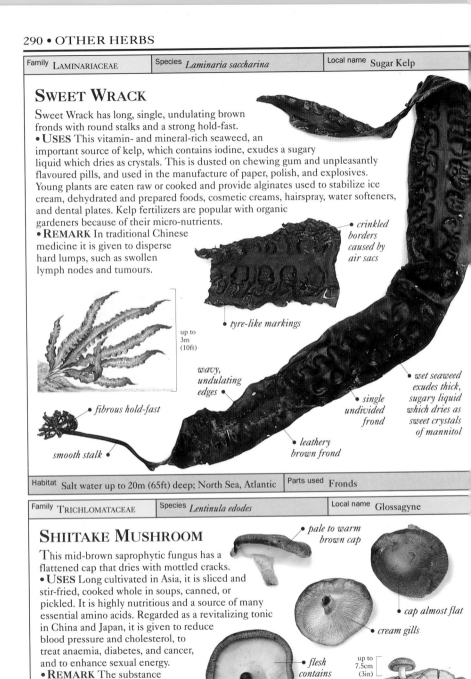

• *crinkled borders caused by air sacs*

• *tyre-like markings*

up to 3m (10ft)

wavy, undulating edges •

• *fibrous hold-fast*

smooth stalk •

• *single undivided frond*

• *wet seaweed exudes thick, sugary liquid which dries as sweet crystals of mannitol*

• *leathery brown frond*

| Habitat Salt water up to 20m (65ft) deep; North Sea, Atlantic | Parts used Fronds |

| Family TRICHLOMATACEAE | Species *Lentinula edodes* | Local name Glossagyne |

SHIITAKE MUSHROOM

This mid-brown saprophytic fungus has a
flattened cap that dries with mottled cracks.
• **USES** Long cultivated in Asia, it is sliced and
stir-fried, cooked whole in soups, canned, or
pickled. It is highly nutritious and a source of many
essential amino acids. Regarded as a revitalizing tonic
in China and Japan, it is given to reduce
blood pressure and cholesterol, to
treat anaemia, diabetes, and cancer,
and to enhance sexual energy.
• **REMARK** The substance
lentinan, extracted from Shiitake
Mushrooms, resists carcinogens.
Carbohydrates from many edible
mushrooms share anti-cancer activity.

• *pale to warm brown cap*

• *cap almost flat*

• *cream gills*

• *flesh contains carbohydrates, protein, and vitamins*

up to 7.5cm (3in)

| Habitat On hardwood logs; China, Japan | Parts used Fruit-body cap |

| Family CACTACEAE | Species *Lophophora williamsii* | Local name Mescal Button |

PEYOTE

This small, clustered cactus has a carrot-like root, a spineless body (the stem), and pink or white flowers.
• **USES** In Mexico the bodies have been dried as "buttons" for use as ceremonial, mind-expanding food or drink for 3,000 years. Peyote is used in the quest for greater knowledge, in prophecy, and in healing as it is considered a panacea for physical and emotional ills. The buttons contain alkaloids, giving a complex experience, with the most spectacular visionary phase created by mescaline. Peyote is applied to painful joints.
• **REMARK** Usage spread into North America and it is now part of the native American Church ceremony.

• spineless, swollen, segmented stem

up to 6cm (2⅓in)

grey-green, slow-growing cactus with tufted hairs and ribbed stem •

| Habitat Deserts; N. Mexico, S. Texas | Parts used |

| Family LYCOPODIACEAE | Species *Lycopodium clavatum* | Local name Ground Pine |

STAG'S HORN CLUBMOSS

This toxic, evergreen, moss-like herb has trailing stems, upright branches, and developing cones encasing ripe spores.
• **USES** The spores were once used for gastric and urinary disorders, as an anti-spasmodic sedative, and to coat pills. Blackfoot Indians knew of the spores' blood-staunching, wound-healing, and moisture-absorbing properties and inhaled them for nose-bleeds and dusted them on cuts. They are still used on wounds and eczema.
• **REMARK** The spores are explosive when set alight, and used to create theatrical lightning and added to fireworks.

• 1–3 elongated cones carrying yellow spores

• upright branch

up to 12cm (5in)

| Habitat Acidic soils, mountains; Europe, North America | Parts used Spores |

| Family USNEACEAE | Species *Pseudevernia prunastri* | Local name Lungs of Oak |

OAK MOSS

Oak Moss is a whitish blue to green, shrubby lichen. A lichen is an alga (which photosynthesizes) and a fungus operating together in a symbiotic relationship.
• **USES** The Arabs use ground Oak Moss to leaven bread. It is collected as a violet-scented fragrance fixative and an oleo-resin, extracted for perfumes and soap. Native Americans used it when binding wounds; it is a stomach tonic and an expectorant, and soothes coughs.
• **REMARK** Oak Moss yields a purple wool dye, but air pollution has made it scarce.

• Oak Moss grows on deciduous tree bark

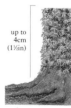

up to 4cm (1½in)

• forked fronds

| Habitat Deciduous trees, humidity; Europe, North America | Parts used Whole plant |

Family SPHAGNACEAE	Species *Sphagnum recurvum*	Local name Curved Leaf Moss

GARDEN SPHAGNUM MOSS

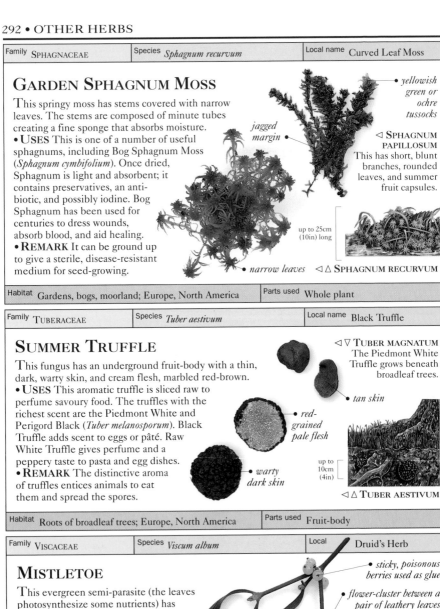

This springy moss has stems covered with narrow leaves. The stems are composed of minute tubes creating a fine sponge that absorbs moisture.
• **USES** This is one of a number of useful sphagnums, including Bog Sphagnum Moss (*Sphagnum cymbifolium*). Once dried, Sphagnum is light and absorbent; it contains preservatives, an anti-biotic, and possibly iodine. Bog Sphagnum has been used for centuries to dress wounds, absorb blood, and aid healing.
• **REMARK** It can be ground up to give a sterile, disease-resistant medium for seed-growing.

yellowish green or ochre tussocks

◁ **SPHAGNUM PAPILLOSUM**
This has short, blunt branches, rounded leaves, and summer fruit capsules.

jagged margin

up to 25cm (10in) long

narrow leaves ◁△ **SPHAGNUM RECURVUM**

Habitat Gardens, bogs, moorland; Europe, North America	Parts used Whole plant

Family TUBERACEAE	Species *Tuber aestivum*	Local name Black Truffle

SUMMER TRUFFLE

This fungus has an underground fruit-body with a thin, dark, warty skin, and cream flesh, marbled red-brown.
• **USES** This aromatic truffle is sliced raw to perfume savoury food. The truffles with the richest scent are the Piedmont White and Perigord Black (*Tuber melanosporum*). Black Truffle adds scent to eggs or pâté. Raw White Truffle gives perfume and a peppery taste to pasta and egg dishes.
• **REMARK** The distinctive aroma of truffles entices animals to eat them and spread the spores.

◁▽ **TUBER MAGNATUM**
The Piedmont White Truffle grows beneath broadleaf trees.

tan skin

red-grained pale flesh

up to 10cm (4in)

warty dark skin

◁△ **TUBER AESTIVUM**

Habitat Roots of broadleaf trees; Europe, North America	Parts used Fruit-body

Family VISCACEAE	Species *Viscum album*	Local Druid's Herb

MISTLETOE

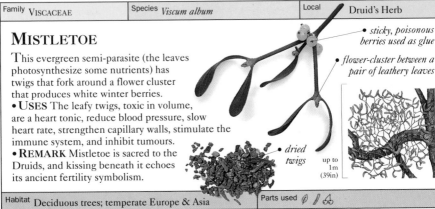

This evergreen semi-parasite (the leaves photosynthesize some nutrients) has twigs that fork around a flower cluster that produces white winter berries.
• **USES** The leafy twigs, toxic in volume, are a heart tonic, reduce blood pressure, slow heart rate, strengthen capillary walls, stimulate the immune system, and inhibit tumours.
• **REMARK** Mistletoe is sacred to the Druids, and kissing beneath it echoes its ancient fertility symbolism.

sticky, poisonous berries used as glue

flower-cluster between a pair of leathery leaves

dried twigs

up to 1m (39in)

Habitat Deciduous trees; temperate Europe & Asia	Parts used

GLOSSARY

Many plant parts and active ingredients are explained in the introduction on pages 10–27. Words printed in **bold** type are defined elsewhere in the glossary.

- **ANALGESIC**
A pain reliever.
- **ANTIBIOTIC**
That which destroys or inhibits the growth of micro-organisms.
- **ASTRINGENT**
A substance that causes contraction of tissues by binding proteins.
- **BALSAMIC**
Having a resinous scent.
- **BASAL**
Of the base; leaf or **inflorescence** joined at ground level.
- **BERRY**
A one- to many-seeded fruit with pulpy flesh and skin.
- **BIPINNATE**
When the divisions of a **pinnate** leaf are, themselves, **pinnate**.
- **BRACT**
A small modified protective leaf at the base of a flower.
- **CALYX**
Sterile flower parts, called **sepals**, that surround the petals.
- **CAPSULE**
A dry fruit enclosing one or more seeds. When ripe it splits open and seeds escape through pores or slits.
- **CATKIN**
A pendulous **inflorescence** made up of tiny stalked flowers.
- **COMPOUND**
A leaf or flower cluster with a branched main axis.
- **CORYMB**
Flat-topped **inflorescence** where outer flowers open first.
- **COUMARIN**
A plant substance that gives the scent of new-mown hay when dried. Anti-coagulant, it may cause haemorrhaging if taken internally.
- **CYME**
A broad flower cluster in which the main stem and side branches grow flowers; it may form a curve.
- **DECIDUOUS**
A plant that sheds its leaves at the end of the growing season.
- **DEMULCENT**
A substance that soothes inflamed internal body tissue. Used externally, it is called an **emollient**.

- **DISK FLORET**
Small, tubular, central florets of a daisy-like flower.
- **DISSECTED LEAF**
A leaf with deeply cut margins.
- **ELLIPTIC**
An oval leaf, pointed at both ends.
- **EMOLLIENT**
See **Demulcent**.
- **EXPECTORANT**
A substance that assists lungs to cough up phlegm.
- **FILAMENT**
Either the stalk of a stamen, or any thread-like part of a plant.
- **FLORET**
A flower unit in an **inflorescence** such as grass spikes or daisies.
- **FLOWER-HEAD**
Compact terminal cluster of stalkless flowers.
- **FREE RADICALS**
Loose oxygen atoms that cross-link molecules to create non-elastic bonds. They may age skin.
- **FROND**
The leaf of a fern or palm tree.
- **FRUIT-BODY**
Visible spore-producing part of a fungus. In mushrooms it is made up of the cap and stipe (stem).
- **HALF-HARDY**
A plant that may not survive extremely cold weather.
- **HARDY**
A plant capable of surviving winter outdoors without protection.
- **INFLORESCENCE**
The arrangement of flowers and their leaves on a stem.
- **LANCEOLATE**
Lance-like leaf, wider at the base.
- **LEGUME**
The seed-pod or the plant of the Leguminosae family, which yields nitrogen **nodes** on its roots.
- **LOBED**
Leaves that are slightly divided; each division is rounded in shape.
- **MORDANT**
A chemical applied to fabrics to bind with, and fix, dye colours.
- **NODE**
A point on a stem from which leaves or shoots arise.
- **OBOVATE**
Leaves that are paddle-shaped, widest above the middle.
- **OVATE**
Leaves that are egg-shaped.

- **PALMATE**
Three or more leaflets arising from the same point.
- **PANICLE**
A branched cluster of stalked flowers.
- **PINNATE**
Three or more pairs of leaflets in two opposite rows along a common stalk. May have a terminal leaflet.
- **POD**
A dry fruit, usually a long cylinder enclosing several seeds, which splits down two sides when ripe.
- **PROSTRATE**
Growing flat along the ground.
- **RACEME**
Unbranched flower cluster, usually pyramid shaped with stalked flowers on an elongated axis.
- **RAY FLORET**
Outer ring of petals on a daisy-like **flower-head**.
- **RECEPTACLE**
Enlarged end of a stem that bears the flower parts.
- **ROOTSTOCK**
The entire root system.
- **SEPAL**
A petal-like leaf. A ring of sepals surrounds and protects the flower-bud, forming the **calyx**.
- **SPIKE**
An elongated **inflorescence** of stalkless individual flowers.
- **SUBSHRUB**
A low-growing shrub with a woody base and soft stems.
- **SUBSPECIES**
A species subdivision; distinct in structure but can interbreed.
- **SUCCULENT**
Thickly cellular and fleshy.
- **TENDER**
A plant that is not frost-hardy.
- **TENDRIL**
A slender, twining organ formed to help the plant cling to a support.
- **UMBEL**
An **inflorescence** where flowers arise from the same point and have stalks the same length.
- **VARIEGATED**
Leaves with secondary markings.
- **VEIL**
A mushroom membrane that encloses the young fruit-body.
- **VERMIFUGE**
A substance that kills or eliminates intestinal worms.

INDEX

ACKNOWLEDGMENTS

THE AUTHOR would like to pay the highest tribute to the DK team for its focus on quality, with special thanks to Charlotte Davies, Mustafa Sami, and Colin Walton; to Dr. Pat Griggs and Holly Shimizu for their botanical knowledge; and to Neil Fletcher and Matthew Ward. Thanks also to my assistant Catriona MacFarlane for correlating the research; and to Louisa Bird for supervising my herb garden.

Many people around the world contributed to the collection of this herbal information: special thanks to Prof. Kaminee Vaidya and Judith Chase in Nepal; W. K. Premawansa of Peradeniya Botanical Garden, Sri Lanka; the remarkable herbalist/driver "Lucky", and Dr. Danister Perera of the Siddhayurvedic Pharmaceutical Co. Ltd., Sri Lanka; Ibu Gedong Bagoes Oka, Bali; Dr. Wee Yeow Chin and Prof. N. B. Abdul Karim of the University of Singapore; Mr Lim of PTE Chinese Medicine Co.; Cao Heng of Hangzou, China; Mina and Shiro Mishima, Ma Suo Shimota, and Seizaburo Hemmi, the Medicinal Plants Garden, Japan; Sumaia and Umaia Farid Ismail of Manaus, Amazonas, Brazil; Godsman Ellis and the Mayan healer Don Eligio of Belize; Anamette Olsen of Denmark; Grethe Gerhardsen Træland of Norway; Vivienne Boulton for Southern Africa; Dr. Anne Anderson of the Cree Nation, Alberta, Canada.

Thanks to my husband J. Roger Lowe for his unfailing support and wisdom, and to my four sons, each for their unique contribution.

I would like to dedicate this book to Manuel Incra Mamani, an Aymara Indian of Bolivia who was killed for revealing the secrets of the best quinine tree to foreigners, thereby saving millions of lives from malaria.

DORLING KINDERSLEY would like to thank: Julia Pashley for picture research; Michael Allaby for compiling the index; Damien Moore for additional editorial assistance; Neal Cobourne for the jacket design; East West Herbs Ltd; David Sleigh, Wellingham Walled Herb Garden; Compton & Compton; Tony Murdock, "Overbecks" Museum and Garden; Selsey Herb Farm; Dr. Richard N. Lester, The University of Birmingham; the staff of the University Botanic Garden, Cambridge, The Royal Botanic Gardens, Kew, Chelsea Physic Garden, and The Botanic Garden, Singapore; Dr. D. B. Sumithraarachchi, Peradeniya Botanical Garden, Sri Lanka; The Lindley Library, Royal Horticultural Society.

Photographs by Neil Fletcher and Matthew Ward, except: Peter Anderson: 23cr; 56bl; 63cb fruit; 70br; 96tr; 96br; 102br; 104t; 145b; 155br; 179bc; 186t; 223tr; 232br; 238b; 246cl; 247l; 247r; 253b; 258t; 281cl; 281cr; 284b; 287br; Kathie Atkinson: 92cl; 93bl; Lesley Bremness: 7tr; 31b; Bridgeman Art Library/Bodleian Library Ash 1431 folio 15v-16r: 6b; Martin Cameron: 13bl; 17br; 19bl; 25bl; 27b steps; Bruce Coleman/Gerald Cubitt: 194bc flower; Bruce Coleman: 253tc stem; Compix/A&J Somaya: 29tc; Eric Crichton: 7bl; Andrew de Lory 29bc flower; Philip Dowell: 13c; 25tr; 122 except cl; 230b; 241tr seeds; 251bl seeds; 253tr seeds; 263c dried; Steve Gorton: 11cl; 21cl; 23b bottle; 27cl; 28bcl; 54tr; 81tr; 109tr dried; 114bl dried; 118 tr dried; 128tr pods; 130cl; 149tc dried; 149br dried; 152c dried; 160bc; 168br; 187tr dried; 199bc root; 199bl leal; 203cr seeds; 233cr; 246tc seeds; 253tcr seed stem; 255bc; 267bc seeds; 278br dried; 286br dried; 288t; Derek Hall: 179tr, Robert Harding Picture Library/ European Magazines Ltd.: 22br; Dave King: 9; 11br; 14cr; 15c petals; 17cl; 27c; 61b; 82bl; 87cr beans; 97br; 108 except bc variegated; 112-113 except br; 116b; 120cl dried petals; 120br hips; 124-125; 126t; 127t; 127c; 132; 133 except tr; 136c; 139bcr salt stems; 140b; 141tr; 142 except bl; 143 except tc; 145tc; 148bc; 150; 151t; 151br; 159b; 160cl; 166t; 168bl; 170cr; 171; 172tr; 182b except dried; 184br; 185tc flower; 189t; 190 except tc, bl; 191 except tc, tr, c, bl; 192bl;

195tc; 196b; 197; 199t, 200b; 214b; 215b; 212cl; 218t; 219cr flowers; 220tr; 220b; 221; 223tcc; 226tc; 229br; 230tc; 231t; 233b; 234bl; 236t; 239t; 241b; 244tc; 252b; 255cl; 255bl; 256 br; 257tc; 259tr; 259b; 262cr; 263br; 264bl; 264br; 266tc; 270t; 272tr; 273br; 274t; 274bl; 274br; Colin Leftley: 46cl; 47bl; 234br; 235br; 264c; 265b; Rory Lowe: back flap; 30bl; 30br; David Murray: 12cr; 15br; 18l; 24cr; 30tr; 30cl; 59tr dried; 60tc berries; 69br fruit; 83bc bark; 86cr pod; 96bl dried; 127bl; 127br; 148br root; 164tr; 193b; 234 seeds; 237cr dried; 237bl dried; 244cl; 244cr; 251bc paste; 260cl; 260c; 260cr; 261tr; 266cl seeds; 273bl seeds; 283cr dried; Martin Norris: 16cl seeds; 19l; 24b dried; 46b; 68bcr; 119bl seeds; 144b roots; 169c seeds; 169br; 226br paste; 239cl seeds; 259c seeds; 263bl; 269c seeds; 283cl dried; 283bl dried; 285c dried; Roger Phillips: 87c butter; 115tl; 118bl fruit; 134tr fruit; Potter's Herbal Supplies, Wigan: 8tr; Still Pictures/Bojan Brecelj: 8b, Still Pictures/Edward Parker: 21br; Colin Walton: 8cl; 12cl; 12c; 13cl; 13tr; 14c; 15tc; 16bl; 17tc; 17cr; 17br; 18cl; 18cr; 19tc; 19tr; 19cl; 19cr; 19r; 20cr; 21tc; 21tr; 21cl; 21cr; 21r; 22c dried; 24tr equipment; 25tl; 25c dried; 25br; 28tr; 28bcr; 28cr; 29tl; 29tr; 29cr; 29br; 31t; 129tc seeds; 152cr; 152b; 158tr; 188br sprouts & seeds; 193tc bulb; 196 tr roots; 216b; 229cr seeds; 243cl seeds; 244b; 244b; 249c seeds; 253cl straw; 269tr; 269bl dried; 272cl seeds; 280cr seeds; 284t flower; 284b seeds. **Illustrations by** Laura Andrew; 168; 170; 203; 204t; 205t; 211t; 212; 213t; 242b; 271b; 272t; 273; Evelyn Binns; 9; 95b; 124b; 125; 126; 127; 146; 171; 172b; 181t; 182t; 185b; 195; 209b; 218b; 219t; 220; 221; 230; 231; 232; 234; 236b; 238t; 238b; 239t; 240t; 241t; 250b; 254b; 266t; 267b;Julia Cobbold; 97b; 101b; 104b; 118t; 128t; 130b; 138b; 193b; 196b; 197; 198b; 199t; 228t; 229; 235; 264; 270t; 275t; Joanne Cowne; 145; 147t; 148t; 153b; 154t; 157t; 186t; 214b; 215b; 216t; 222; 255t; Myra Giles; 267t; 277t; 292c; Ruth Hall; 117b; 157b; 175t; 214t; 215t; 219b; 223b; 252t; 258b; 268b; 270b; 274t; 282b; Tim Hayward: 36t; 38b; 39; 40t; 46; 48; 49; 50t; 53; 55; 56; 57; 58b; 62; 63; 71; 72; 74; 75; 76; 77; 78t; 79b; 82; 84t; 85b; 86t; 87t; 90t; 93b; 94b; 95t; 103b; 105b; 107b; 110t; 115b; 131b; Philippa Lumber; 268t; 280; 284; 291b; Stephen McLean; 10br *Langermannia*; 277b; 281; 289b; David More; 10cl *Alnus*; 34; 35; 37; 38t; 41; 42; 43t; 44b; 51b; 54; 58t; 59b; 64; 65; 66; 67t; 68; 69; 70; 71; 80t; 81t; 83t; 90b; 91; 92; 93; 99b; 100; 103t; 132; 133; 140b; 141; 148b; 149b; 156b; 158b; 159b; 161b; 238c; Leighton Moses; 10bcl *Piper*; 276b; 278t; 283; 288b; 290t; Sue Oldfield; 32; 33; 36b; 40b; 43b; 44t; 45; 50b; 51t; 52; 59t; 60; 61; 67b; 68b; 73; 78b; 79t; 80b; 81b; 83b; 84b; 85t; 86b; 87b; 88; 89; 97t; 98; 99t; 101t; 102t; 103t; 109t; 111; 114; 116t; 119; 129b; 130t; 131t; 153t; 202b; Liz Pepperell; 12; 14 line; 16; 18; 20; 128b; 136; 142; 150; 151; 154b; 158t; 166c; 172t; 173; 179; 180; 181b; 182b; 183b; 189b; 192; 202t; 228b; 240b; Valerie Price; 102b; 147b; 149t;159t; 160b; 183t; 184t; 201; 211b; 226b; 239b; 241b; 243; 244t; 245b; 246; 247; 248; 249t; 250t; 251t; 252b; 253b; 257t; 257c; 259b; 262t; 263b; 265t; 266b; Michelle Ross; 10c *Camellia*; 10bl *Lycopersicon*; 14 colour; 94t; 96; 106; 104t; 109b; 110b; 118b; 120; 122; 123; 124t; 129t; 134t; 135; 137; 138t; 139b; 140t; 155b; 162t; 163; 166b; 174 175b; 176b 177 178; 186b; 187t;189t; 190t; 194t; 196t; 198t; 200t; 206b; 223t; 233; 236t; 244b; 245t; 253c; 256; 257b; 260; 263t; 269t; 275b; 276t; 286b; 289t; 290b; Hayley Simmons; 10bcr *Dryopteris*; 285t; 286t; 287b; 292t; Catherine Slade; 112; 115t; 116b; 117t; Jenny Steer; 279b; 282t; 287t; 288t; 292b; Rebekah Thorpe; 274b; 278b; 279t; 291c; Jonathon Tyler; 285b; Barbara Walker; 10cr; 105t; 107t; 134b; 139t; 144; 152t; 155t; 156t; 162b; 169b; 176t; 185t; 193t; 194b; 199b; 200b; 207; 208; 209t; 216b; 217t; 218t; 224; 225; 226t; 227; 242t; 249b; 254t; 255b; 258t; 259t; 262b; 268c; 269b; 291t; Wendy Webb; 10cbr; Debra Woodward; 160t; 161t; 164; 165; 167; 169t; 187b; 188; 204b; 205b; 206t; 210; 213b; 217b; 237; 251b; 265b; 266b; 271t; 272b. **Endpaper illustrations** by Caroline Church.